Myelodysplastic Syndromes

Clinical and Biological Advances

Myelodysplastic Syndromes: Clinical and Biological Advances stands out as the definitive text on the genetics, pathophysiology, and clinical management of this wide-range of syndromes. Written by international experts, this book provides a state-of-the-art update of the current status and recent advances in the field. The chapters cover all aspects of the myelodysplastic syndromes, from an in-depth analysis of the multifactorial nature of this disease, including a careful assessment of stromal, immunological, and stem cell abnormalities, to a review of recent molecular and cytogenetic discoveries and insights. This book will be a valuable resource for clinicians and researchers who wish to learn more about myelodysplastic syndromes.

Peter L. Greenberg is Professor of Medicine at Stanford University Cancer Center, Stanford, and Chief, Hematology Section, VA Palo Alto Health Care System, Palo Alto, California, USA.

T0210522

Myelodysplastic Syndromes

Clinical and Biological Advances

Edited by

Peter L. Greenberg

Stanford University Cancer Center, Stanford and
VA Palo Alto Health Care System, Palo Alto

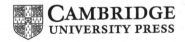

CAMBRIDGE
UNIVERSITY PRESS

CAMBRIDGE UNIVERSITY PRESS
Cambridge, New York, Melbourne, Madrid, Cape Town, Singapore,
São Paulo, Delhi, Dubai, Tokyo, Mexico City

Cambridge University Press
The Edinburgh Building, Cambridge CB2 8RU, UK

Published in the United States of America by Cambridge University Press, New York

www.cambridge.org
Information on this title: www.cambridge.org/9780521182287

© Cambridge University Press 2006

First published 2006
First paperback edition 2010

A catalogue record for this publication is available from the British Library

ISBN 978-0-521-49668-1 Hardback
ISBN 978-0-521-18228-7 Paperback

To Suzanne, Sarah, Daniel, Miriam, and, of course, Simi, whose love, encouragement, and support have been critical beacons for my worlds; to my MDS colleagues for their spirited camaraderie and scientific stimulation; to my patients with MDS who have permitted me the privilege of participating in their lives and struggles, who have taught me much of the eternal odds they/we face. All have been vital for my ongoing exploration to better comprehend and treat this distinctively problematic disease.

Contents

Contributors

A. John Barrett MD
Hematology Branch
National Heart, Lung and Blood Institute
National Institutes of Health
9000 Rockville Pike, Bldg 10, Room 7C103
Bethesda MD 20892
USA

Richard D. Brunning MD
University of Minnesota Hospital
Department of Laboratory Medicine
and Pathology
Box 609
Minneapolis MN 55455
USA

Andrew J. Buresh MD
University of Arizona Medical Center
Hematology Unit
1515 N. Campbell Ave
Tucson AZ 85724
USA

H. Joachim Deeg MD
Fred Hutchinson Cancer Research Center
1100 Fairview Avenue North, D1-100
P O Box 19024
Seattle WA 98109-1024
USA

Jason Gotlib MD MS
Stanford University Cancer Center
Division of Hematology
875 Blake Wilbur Drive
Room 2335
Stanford CA 94305
USA

Peter L. Greenberg MD
Stanford University Cancer Center
Division of Hematology
875 Blake Wilbur Drive
Stanford CA 94305-5821
USA and Hematology Section
VA Palo Alto Health Care System
Palo Alto CA 94304
USA

Wolf-Karsten Hofmann MD
University Hospital "Benjamin
Franklin"
Department of Hematology,
Oncology and Transfusion
Medicine
Hindenburgdamm 30
12203 Berlin
Germany

H. Phillip Koeffler MD
UCLA School of Medicine
Division of Hematology/Oncology
Cedars Sinai Research Institute
8700 Beverly Blvd, B-208
Los Angeles CA 90048
USA

Michelle M. Le Beau PhD
University of Chicago
Section of Hematology/Oncology
5841 S. Maryland, MC2115
Chicago IL 60637
USA

Alan F. List MD
University of South Florida
Moffitt Clinic Center, Hematologic
Malignancies Program
Department of Interdisciplinary Oncology
12902 Magnolia Drive
Tampa FL 33612-9497
USA

Harold J. Olney MD CM
Université de Montréal
CHUM Hôpital Notre-Dame
1560 Sherbrooke Street East
Montreal
Quebec H2L 4M
Canada

Bart Scott MD
Fred Hutchinson Cancer Research Center
825 Eastlake Ave E, PO Box 19023
Seattle WA 98109-1023
USA

Elaine Sloand MD
Hematology Branch
National Heart, Lung and Blood
Institute
National Institutes of Health
9000 Rockville Pike, Bldg 10, Room
7C103
Bethesda MD 20892
USA

Mary Laudon Thomas RN MS AOCN
Veterans Affairs Palo Alto Health Care
System
3801 Miranda Avenue
Palo Alto CA 94304
USA

Neal S. Young MD
Hematology Branch
National Heart, Lung and Blood Institute
National Institutes of Health
9000 Rockville Pike, Bldg 10, Room
7C103
Bethesda MD 20892
USA

Preface

Myelodysplastic syndrome (MDS) is a particularly problematic disease. This myeloid clonal hemopathy is heterogeneous, with varying stages having differing clinical problems that require specific yet disparate therapeutic approaches. Major morbidity relates to the patients' symptomatic cytopenias and their potential for progression to acute myeloid leukemia (AML). The patients' generally elderly ages complicate management of the illness due to attendant comorbidities. Beyond standard supportive care with transfusions, virtually all treatments for MDS are currently experimental. This combination of characteristics has contributed to the difficulty in determining appropriate therapy for MDS patients. Fundamental to improving the care for these individuals is a more thorough clinical characterization and basic understanding of mechanisms causing the marrow hemopoietic dysfunction central to this disorder.

Given these features and the increasing incidence of MDS as our populations age, this book is quite germane in providing a comprehensive state-of-the-art update of the current status and recent advances in the field. It describes major treatises by an international group of MDS experts on the clinical classification, underlying pathogenetic mechanisms, and biologically targeted treatments of the disease. Each of the book's 10 chapters provides critical insights into specific topics, demonstrating interconnections between subjects.

Chapter 1 reviews the current clinical and prognostic categorizations of MDS, describing the complexity of establishing disease diagnosis and the critical clinical and biological features used to categorize MDS prognostically so that effective management strategies may be undertaken. Chapter 2 provides more extensive descriptions and photomicrographs of the major criteria for the morphologic classifications of MDS, including those for both adult and pediatric patients.

In order to understand basic pathogenetic mechanisms underlying MDS, an indepth analysis of the multifactorial nature of the biological derangements causing marrow dysfunction in this disorder is provided in Chapter 3, including careful assessment of marrow stromal, immunologic, as well as stem cell abnormalities and dysregulation. Particular focus in this discourse depicts the changing patterns of the aberrant biology associated with evolving stages of MDS. This evaluation examines the molecular lesions and their influences which generate the initially slow but insidious course of the disease, with a subsequent frequent triggering to more active disease progression. The role of the senescence process in enhancing the vulnerability of aging itself for susceptibility to MDS is also discussed in detail.

Chapters 4 and 5 are critical extensions of the analysis of MDS pathobiology, evaluating recently determined major cytogenetic and molecular discoveries involved in the syndrome. These treatises review current insights into disease biology using novel investigative techniques, including microarray analysis of differential gene expression profiles.

A growing plethora of therapeutic options for MDS is becoming available, particularly using biologically specific targeted drugs for treating the disease. Clinical subsets of MDS patients have been defined and discussed in Chapter 6 wherein immunologic mechanisms and immune-modulating therapy may be effective. Chapter 7 comprehensively updates results of experimental clinical trials using the many and various new agents targeting specific pathogenetic features in MDS and the strategies being used for managing differing subtypes of MDS. Treatment with hemopoietic cytokines for management of the patients' symptomatic cytopenias is reviewed in Chapter 8. Due to recently improved appreciation of the negative clinical consequences of iron overload for multiply transfused MDS patients and the current availability of novel oral iron chelators, interest has been rekindled for use of iron chelation therapy. The current management of iron overload, as well as the biologic derangements caused by tissue siderosis, are also discussed in this chapter.

The only potentially curative therapy for MDS is hemopoietic stem cell transplantation (HSCT). However, age limitations for this high-intensity form of treatment and its relative toxicity require careful consideration of eligibility criteria prior to application of this procedure. Results of HSCT investigations using risk-based categorization of MDS patients and the newer preparative regimens (including reduced-intensity conditioning) are discussed in Chapter 9.

The complexity of the disease's clinical course and the multiple options for management approaches engender an element of uncertainty in the minds of many, patients and clinicians alike. These disconcerting issues have a particularly prominent impact on each MDS patient's quality of life. Such effects on the various domains comprising this component of the patients' lives (functional, emotional, physical, spiritual, and social) are reviewed in Chapter 10.

An important property of this book is the interconnectedness between chapters, engendering cross-fertilization for improved understanding of this disease. Numerous unique aspects of MDS have been incorporated into each chapter and the co-authors provide proposals for major future directions for the field. These comprehensive features should permit valuable insights for the reader into this potentially life-threatening illness and its effective management.

Clinical and prognostic characterization of myelodysplastic syndromes

Peter L. Greenberg

Stanford University Cancer Center, Stanford, and VA Palo Alto Health Care System, Palo Alto, CA, USA

The myelodysplastic syndromes (MDS) provide a clinical model for evaluating the evolution of a relatively indolent malignancy into one which is frankly aggressive. The morbidity and mortality in this myeloid clonal hemopathy relate to either marrow dysfunction associated with ineffective hematopoiesis and its peripheral blood cytopenias or to disease evolution into a variant of acute myeloid leukemia (AML-MDS). MDS may arise de novo or is therapy-related (secondary, t-MDS) following treatment with chemotherapy or chemoradiotherapy for other illnesses. The disease is generally relatively indolent, with a rate of progression related to a number of defined clinical features.[1]

Morphologic classifications

The morphologic findings in MDS consist of variable degrees of dysplasia and generally increased or normal marrow hemopoietic cellularity associated with peripheral blood cytopenias and cytopathies. There are currently two morphological classification systems used to categorize MDS patients: the initial French–American–British (FAB) and the more recently proposed World Health Organization (WHO) classification.

French–American–British

The FAB group provided a marrow-based morphologic method for systematically characterizing MDS patients. These features include assessment of the proportion of myeloblasts and degree of dysplasia in the hemopoietic cells, within at least two of the three hemopoietic cell lines.[2] The characteristic

Myelodysplastic Syndromes: Clinical and Biological Advances, ed. Peter L. Greenberg. Published by Cambridge University Press. © Cambridge University Press 2006.

MDS features include megaloblastoid erythropoiesis, nucleocytoplasmic asynchrony in the early myeloid and erythroid precursors, and dysmorphic megakaryocytes.

The FAB morphologic classification method separates patients into five subgroups: (1) refractory anemia (RA); (2) refractory anemia with ringed sideroblasts (RARS); (3) refractory anemia with excess blasts (RAEB); (4) refractory anemia with excess blasts in transformation (RAEB-T); and (5) chronic myelomonocytic leukemia (CMML). The first four entities are characterized by abnormal marrow myeloid cell differentiation patterns with RA or RARS patients having less than 5% blasts, associated with dysplasia, RAEB having between 5 and 20% blasts and RAEB-T having 20–30% blasts. RARS patients have ≥ 15% ringed sideroblasts. In contrast, AML is considered to be present if marrows have > 30% blasts. However, to diagnose MDS more accurately, it is important to assess the relative stability (or lack thereof for at least several months) of blood counts, in addition to enumerating the marrow blast percentage and degree of dysplasia, as the patients may have an evolving form of AML. The criteria for CMML include a peripheral monocytosis exceeding 1000/mm^3, increased numbers of monocytic cells in the bone marrow, dysplasia in the erythroid, megakaryocytic or granulocytic series, and 1–20% marrow blasts.

For a generation, this classification system was quite useful clinically, particularly permitting consistent diagnostic approaches to be applied worldwide for these patients. However, difficulties emerged with the somewhat limited ability of this method to provide precise prognostic information regarding clinical outcomes in a substantial portion of patients. This limitation related to the relatively wide proportion of marrow blasts in RAEB and CMML subgroups (i.e., 5–20% and 1–20% blasts, respectively) and sole reliance of the system on marrow morphology (blast percentage) for its classification. Subsequently CMML has been usefully separated into two subgroups – proliferative and non-proliferative. The proliferative form of CMML (i.e., with leukocyte counts > 12 000/mm^3, hepatosplenomegaly, constitutional symptoms) is more akin to a myeloproliferative disorder (MPD) than to MDS.[3,4] This form of CMML differs in its major clinical features from the non-proliferative (dysplastic) subtype of the disorder, which has monocytosis but relatively low leukocyte counts. These patients were previously considered to have RAEB or RA subtypes of MDS with monocytosis.

Table 1.1 Classification of myelodysplastic syndrome (MDS)

French–American–British (FAB)[2]	World Health Organization (WHO)[5–7]
NC^a	RA (unilineage)^b
NC^a	RARS (unilineage)^{b,c}
RA	5q– syndrome^d
RA	RCMD
RARS	RCMD (w/RS)
RAEB	RAEB-1
RAEB	RAEB-2
RAEB-T	AML
CMML	MDS/MPD^e
NC^a	MDS unclassified

^{a} NC, category not considered to be MDS by FAB.

^{b} Requires 6 months, persisting anemia without other cause to establish the diagnosis.

^{c} Pure sideroblastic anemia/idiopathic sideroblastic ineffective erythropoiesis.

^{d} < 5% marrow blasts, micromegakaryocytes, and thrombocytosis; included in RA within FAB.

^{e} MDS if white blood cells (WBC) $\leq 12\,000/mm^3$ (in relevant FAB category)/MPD if WBC $> 12\,000/mm^3$.

RA, refractory anemia; RARS, RA with ringed sideroblasts; RAEB, RA with excess blasts; RAEB-T, RAEB in transformation; CMML, chronic myelomonocytic leukemia; RCMD, RA with multilineage dysplasia; AML, acute myeloid leukemia; MDS/MPD, MDS/myeloproliferative disease.

Thus, CMML in this classification is a disorder which encompassed features of both chronic MPD and MDS.

World Health Organization

A group of hematopathologists convened by WHO recently proposed a new classification for MDS,[5–7] modifying the FAB definitions of MDS (Table 1.1). Although most prior data required at least two-line dysplasia to diagnose MDS, the WHO guidelines accept unilineage dysplasia for the diagnosis of refractory anemia and refractory anemia with ringed sideroblasts, so long as other causes of the dysplasia are absent and the dysplasia persists for at least 6 months. The latter caveat relates to the fact that a number of toxins (e.g., arsenic, alcohol) and viral infections (e.g., human immunodeficiency virus (HIV) infection) may cause morphologic changes similar to MDS in marrow cells.[8,9]

Other categories within the WHO proposal include: (1) refractory cytopenia with multilineage dysplasia (RCMD); (2) separation of RAEB patients into those with < 10% blasts (RAEB-1) or ≥ 10% marrow blasts (RAEB-2); (3) 5q minus (5q−) syndrome; and (4) MDS unclassified. The category MDS/MPD was proposed for patients who had previously been classified as CMML.

The WHO proposals included the 5q− syndrome as a separate entity, so long as the classical features of the syndrome were met. This category requires 5q− as the sole chromosomal abnormality, RA morphologic subtype, and characteristic morphologic features, i.e., macrocytic anemia, normal or high platelet counts, hypolobulated micromegakaryocytes. The patients generally had a relatively indolent clinical course, in which evolution to AML was uncommon.[10,11] Superimposed cytogenetic lesions in addition to 5q−, however, were associated with a poorer prognosis and more progressive course.[12]

The WHO panel also suggested excluding RAEB-T patients from being considered as MDS. They proposed that patients with ≥ 20% marrow blasts should now be included as AML, rather than using the previous > 30% blast cutpoint which had been recommended by the FAB group. However, the diagnosis of MDS is not only related to blast quantitation, as these patients possess a more indolent pace of disease related to distinctive biologic features which differ from those of de novo AML.[13,14] In addition, therapeutic responses generally differ for patients in these two patient groups. AML evolving from MDS (AML-MDS) and high-risk MDS (RAEB-T) are often more resistant to standard cytotoxic chemotherapy than is de novo AML. Investigational therapy is preferable for the former patient groups.

The decision to classify and then manage patients having marrow blasts in the range of 20–30% as either AML or high-risk MDS is thus complex and needs consideration of other clinical features such as age, antecedent factors, cytogenetics, comorbidities, pace of disease, and performance status.[14] Although the WHO classification is quite useful, studies have provided conflicting evidence regarding the distinguishing features of certain subgroups in these proposals.[15,16]

Several national panels of MDS investigators and clinicians (US, Italian, and British) have provided management guidelines for the disease.[17–19] While awaiting further data needed to clarify WHO proposals, the US National Comprehensive Cancer Network (NCCN) panel for MDS Practice Guidelines has recommended reporting both the FAB and the WHO morphologic descriptions of MDS marrow.[17] This approach permits flexibility for patient management and their entry into relevant therapeutic clinical protocols. Given the longstanding experience with FAB categorization, the British MDS Guidelines Committee recommended use of the FAB morphologic criteria, whereas the Italian Guidelines Group suggested following the WHO recommendations.[18,19]

Clinical variants

Hypocellular MDS

Although most patients with MDS have hypercellular or normocellular bone marrows, a small subgroup of MDS patients (< 15%) have marrow hypoplasia at the time of diagnosis.[20–22] Differentiation of these patients from those with either aplastic anemia or hypoplastic AML may be difficult. Most hypocellular MDS cases fit into the categories of RA and RAEB. A potentially useful means of identifying hypocellular MDS, in distinction to aplastic anemia, is the finding of an associated clonal cytogenetic abnormality.[22] In a series of patients with aplastic anemia, clonal chromosomal abnormalities were present in only 4% of individuals, and were those also seen in MDS or AML.[23]

MDS with fibrosis

Mild to moderate myelofibrosis occurs in up to 50% of all MDS subtypes, with marked fibrosis occurring in < 15% of cases, a higher proportion having these features in therapy-related MDS (t-MDS).[24] Myelofibrotic MDS is characterized by the abrupt onset of pancytopenia without organomegaly, but with substantial red blood cell anisopoikilocytosis, trilineage dysplasia, atypical megakaryocyte proliferation with hypolobated forms, and increased numbers of marrow blasts.[24,25] Occasionally a leukoerythroblastic peripheral blood picture is evident. The clinical course is generally progressive.

Secondary MDS

Secondary (i.e., therapy-related and toxic chemical-related) MDS (t-MDS) causes morbidity and mortality with or without progression to AML.[26–28] The increasing incidence of t-MDS and t-AML reflects a number of factors:

the increased longevity of many patients following more successful treatment of certain solid tumors, more intensive treatment regimens combining high-dose chemotherapy and irradiation, broader utilization of adjuvant chemo-irradiation in solid tumor therapy, environmental pollution and increased exposure to chemicals and carcinogens (particularly organic solvents).[26–28] Generally these patients have poorer prognoses than those with primary MDS. The major organic solvent implicated in leukemogenesis is benzene, with disease occurrence related to the intensity and duration of exposure to this chemical. Recent studies have indicated that polymorphisms in enzymes which detoxify benzene (e.g., NQO1), with concomitant increases in toxic metabolites capable of damaging DNA, are associated with enhanced vulnerability to benzene poisoning and development of leukemia.[26]

In t-MDS, abnormal karyotypes are evident in virtually all patients, generally with multiple chromosome aberrations, most frequently involving chromosomes 5 and 7 (85%).[29–31] The classical therapy-related MDS/leukemia involving chromosome 5 and 7 abnormalities, related to alkylating agents and irradiation, is the most common form.[27] Two additional forms of t-AML have been described: one type attributed to exposure to topoisomerase II-active chemotherapeutic agents (e.g., etoposide) and involving the chromosome 11q23 locus, and the other involving the chromosome 21q22 locus.[29,32] The benzene-induced cytogenetic abnormality is frequently trisomy 9.[33]

Prognostic determinations

Morphologic assessment: FAB

Mortality in MDS relates to the patient's morphologic subtype and is due to a variety of causes, including evolution to AML, infection, or bleeding complications associated with the patient's dominant cytopenia(s). Since most MDS patients are elderly, concomitant non-hematologic diseases also substantially contribute to their morbidity and mortality. Utilizing FAB subgroup morphologic criteria, there was a moderate degree of precision regarding prognostic findings for survival and AML evolution (Table 1.2, Fig. 1.1).[34–38] Patients with RAEB and RAEB-T had relatively poor prognoses, with median survivals generally ranging from 5 to 12 months, in contrast to RA or RARS patients with median survivals of 3–6 years. The proportion of these individuals who transformed to AML varied similarly: in the higher-risk RAEB

Table 1.2 Myelodysplastic syndrome: survival and leukemic evolution related to FAB morphologic subgroups[a]

	FAB subgroups				
	RA	RARS	RAEB	RAEB-T	CMML
Median survival (months)	43	73	12	5	20
Transformation to AML (percent)	15	5	40	50	35
Proportion of patients (percent)	25	15	35	15	10

[a] Meta-analysis.

Reproduced with permission from Greenberg.[1]

FAB, French–American–British; RA, refractory anemia; RARS, RA with ringed sideroblasts; RAEB, RA with excess blasts; RAEB-T, RAEB in transformation; CMML, chronic myelomonocytic leukemia; AML, acute myeloid leukemia.

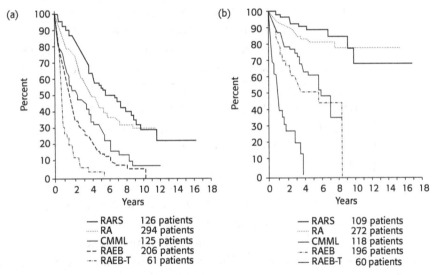

	RARS	126 patients		RARS	109 patients
RA	294 patients		RA	272 patients
CMML	125 patients		CMML	118 patients
RAEB	206 patients		RAEB	196 patients
RAEB-T	61 patients		RAEB-T	60 patients

Fig. 1.1   (a) Survival and (b) freedom from acute myeloid leukemia evolution in patients with myelodysplastic syndrome who were evaluated by the International MDS Workshop, in relation to their French–American–British classification subgroup (Kaplan–Meier curves). RA, refractory anemia; RARS, RA with ringed sideroblasts; RAEB, RA with excess blasts; RAEB-T, RAEB in transformation; CMML, chronic myelomonocytic leukemia. This research was originally published in Blood[46]. Greenberg, P., Cox, C., Le Beau, M. M. *et al.* International Scoring System (IPSS) for evaluating prognosis in myelodysplastic syndrome. *Blood*, 1997; **89**, 2079–88. © the American Society of Hematology.

and RAEB-T patients this incidence was 40–50%, whereas in the remainder of the patients it was 5–15%. Regarding time to disease evolution, 25 and 55% of patients with RAEB and RAEB-T, respectively, underwent transformation to AML at 1 year, and 35 and 65% at 2 years. In contrast, for patients with RA this incidence was 5 and 10% at 1 and 2 years, whereas none of the RARS patients underwent leukemic transformation within 2 years. Patients with higher marrow blast percentages had poorer prognoses, with specific cutpoints of > or < 10% marrow blasts having major impact on survival.[34]

For CMML patients, the major prognostic feature for their survival (as for the other MDS subgroups) was their marrow blast percentage.[39–42] Median survival of CMML patients with < 5% marrow blasts was 53 months, versus 16 months (similar to RAEB) for those with 5–20% blasts. Monocytosis greater than 2600/mm^3 and abnormal cytogenetics also correlated with poor survival. The separation of these patients into proliferative and nonproliferative/dysplastic subgroups (based on their leukocyte counts) is supported by evaluation of their clinical outcomes.[3,41] CMML patients have also been further subdivided into four prognostic risk groups based on a combination of independent predictive factors: (1) level of marrow blasts; (2) degree of anemia; (3) peripheral blood immature mononuclear cells; and (4) lymphocytes.[43] In CMML and other MDS patients, the presence of a number of gene mutations (e.g., *ras, fms, flt3*), high lactate dehydrogenase, and high beta$_2$-microglobulin levels were also associated with poorer prognoses (see below).[44,45]

Other suggested independent morphologic prognostic indicators are the presence of myelofibrosis or of Auer rods. MDS patients with myelofibrosis generally have poorer survivals than those without fibrosis.[24] In the FAB classification, the presence of Auer rods in myeloid cells implied the diagnosis of RAEB-T. However, the adverse prognostic influence of Auer rods per se has not been clearly demonstrated.

Morphologic assessment: WHO

The WHO classification has helped to morphologically stratify the prior heterogeneous histologic subtypes of some FAB-categorized MDS patients. Prognostic data have been obtained with this categorization, although the degree of inconsistency in reported clinical outcomes warrants further evaluation.[14–16] Those patients with uni- versus multilineage dysplasia (refractory cytopenia with multilineage dysplasia – RCMD) have differing prognoses, with RCMD generally having poorer clinical outcomes.[15] Clear previous evidence has demonstrated the importance of separating RAEB patients into those with < or > 10% marrow blasts,[34,46] thus the RAEB-1 and -2 WHO categories appear clinically useful.

The classical 5q– syndrome has a generally low risk of transformation to acute leukemia, and favorable prognosis.[11,47] The better survival of 5q– syndrome patients compared to other MDS patients is also associated with a low incidence of deaths from infection and bleeding. Non-hematologic illnesses and hemosiderosis from red blood cell transfusion dependence constitute major causes of morbidity and mortality in this group of patients. The presence of karyotypic abnormalities in addition to 5q– or > 5% marrow blasts is associated with a worse prognosis.[12] Of interest is the distinctive responsiveness of this subgroup of MDS patients to a recently evaluated biologic agent, Revlimid (CC5013).[48]

Atypical localization of immature precursors

Studies analyzing marrow biopsies have demonstrated that some MDS patients had clusters of blast cells in central marrow regions, rather than being normally paratrabecular, referred to as abnormal localization of immature myeloid precursors (ALIP). Patients with these morphologic findings had significantly shorter survival in all subtypes of MDS.[49,50] ALIP-positive cases were more common in RAEB, RAEB-T, and CMML.

Biologic assessment

In vitro hemopoietic clonogenic assays

Despite the more indolent nature of MDS than AML, many in vitro hemopoietic clonogenic abnormalities evident in AML are also present in MDS. These biological parameters have been useful for evaluating pathogenetic mechanisms and prognosis in MDS patients.[51] The colony-forming capacities of all of the marrow hemopoietic precursor cells (CFU-GEMM, BFU-E, CFU-E, CFU-GM, CFU-Meg) are quite low or absent in the majority of MDS patients, as found in most AML patients. Also similar to leukemic patients, an increased proportion of CFU-GMs are of light buoyant density, have abortive myeloid cluster formation, and defective cellular maturation occurs within the colonies.

Table 1.3 Prognosis of myelodysplastic syndromes: utility of in vitro marrow myeloid clonogenic culture studies

Growth patterns	Incidence (%)	Transformation AML (%)	Median survival (months)
RAEB-T ($n = 80$)[52,53]		51 (45–60)	9 (7–11)
Non-leukemic growth	33 (27–38)	31 (29–33)	20 (15–25)
Leukemic growth	68 (62–73)	60 (50–70)	7 (5–8)
RAEB ($n = 17$)[54,55]		41	14
Non-leukemic growth	70	29	21
Leukemic growth	30	100	10
RA ($n = 82$)[53,56,57]		39 (35–44)	24 (9–20)
Non-leukemic growth	54 (30–74)	20 (21–40)	47 (9–50)
Leukemic growth	46 (26–70)	60 (50–80)	8 (4–10)

Mean values and ranges of means for cited studies.

Reprinted from *Seminars in Hematology*, 33, Greenberg, P. L. Biological and clinical implications of marrow culture studies in the myelodysplastic syndrome, 163–75, copyright (1996), with permission from Elsevier.

AML, acute myeloid leukemia; RAEB-T, refractory anemia with excess blasts in transformation; RA, refractory anemia.

In vitro marrow myeloid (CFU-GM) clonal growth in MDS may be divided into leukemic and non-leukemic patterns.[51] Leukemic-type growth includes micro- or macrocluster formation with defective maturation or blasts within the aggregates, single persisting blasts, or very low colony formation (< 2 colonies per 10^5 marrow cells). Non-leukemic growth is marked by having persisting colony formation, even if moderately decreased in frequency. As shown in Table 1.3, six studies involving 179 MDS patients with differing FAB morphologic subtypes demonstrated correlation between clinical outcome and in vitro marrow growth.[51–57] When patients were stratified according to their in vitro myeloid growth patterns, subgroups of MDS patients with non-leukemic growth patterns had a 20–31% incidence of transformation to AML and 20–47-month median survivals. In contrast, MDS patients with leukemic growth patterns had a 60–100% incidence of transformation and 7–10-month median survivals. MDS patients with single hemopoietic cell line defects, such as idiopathic sideroblastic ineffective erythropoiesis and idiopathic neutropenia with a low propensity to leukemic evolution, had normal marrow granulopoietic growth parameters.[51] Such patients who died without undergoing transformation generally did so as a result of infectious or bleeding complications. Factors other than in vitro hemopoietic growth patterns contribute to transformation, as not all patients with abnormal clonal growth had poor prognoses. Correlation has been demonstrated between in vitro myeloid growth patterns, abnormal marrow cytogenetics, and poor prognoses.[51] The findings of decreasing CFU-GM incidence, a higher proportion of light-density CFU-GM, and increased cluster/colony ratios provide functional evidence of clonal evolution and prognostic information as these diseases progress towards acute transformation.

Combined assessment – morphologic, clinical, and biologic

Additionally, other methods have been utilized beyond solely using morphologic criteria to attempt to improve the prognostic classification of MDS. A variety of investigations incorporated individual parameters such as cytogenetics, lactate dehydrogenase, cytopenias, and patient age into FAB-type morphologic categories.[34–39,45] Each of these studies provided useful clues regarding the need for combining morphologic, clinical, and biologic features to refine the MDS classification system.

International Prognostic Scoring System

As a result of this expanding array of potential classification methods, an International MDS Risk Analysis Workshop (IMRAW) was convened, which brought together a group of investigators who had previously developed independent risk-based prognostic systems for MDS patients.[46] In this workshop, morphologic criteria (using FAB criteria), cytogenetics, and clinical data were combined and collated from 816 patients with primary MDS from seven previously reported studies. As a result of combining these data and extensive analysis, a consensus classification system for MDS was developed – the International Prognostic Scoring System (IPSS). Analysis of these data permitted determination of variables critical for improving prognostic assessment of clinical outcomes. Specific features, defined by multivariate analysis, were associated with differing clinical outcomes: percent marrow blasts, cytogenetic risk group, number of cytopenias, and patient's age. The marrow cytogenetic risk subgroups were shown be: good (normal, -y, 5q− alone,

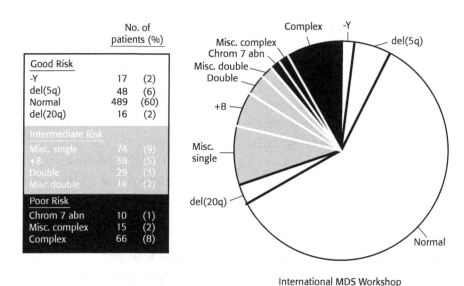

	No. of patients (%)	
Good Risk		
-Y	17	(2)
del(5q)	48	(6)
Normal	489	(60)
del(20q)	16	(2)
Intermediate Risk		
Misc. single	74	(9)
+8	38	(5)
Double	29	(3)
Misc.double	14	(2)
Poor Risk		
Chrom 7 abn	10	(1)
Misc. complex	15	(2)
Complex	66	(8)

International MDS Workshop

Fig. 1.2   Marrow cytogenetic abnormalities in myelodysplastic syndrome (MDS). Analysis of clinical outcome data from 816 patients in the International MDS Risk Analysis Workshop (IMRAW)[46] depicts three cytogenetic prognostic risk groups: (1) good risk: normal, del(5q) only, del(20q) only, or –Y only; (2) poor risk: complex karyotype (i.e., ≥ 3 anomalies) or chromosome 7 abnormalities; and (3) intermediate risk: other abnormalities. The number and percentage of patients with the specific karyotypic abnormality are shown.

20q– alone), Poor (chromosome 7 anomalies and complex, i.e., ≥ three abnormalities) and intermediate (other abnormalities) (Fig. 1.2). CMML patients with white blood cell counts $>12 \times 10^3/mm^3$ were excluded from IMRAW evaluation as they were believed to be best categorized as MPD rather than MDS.

Statistical weighting of these clinical and biologic variables was performed and these features were combined in an additive fashion, placing patients into one of four clinical risk groups: low, intermediate 1, intermediate 2, and high (Table 1.4). This subgrouping provided useful information regarding the patients' survival and freedom from AML evolution (Table 1.5, Fig. 1.3). In addition, patient's age was found to have a major impact on survival but not on AML evolution (Table 1.5, Fig. 1.4). As the majority of MDS patients are relatively elderly (median age 65–70 years in most studies), their associated medical comorbidities often impacted negatively on their longevity. The IMRAW data extended that from prior studies and demonstrated differing

Table 1.4 International Prognostic Scoring System (IPSS) for myelodysplastic syndromes

	Score value				
Prognostic variable	0	0.5	1.0	1.5	2.0
Marrow blasts (%)	< 5	5–10	–	11–20	21–30
Karyotype[a]	Good	Intermediate	Poor		
Cytopenias[b]	0/1	2/3			

[a] Good, normal, -y, del(5q), del(20q); poor, complex (≥ three abnormalities) or chromosome 7 anomalies; intermediate, other abnormalities.
[b] Absolute neutrophil count < 1800/mm^3; platelet count < 100 000/mm^3; hemoglobin < 10 g/ml.

Risk group	Score
Low	0
Intermediate 1	0.5–1.0
Intermediate 2	1.5–2.0
High	≥ 2.5

This research was originally published in *Blood*. Greenberg, P., Cox, C., Le Beau, M. M. *et al*. International scoring system (IPSS) for evaluating prognosis in myelodysplastic syndrome. *Blood*, 1997; **89**: 2079–88. © the American Society of Hematology.

prognoses for patients with > or <10% marrow blasts.[34] The IPSS was able to recategorize the RAEB patients into intermediate 1 and intermediate 2 subtypes; RA patients were generally in low and intermediate 1 categories, whereas RAEB-T patients were generally in the high IPSS category (Fig. 1.5). These data also demonstrated that being in more advanced IPSS risk groups was associated with a higher proportion of patients who died with leukemia rather than due to complications of their dominant cytopenias (Table 1.6).

The IMRAW data,[46,58] and those of others[35,38,59,60] demonstrated the importance of cytogenetic subtypes as a major variable in determining clinical outcome, particularly in the low and intermediate risk categories. For workshop patients evaluated with and without cytogenetic evaluation, the percentage of patients within the high-risk subgroups was similar when using the complete IPSS (7% of patients) versus the partial model (i.e., without cytogenetics) (6%), driven mainly by marrow blast percentage and associated

Table 1.5 Age-related survival and acute myeloid leukemia (AML) evolution of myelodysplastic syndrome patients within the International Prognostic Scoring System (IPSS) subgroups

	No. of patients	Low	Intermediate 1	Intermediate 2	High
Total patients: n (%)	816	267 (33%)	314 (38%)	176 (22%)	59 (7%)
		5.7	3.5	1.2	0.4
Median survival (years)					
Age					
≤ 60 years	205 (25%)	11.8	5.2	1.8	0.3
> 60 years	611	4.8	2.7	1.1	0.5
≤ 70 years	445 (54%)	9.0	4.4	1.3	0.4
> 70 years	371	3.9	2.4	1.2	0.4
Total patients: n (%)	759	235 (31%)	295 (39%)	171 (22%)	58 (8%)
		9.4	3.3	1.1	0.2
25% AML evolution (years)					
Age					
≤ 60 years	187 (25%)	> 9.4 (NR)	6.9	0.7	0.2
> 60 years	572	9.4	2.7	1.3	0.2
≤ 70 years	414 (55%)	> 9.4 (NR)	5.5	1.0	0.2
> 70 years	345	> 5.8 (NR)	2.2	1.4	0.4

NR, not reached.

This research was originally published in Blood. Greenberg, P., Cox, C., Le Beau, M. M. *et al.* International scoring system (IPSS) for evaluating prognosis in myelodysplastic syndrome, *Blood*, 1997; **89**: 2079–88. © the American Society of Hematology.

cytopenias. However, much less discriminating power for the intermediate and low-risk patients was demonstrated when cytogenetics were omitted from the classification method.[58] With incorporation of cytogenetics, a redistribution of patients occurred, generally shifting the patient's risk category to a more advanced stage, i.e., from low into intermediate 1 and intermediate 2 risk groups. The proportion in the low category changed to 33% (complete IPSS) from 70% (partial); intermediate 1: to 38% from 16%; intermediate 2: to 22% from 8%. Thus, cytogenetic features contributed substantially to patients' intermediate 1 and 2 categorizations, the patients generally most difficult to classify prognostically.

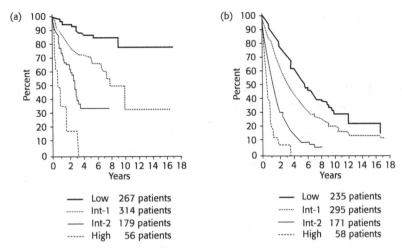

Fig. 1.3   (a) Survival and (b) freedom from acute myeloid leukemia evolution in patients with myelodysplastic syndrome (MDS), in relation to their classification by the International Prognostic Scoring System (IPSS) for MDS: low, intermediate 1 (Int-1), intermediate 2 (Int-2), or high (Kaplan–Meier curves). This research was originally published in *Blood*. Greenberg, P., Cox, C., Le Beau, M. M. *et al.* International Scoring System (IPSS) for evaluating prognosis in myelodysplastic syndrome. *Blood*, 1997; **89**, 2079–88. © the American Society of Hematology.

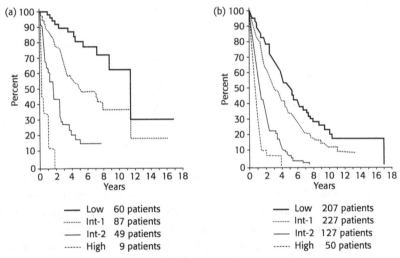

Fig. 1.4   Survival according to age (a) ≤ 60 years or (b) > 60 years of myelodysplastic syndrome (MDS) patients in relation to their classification by the International Prognostic Scoring System (IPSS) for MDS: low, intermediate 1 (Int-1), intermediate 2 (Int-2), or high (Kaplan–Meier curves). This research was originally published in *Blood*. Greenberg, P., Cox, C., Le Beau, M. M. *et al.* International Scoring System (IPSS) for evaluating prognosis in myelodysplastic syndrome. *Blood*, 1997; **89**, 2079–88. © the American Society of Hematology.

Table 1.6 Survival of myelodysplastic syndrome patients with or without acute myeloid leukemia evolution: leukemia-free survival

Subgroups	Number of patients	Patients died: number (%)	Patients died with leukemia (%)	Patients died without leukemia (%)
Low	235	113 (48)	22 (19)	91 (81)
Intermediate 1	295	181 (61)	55 (30)	126 (70)
Intermediate 2	171	147 (86)	49 (33)	98 (67)
High	58	51 (88)	23 (45)	28 (55)
Total	759	492 (65)	149 (30)	343 (70)

This research was originally published in Blood. Greenberg, P., Cox, C., Le Beau, M. M. *et al.* International scoring system (IPSS) for evaluating prognosis in myelodysplastic syndrome. *Blood*, 1997; **89**: 2079–88. © the American Society of Hematology.

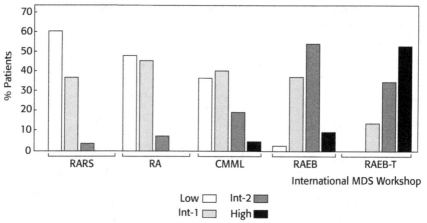

Fig. 1.5   Relationship between French–American–British (FAB) and International Prognostic Scoring System (IPSS) classifications for 816 patients evaluated in the International MDS Risk Analysis Workshop.[46] FAB classifications are: RA, refractory anemia; RARS, RA with ringed sideroblasts; RAEB, RA with excess blasts; RAEB-T, RAEB in transformation; CMML, chronic myelomonocytic leukemia. IPSS classifications are: low, intermediate 1 (Int-1), intermediate 2 (Int-2), or High.

To determine whether the depth of cytopenias was associated with differing patient survivals in MDS, data from IMRAW patients were further analyzed.[61] Shorter survival was associated with patients having lower depths of their cytopenias: median survivals for patients with neutrophil counts $(\times 10^3/\text{mm}^3)$ < 1.5, < 1.0, < 0.5 were 2.5, 1.7, 1.4 years, respectively; for platelets $(\times 10^3/\text{mm}^3)$ < 100, < 75, < 50 the survivals were 1.6, 1.0, 1.0 years,

Table 1.7 Post International Prognostic Scoring System (IPSS) classification: proposed refinements

Morphology	ALIP, hypoplasia, fibrosis
Cytogenetics	Additional subgroups: 5q−, 8+, 1q, 12p
Angiogenesis	Microvascular density, cytokine levels
Immunophenotype	CD34 coexpression: aberrant antigenic markers; CD117/7 v 15
Immunologic markers	PNH clonality, HLA-DR15 histocompatability type
Molecular anomalies	Apoptosis levels, markers (pro: antiapoptotic gene expression)
	Gene mutations: *ras, fms, p53, WT1, bcl-2, AML1, flt3*
	Hypermethylation: *p15*
	Telomere dynamics: telomere length, telomerase levels

ALIP, atypical localization of immature precursors; PNH, paroxysmal nocturnal hemoglobinuria; HLA, human leukocyte antigen.

respectively. These data indicate that assessment of the depth of peripheral blood counts is a useful adjunct to the IPSS for determining MDS clinical outcomes.

A number of investigations from different international regions have applied the IPSS, confirming good correlation of this categorization with clinical outcome of their MDS patients.[62–66] Investigations using this classification system have also confirmed and extended its relevance for assessing prognosis and its potential for the design and analysis of therapeutic trials in MDS. Several studies of allogeneic hemopoietic stem cell transplantation (HSCT) in MDS patients have shown good correlation of clinical outcomes with IPSS scores, particularly with the IPSS-defined cytogenetic risk groups.[67,68]

Post-IPSS classification refinement

The IPSS system has provided a framework for prognostic classification and to add further refinements using newly developed relevant criteria. Subsequently, certain other features of MDS marrow have been shown to complement the IPSS and impact on clinical outcome. These features include cytogenetics, morphologic characteristics (e.g., ALIP), angiogenic markers, immunophenotype, molecular abnormalities, in vitro clonogenic myeloid assays, and telomere dynamics (Table 1.7).

Cytogenetics

Modification of the IPSS cytogenetic risk groups has been suggested by data from several large studies.[69,70] In univariate analyses with a large number of MDS patients in which cytogenetics were assessed, individuals with 1q abnormalities alone experienced poor survival, whereas those with trisomy 8 had a higher risk of acute leukemic transformation than the remaining patients.[69] Patients with del(12p) alone had a similar survival to patients with a normal karyotype and showed a trend for better survival than other cases belonging to the IPSS intermediate-risk cytogenetic subgroup. These data indicate that evaluation of larger numbers of patients with relatively uncommon cytogenetic anomalies may permit further refinement of the IPSS cytogenetic risk categories.

Morphologic features

ALIP

The presence of ALIP significantly added to the prognostic value of the IPSS, with poorer overall and leukemia-free survival in patients with this feature, particularly within the lower-risk categories.[71] ALIP was also predictive of outcome within a group of intensively treated MDS patients.

Angiogenesis

Autocrine production of vascular endothelial growth factor has been linked to the promotion of leukemia colony formation and ALIP in MDS.[72] Microvascular density (MVD) was significantly elevated in MDS patients compared with normal controls, but lower than that seen in AML or MPD.[73,74] Among MDS FAB subtypes, MVD was higher in patients with RAEB-T, CMML, and fibrosis compared with RA, RARS, or RAEB, which were associated with poorer prognoses.

Immunophenotype

Flow cytometric analysis of blasts has provided a potentially valuable additive prognostic tool for MDS patients. Investigators showed that marrow blasts from most MDS patients possess a specific immunophenotypic signature distinct from AML and normal blasts.[75] A high percentage of enriched MDS blast cells had an immunophenotype descriptive of committed progenitor cells (i.e., were positive for CD34, 33, 13, 38, human leukocyte antigen

(HLA)-DR). In addition, differential expression of other surface markers on these blasts correlated with stage of disease and prognosis. The immature-type CD7 and CD117 markers were generally positive on blasts from late-stage MDS patients who had poor clinical outcomes. In contrast, the more mature CD15 marker was generally positive on blasts from MDS patients with earlier-stage disease and better prognoses. A shift occurred to a more immature phenotype accompanying disease progression. These investigators also demonstrated that RAEB-T blasts possessed immunophenotypic markers more closely related to MDS than to de novo AML, indicating that biologic differences exist between these entities. Although CD34 immunore-activity was also found to be associated with clinical outcomes in the patients, the CD34 positivity reflects marrow blast count and thus is unlikely to be an independent prognostic marker.

A different flow cytometric scoring system (FCSS) was used by other workers to condense multiple flow cytometric abnormalities of marrow cells from MDS patients into numerical scores.[76] Scores were calculated based on types of abnormality in the maturing myeloid cells and monocytes, flow cytometric blast counts, and degree of impaired myelopoiesis based on the lymphoid-to-myeloid ratio. Additional weight was given to marrows showing lineage infidelity (i.e., presence of lymphoid antigens on myeloid or monocytic cells) or marked maturational asynchrony, as evidenced by CD34 expression on maturing myeloid cells or monocytes. These two abnormalities are believed to result from significant gene dysregulation. The FCSS correlated directly with IPSS scores and cytogenetic risk categories and inversely with leukocyte and absolute neutrophil counts.

In MDS patients who underwent allogeneic HSCT, the FCSS correlated with posttransplantation outcome.[76] In multivariate analyses, there was a significant contribution of the FCSS independent of the IPSS for predicting survival and relapse. Thus, with further validation of these methods, incorporation of marrow immunophenotypic analyses into the IPSS system should further refine the ability to provide useful prognostic information in MDS.

Immunologic markers

A portion of MDS patients have had their cytopenias respond to immuno-suppressive therapy (e.g., antithymocyte globulin, ciclosporin). The predominant responders have been those with the following characteristics: relative

Table 1.8 Altered gene expression associated with disease progression and poor prognosis in myelodysplastic syndromes[a]

Gene abnormally expressed[b]	Function	Chromosome	MDS incidence	References
N-ras	Cell proliferation	1p13	16% (7–48%)	80–83
fms	M-CSF receptor tyrosine kinase	5q33	15% (12–20%)	80,84,85
flt3	Receptor tyrosine kinase	13q12	4% RAEB, CMML, 0 RA	81,105
p53	Tumor suppressor	17p13	12% (7–20%)	80,87–96
			44% t-MDS	88,94
WT1	Transcription factor	11p13	65% RA	97
			100% RAEB, t-AML	
AML1	Transcription factor	21q22	8% (5–11%)	103,104
			19% RAEB, RAEB-T	
			2% RA, RARS	
p15	Cell cycle activator	9p21	38% (83% > 10 blasts)	102

[a] Mean (range) percentage values cited collated from meta-analysis of listed references.
[b] Mutations present in expressed genes except hypermethylation of p15.
MDS, myelodysplastic syndrome; M-CSF, macrophage-colony-stimulating factor; RAEB, refractory anemia with excess blasts; CMML, chronic myelomonocytic leukemia; RA, refractory anemia; t-AML, therapy-related acute myeloid leukemia; t-MDS, therapy-related myelodysplastic syndrome; RAEB-T, RAEB in transformation; RARS, RA with ringed sideroblasts.

youth, IPSS low-risk disease, morphologic RA subtype, hypoplastic MDS, normal cytogenetics, evidence of a paroxysmal nocturnal hemoglobinuria (PNH) clone or those having the HLA-DR15 subtype.[77–79]

Molecular abnormalities

A number of lesions in gene expression have been associated with poor prognoses in MDS. These anomalies have provided complementary information which was additive to the patient's IPSS category. Individual oncogene mutations, indicative of genetic instability, were associated with disease progression and poor survival in MDS. The implicated genes include *ras, fms, p53,* Wilms tumor (*WT1*), *bcl-2, p15, AML1,* and *flt3* (Table 1.8).

Ras   The frequency of Ras oncoprotein mutations in MDS ranged from 3 to 33%, most commonly in CMML (32–65%).[80–83] Data have generally been consistent regarding the association of such mutations with poor survival or progression to AML. A cohort of 75 MDS patients were investigated for *ras*, *fms*, and *p53* mutations. These molecular alterations were found to correlate with cytogenetics, IPSS status, transformation to acute leukemia, and survival.[80] A mutation incidence of 57% was found, with 48% *ras* mutations, 12% *fms* mutations, and 8% *p53* mutations. The mutation status for *ras* and *fms* was associated with IPSS subgroup, increasing with poor-risk disease. The highest incidence of these lesions was in the CMML subgroup. A statistically significant increased frequency of transformation to AML and poor survival was observed in MDS patients harboring *ras* or *fms* mutations. Patients with these oncogene mutations had a significantly poorer survival compared with those without mutations.[82] Multivariate analysis showed that combining the IPSS subgroup, mutation status, and age provided the best predictive model of a poor outcome.

fms   The *fms* proto-oncogene encodes the receptor for monocyte-colony-stimulating factor (M-CSF) and point mutations within the gene can confer transforming activity.[84, 85] *fms* mutations occur at a frequency of < 20% in MDS patients, and, similar to *ras*, are preferentially observed in CMML.[80,84] Neither *ras* nor *fms* mutations were present in the low-risk patients with 5q− cytogenetic lesions.[86]

p53   Patients with *p53* (TP53) or *WT1* mutations or those with *bcl-2* coexpression in CD34+ blasts were more frequently found in more advanced MDS categories and had poorer clinical outcomes than in those with the earlier IPSS subgroups. The frequency of mutations of the *p53* tumor suppressor gene in de novo MDS patients has generally been reported to be in the 5–20% range, with higher rates observed in t-MDS/AML.[80,87,88] The development of a new *p53* mutation or loss of the wild-type allele was associated with progression of disease and poor survival.[89–93] Mutations of *p53* correlated with resistance to chemotherapy, evolution to leukemia, and shorter survival. In studies of t-MDS/AML, *p53* mutations were associated with complex karyotypes and microsatellite instability, suggesting a mutator phenotype.[94,95] Multivariate analysis demonstrated that patients with *p53* mutation within each IPSS subgroup had a significantly worse survival than those without the mutation.[95] The 17p deletion is strongly correlated with the presence of $p53$ mutations, and has been associated with a particular type of dysgranulopoiesis which combines the pseudo-Pelger–Huët anomaly and small vacuolated neutrophils.[96]

WT1 Quantitative assessment of the *WT1* tumor suppressor transcript levels demonstrated that these values correlated with the marrow blast percentage, cytogenetic abnormalities, and IPSS score.[97] The degree of *WT1* expression was much higher in RAEB and t-AML compared with RA, and increased during disease progression. However, whether this marker is merely linked to blast differentiation stage requires clarification.

bcl-2 Flow cytometric analyses demonstrated that CD34 and Bcl-2 were usually coexpressed in the same immature cells. Levels of Bcl-2 protein expression was demonstrated to be well correlated with the patient's IPSS category.[98] Higher expression of proapoptotic Bcl-2-family proteins (*Bak, Bad, Bcl-x$_S$*) and higher pro versus antiapoptotic ratios (e.g., *Bcl-x$_S$/Bcl-x$_L$*) were associated with early MDS stages, longer survival, and decreased risk of leukemic transformation, whereas increased expression of antiapoptotic proteins (*Bcl-2, Bcl-x$_L$*) was associated with later-stage disease and decreased survival.[99,100] Early myeloid precursors, mainly myeloblasts, were identified in marrow biopsies after immunostaining. Bcl-2 expression (in both proportion and absolute number) within these cells correlated with initial MDS stage (i.e., had significantly lower positivity in morphologically early MDS than in later stages of the disease). Moreover, this expression progressed over time, and was associated with increased levels upon disease evolution to AML.[101]

p15 $p15^{INK4b}$ gene is an inhibitor of cyclin-dependent kinase (CDK) 4 and CDK6, whose expression is induced by transforming growth factor-β (TGF-β). Reports indicate frequent epigenetic effects (i.e., hypermethylation) of the $p15^{INK4b}$ gene promoter in leukemias. Investigation of the methylation status of $p15^{INK4b}$ gene in MDS patients demonstrated that methylation of this gene was observed in 38% of patients and was associated with a poorer prognosis.[102] Methylation of the $p15^{INK4b}$ gene in MDS correlated with advanced-stage blastic bone marrow involvement and increased with disease evolution toward AML. These data further suggest that proliferation of leukemic cells may require escape of cell cycle regulation, and possibly of the TGF-β-inhibitory effect.

AML1   A high incidence of somatically acquired point mutations in the *AML1* gene has been reported in poorly differentiated AML and in radiation-associated t-MDS or t-AML.[103,104] *AML1* point mutations were found predominantly in high-risk MDS patients and AML-MDS. Patients with AML-MDS with an *AML1* mutation had a significantly worse prognosis than those without such mutations.

flt3   Analysis of *flt3* mutations in MDS (3%; 6% in CMML) showed that *flt3*/ITD (internal terminal duplication) was associated with a high risk of transformation to AML and poor survival in patients with MDS.[81] One-third of these MDS patients acquired activating mutations of *flt3* or *N-ras* gene during AML evolution and *Flt3*/ITD predicted poor outcome in MDS.[105] These data were independent of the patient's IPSS category.

Telomere dynamics

To clarify the possible association between genomic instability and clinical outcome in MDS patients, telomere dynamics have been compared in patients within different IPSS risk groups.[106] MDS patients with shortened terminal restriction fragments (TRFs) of their telomeres had a significantly higher percentage of marrow blasts, cytogenetic abnormalities, and advanced IPSS category.[106] The incidence of leukemic transformation was significantly higher in patients with shortened TRF length. The heterogeneous nuclear ribonucleoprotein (hnRNP) B1, a marker for early cancers, is involved in pre-mRNA processing and binds to telomeric cDNA repeats. In MDS, hnRNP B1 levels were higher in RAEB and RAEB-t subtypes than in RA and RARS. Most of the MDS patients had normal-to-low levels of telomerase activity, suggesting that changes in TRF length rather than telomerase activity more accurately reflect prognostic features of MDS. Such abnormal mechanisms of telomere maintenance in subgroups of MDS patients may be an early indication of genomic instability.

Classification as framework for management guidelines

The IPSS has proven useful for aiding management as well as for design and analysis of therapeutic trials for MDS patients. The US NCCN MDS Practice Guidelines Committee has recommended several central clinical parameters for planning therapeutic strategies in MDS: patient's IPSS stage, age, and performance status.[17] This approach for patient management has also been adopted by the British and Italian MDS Guidelines groups.[18,19] Patients in the relatively lower risk IPSS categories (low, intermediate 1) would primarily be recommended to receive relatively low-intensity treatment, whereas those in the higher-risk categories (intermediate 2 and high) would primarily be considered for relatively high-intensity treatment. The major aim of the lower-intensity treatment would be hematologic improvement (mainly using hemopoietic cytokines, biologic response modifiers, and low-intensity chemotherapy), whereas the higher-intensity treatment would attempt to alter disease natural history (using intensive induction chemotherapy or allogeneic HSCT). See Chapters 6–9 for more detailed information about the specific therapies utilized in these patient subgroups.

Summary and future directions

Morphological classification methods such as those reported by the FAB and WHO investigators have been very useful for diagnostic categorization of MDS patients. The IPSS prognostic classification method provides a clinical and biological framework for patient management and design and analysis of therapeutic trials in MDS. Data reviewed herein indicate that future studies are warranted using flow cytometric analysis, molecular and immunophenotypic markers for evaluating prognosis in this disorder to usefully incorporate these additional clinical and biological features to refine further the categorization of MDS patients (Table 1.7). This approach is particularly important as certain patient subtypes defined by these methods have recently been shown to be responsive to specific therapeutic agents. Although individual gene mutations have been informative regarding prognosis in MDS, as the disease is multigenic in nature, and the lesions were non-specific for MDS, evaluation of a more comprehensive set of differential gene expression profiles using microarray analysis in MDS marrow cells will likely provide the next generation of critical markers for this disease and its evolutionary potential.

REFERENCES

1. Greenberg, P. L. (2000). The myelodysplastic syndromes. In *Hematology: Basic Principles and Practice*, 3rd edn, ed. R. B. E. Hoffman, S. Shattil, and H. Cohen. New York: Churchill Livingstone, pp. 1106–29.

2. Bennett, J. M., Catovsky, D., Daniel, M. T. *et al.* (1982). Proposals for the classification of the myelodysplastic syndrome. *Br. J. Haematol.*, **51**, 189.

3. Groupe Français de Cytogénétique Hématologique (1991). Chronic myelomonocytic leukemia: single entity or heterogeneous disorder? A prospective multicenter study of 100 patients. *Cancer Genet. Cytogenet.*, **55**, 57.

4. Bennett, J. M., Catovsky, D., Daniel, M. T. *et al.* (1994). The chronic myeloid leukemias: guidelines for distinguishing chronic granulocytic, atypical chronic myeloid, and chronic myelomonocytic leukemia. *Br. J. Haematol.*, **87**, 746.

5. Harris, N., Jaffe, E., Diebold, J. *et al.* (1999). WHO classification of neoplastic diseases of the hematopoietic and lymphoid tissues: report of the Clinical Advisory Committee meeting – Airlie House, Virginia, November 1997. *J. Clin. Oncol.*, **17**, 3835–49.

6. Bennett, J. M. (2000). WHO classification of the acute leukemias and myelodysplastic syndrome. *Int. J. Hematol.*, **72**, 131–3.

7. Brunning, R. D., Bennett, J. M., Flandrin, G. *et al.* (2001). Myelodysplastic syndromes. In *Tumours of the Hematopoietic and Lymphoid Tissues*, ed. E. S. Jaffe, N. L. Harris, H. Stein, and J. Vardiman. Lyon, France: IARC Press, pp. 62–73.

8. Rosati, S., Anastasi, J., and Vardiman, J. (1996). Recurring diagnostic problems in the pathology of the myelodysplastic syndromes. *Semin. Hematol.*, **33**, 111–26.

9. Katoutsi, V., Kohlmeyer, U., Maschek, H. *et al.* (1994). Comparison of bone marrow and hematologic findings in patients with human immunodeficiency virus infection and those with myelodysplastic syndromes and infectious disease. *Am. J. Clin. Pathol.*, **101**, 123.

10. Sokal, G., Michaux, J., Van den Berghe, H. *et al.* (1975). A new hematological syndrome with a distinct karyotype: the 5q– chromosome. *Blood*, **46**, 519.

11. Mathew, P., Tefferi, A., Dewald, G. W. *et al.* (1993). The 5q– syndrome: a single institution study of 43 consecutive patients. *Blood*, **81**, 1040.

12. Larripa, I., Acevedo, S., Paulau, N. M. *et al.* (1991). Leukemic transformation in patients with 5q– and additional abnormalities. *Haematologica*, **76**, 363.

13. Albitar, M., Manshouri, T., Shen, Y. *et al.* (2002). Myelodysplastic syndrome is not merely "preleukemia". *Blood*, **100**, 791–8.

14. Greenberg, P., Anderson, J., de Witte, T. *et al.* (2000). Problematic WHO reclassification of myelodysplastic syndromes. *J. Clin. Oncol.*, **18**, 3447–9.

15. Germing, U., Gatterman, N., Strupp, C., Aivado, M., and Aul, C. (2000). Validation of the WHO proposals for a new classification of primary myelodysplastic syndromes: a retrospective analysis of 1600 patients. *Leuk. Res.*, **24**, 983–92.

16. Nosslinger, T., Reisner, R., Koller, E. *et al.* (2001). Myelodysplastic syndromes, from French–American–British to World Health Organization: comparison of classifications on 431 unselected patients from a single institution. *Blood*, **98**, 2935–41.

17. Greenberg, P. L., Bennet, J., Bloomfield, C. *et al.* (2003). NCCN practice guidelines for myelodysplastic syndromes, version 2004. *J. Natl Comp. Cancer Network (JNCCN)*, **1**, 456–71.

18. Bowen, D., Culligan, D., Jowitt, S. *et al.* (2003). UK MDS guidelines group. Guidelines for the diagnosis and therapy of adult myelodysplastic syndromes. *Br. J. Haematol.*, **120**, 187–200.

19. Alessandrino, E. P., Amadori, S., Barosi, G. *et al.* Italian Society of Hematology: evidence- and consensus-based practice guidelines for the therapy of primary myelodysplastic syndromes. A statement from the Italian Society of Hematology. *Haematologica*, **87**, 1286–306.

20. Yoshida, Y., Oguma, S., Uchino, H. *et al.* (1988). Refractory myelodysplastic anaemias with hypocellular bone marrow. *J. Clin. Pathol.*, **41**, 763.

21. Maschek, H., Kalousti, V., Rodriguez-Kaiser, M. *et al.* (1993). Hypoplastic myelodysplastic syndrome: incidence, morphology, cytogenetics, and prognosis. *Ann. Hematol.*, **66**, 117.

22. Toyama, K., Ohyashiki, K., Yoshida, Y. *et al.* (1993). Clinical and cytogenetic findings of myelodysplastic syndromes showing hypocellular bone marrow or minimal dysplasia, in comparison with typical myelodysplastic syndromes. *Int. J. Hematol.*, **58**, 33.

23. Tichelli, A., Gratwohl, A., and Nissen, C. (1994). Late clonal complications in severe aplastic anemia. *Leuk. Lymphoma*, **12**, 167.

24. Maschek, H., Georgii, A., Kaloutsi, V. *et al.* (1992). Myelofibrosis in primary myelodysplastic syndromes: a retrospective study of 352 patients. *Eur. J. Haematol.*, **48**, 208.

25. Ohyashiki, K., Sasao, I., Ohyashiki, J. H. *et al.* (1991). Clinical and cytogenetic characteristics of myelodysplastic syndromes developing myelofibrosis. *Cancer*, **68**, 178.

26. Park, D. J. and Koeffler, H. (1996). Therapy-related myelodysplastic syndromes. *Semin. Hematol.*, **33**, 256.

27. Krishnan, A., Bhatia, S., Slovak, M. L. *et al.* (2000). Predictors of therapy-related leukemia and myelodysplasia following autologous transplantation for lymphoma: an assessment of risk factors. *Blood*, **95**, 1588.

28. Pedersen-Bjergaard, J., Aandersen, M., and Christiansen, D. H. (2000). Therapy-related acute myeloid leukemia and myelodysplasia after high-dose chemotherapy and autologous stem cell transplantation. *Blood*, **95**, 3273–9.

29. Le Beau, M. M., Albain, K., Larson, R. A. *et al.* (1986). Clinical and cytogenetic correlations in 63 patients with therapy-related myelodysplastic syndromes and acute nonlymphocytic leukemia: further evidence for characteristic abnormalities of chromosomes no. 5 and 7. *J. Clin. Oncol.*, **4**, 325.

30. Jacobs, R. H., Cornbleet, M. A., Vardiman, J. *et al.* (1986). Prognostic implications of morphology and karyotype in primary myelodysplastic syndromes. *Blood*, **67**, 1765.

31. Pedersen-Bjergaard, J., Philip, P., Larsen, S. O. *et al.* (1990). Chromosome aberrations and prognostic factors in therapy-related myelodysplasia and acute non-lymphocytic leukemia. *Blood*, **76**, 1083.

32. Pedersen-Bjergaard, J. and Philip, P. (1991). Balanced translocations involving chromosome bands 11q23 and 21q22 are highly characteristic of myelodysplasia and leukemia following therapy with cytostatic agents targeting at DNA-topoisomerase II. *Blood*, **78**, 1147.

33. Zhang, L., Rothman, N., Wang, Y. *et al.* (1996). Interphase cytogenetics of workers exposed to benzene. *Environ. Health Perspect.*, **104**, 1325–9.

34. Sanz, G. F., Sanz, M., Vallespi, T. *et al.* (1989). Two regression models and a scoring system for predicting survival and planning treatment in myelodysplastic syndromes: a multivariate analysis of prognostic factors in 370 patients. *Blood*, **74**, 395–408.

35. Morel, P., Hebbar, M., Lai, J. *et al.* (1993). Cytogenetic analysis has strong prognostic value in de novo myelodysplastic syndromes and can be incorporated in a new scoring system: a report on 408 cases. *Leukemia*, **7**, 1315.

36. Mufti, G. J., Stevens, J., Oscier, D. G., Hamblin, T. J., and Machin, D. (1985). Myelodysplastic syndromes: a scoring system with prognostic significance. *Br. J. Haematol.*, **59**, 425.

37. Aul, C., Gatterman, N., Heyll, A., and Germing, U. (1992). Primary myelodysplastic syndromes: analysis of prognostic factors in 235 patients and proposals for an improved scoring system. *Leukemia*, **6**, 52.

38. Toyama, K., Ohyakashi, K., Yoshida, Y., and Abe, T. (1993). Clinical implications of chromosomal abnormalities in 401 patients with MDS: a multicentric study in Japan. *Leukemia*, **7**, 499.

39. Worsley, A., Oscier, D., Stevens, J. *et al.* (1988). Prognostic features of chronic myelomonocytic leukaemia: a modified Bournemouth score gives the best prediction of survival. *Br. J. Haematol.*, **68**, 17.

40. Del Canizo, M. C., Sanz, G., San Miguel, J. F. *et al.* (1989). Chronic myelomonocytic leukemia clinico-biological characteristics: a multivariate analysis in a series of 70 cases. *Eur. J. Haematol.*, **42**, 466.

41. Stark, A. N., Thorgood, J., Head, C. *et al.* (1987). Prognostic factors and survival in chronic myelomonocytic leukaemia (CMML). *Br. J. Cancer*, **56**, 59.
42. Lambertenghi-Deliliers, G., Orazi, A., Luksch, R. *et al.* (1991). Myelodysplastic syndrome with increased marrow fibrosis: a distinct clinico-pathological entity. *Br. J. Haematol.*, **78**, 161.
43. Onida, F. Kantiarjian, H., Smith, T. L. *et al.* (2002). Prognostic factors and scoring systems in chronic myelomonocytic leukemia: a retrospective analysis of 213 patients. *Blood*, **99**, 840–9.
44. Gatto, S., Ball, G., Onida, F. *et al.* (2003). Contribution of beta-2 microglobulin levels to the prognostic stratification of survival in patients with myelodysplastic syndrome (MDS). *Blood*, **102**, 1622–5.
45. Wimazal, F., Sperr, W., Kundi, M. *et al.* (2001). Prognostic value of lactate dehydrogenase activity in myelodysplastic syndromes. *Leuk. Res.*, **25**, 287–94.
46. Greenberg, P., Cox, C., Le Beau, M. M. *et al.* (1997). International scoring system (IPSS) for evaluating prognosis in myelodysplastic syndrome. *Blood*, **89**, 2079–88.
47. Van den Berghe, H. and Michaux, L. (1997). 5q−, twenty-five years later: a synopsis. *Cancer Genet. Cytogenet.*, **94**, 1–7.
48. List, A. F., Kurtin, S., Glinsmann-Gibson, B. *et al.* (2003). Efficacy and safety of CC5013 for treatment of anemia in patients with myelodysplastic syndromes. *Blood*, **102**, abstract 641.
49. Tricot, G., Dewolf-Peeter, C., Vlietinck, R. *et al.* (1984). Bone marrow histology in myelodysplastic syndromes: II. Prognostic values of abnormal localization of immature precursors in MDS. *Br. J. Haematol.*, **58**, 217.
50. Tricot, G., Vlietinck, R., Boogaerts, M. A. *et al.* (1985). Prognostic factors in the myelodysplastic syndromes: importance of initial data on peripheral blood counts, bone marrow cytology, trephine biopsy and chromosomal analysis. *Br. J. Haematol.*, **60**, 19.
51. Greenberg, P. L. (1996). Biologic and clinical implications of marrow culture studies in the myelodysplastic syndromes. *Semin. Hematol.*, **33**, 163–75.
52. Berthier, R., Douday, F., Metral, J. *et al.* (1979). In vitro granulopoiesis in oligoblastic leukemia: prognostic value, characterization, and serial cloning of bone marrow colony and cluster forming cells in agar culture. *Biomedicine*, **30**, 305.
53. Greenberg, P. L., Bax, I., Mara, B. *et al.* (1976). The myeloproliferative disorders: correlation between clinical evolution and alteration of granulopoiesis. *Am. J. Med.*, **61**, 878.
54. Faille, A., Dresch, C., Poirer, O. *et al.* (1978). Prognostic value of in vitro bone marrow culture in refractory anaemia with excess of myeloblasts. *Scand. J. Haematol.*, **20**, 280.
55. Milner, G. R., Testa, N., Geary, C. G. *et al.* (1977). Bone marrow studies in refractory cytopenia and smoldering leukaemia. *Br. J. Haematol.*, **35**, 251.

56. Spitzer, G., Verma, D., Dicke, K. *et al.* (1979). Subgroups of oligoleukemia as identified by in vitro agar culture. *Leuk. Res.*, **3**, 29.

57. Verma, D. S., Spitzer, G., Dicke, K. A. *et al.* (1979). In vitro agar culture patterns in preleukemia and their clinical significance. *Leuk. Res.*, **3**, 41.

58. Greenberg, P., Cox, C., and Bennett, J. (1997). IPSS and other prognostic scoring systems for MDS. *Blood*, **90**, 4232–4.

59. Pierre, R. V., Catovsky, D., Mufti, G. J. *et al.* (1989). Clinical-cytogenetic correlations in myelodysplasia (preleukemia). *Cancer Genet. Cytogenet.*, **40**, 149.

60. Yunis, J. J., Lobell, M., Arnesen, M. A. *et al.* (1988). Refined chromosome study helps define prognostic subgroups in most patients with primary myelodysplastic syndrome and acute myelogenous leukaemia. *Br. J. Haematol.*, **68**, 189.

61. Greenberg, P., Le Beau, M., Fenaux, P. *et al.* (1997). Application of the International Prognostic Scoring System for MDS. *Blood*, **90**, 2843–6.

62. Pfeilstocker, M., Reisner, R., Nosslinger, T. *et al.* (1999). Cross-validation of prognostic scores in myelodysplastic syndromes on 386 patients from a single institution confirms importance of cytogenetics. *Br. J. Haematol.*, **106**, 455–63.

63. Verburgh, E., Achten, R., Maes, B. *et al.* (2003). Additional prognostic value of bone marrow histology in patients subclassified according to the International Prognostic Scoring System for myelodysplastic syndromes. *J. Clin. Oncol.*, **21**, 273–82.

64. Zhao, W. L., Xu, L., Wu, W. *et al.* (2002). The myelodysplastic syndromes: analysis of prognostic factors and comparison of prognostic systems in 128 Chinese patients from a single institution. *Hematol. J.*, **3**, 137–44.

65. Lee, J. H., Lee, J., Shin, Y. R. *et al.* (2003). Application of different prognostic scoring systems and comparison of the FAB and WHO classifications in Korean patients with myelodysplastic syndrome. *Leukemia*, **17**, 305–13.

66. Cermak, J., Vitek, A., and Michalova, K. (2004). Combined stratification of refractory anemia according to both WHO and IPSS criteria has a prognostic impact and improves identification of patients who may benefit from stem cell transplantation. *Leuk. Res.*, **28**, 551–7.

67. Nevill, T. J., Fung, H., Shepherd, J. D. *et al.* (1998). Cytogenetic abnormalities in primary myelodysplastic syndrome are highly predictive of outcome after allogeneic bone marrow transplantation. *Blood*, **92**, 1910–17.

68. Appelbaum, F. R. and Anderson, J. (1998). Allogeneic bone marrow transplantation for myelodysplastic syndrome: outcomes analysis according to IPSS score. *Leukemia*, **12** (suppl. 1), S25–9.

69. Sole, F., Epsinet, B., Sanz, G. F. *et al.* (2000). Incidence, characterization and prognostic significance of chromosomal abnormalities in 640 patients with primary myelodysplastic syndromes. Grupo Cooperativo Español de Citogenética Hematológica. *Br. J. Haematol.*, **108**, 346–56.

70. Maes, B., Meeus, P., Michaux, L. *et al.* (1999). Application of the International Prognostic Scoring System for myelodysplastic syndromes. *Ann. Oncol.*, **10**, 825–9.

71. Lambertenghi Deliliers, G., Annaloro, C., Soligo, D., and Oriani, A. (1998). The diagnostic and prognostic value of bone marrow immunostaining in myelodysplastic syndromes. *Leuk. Lymphoma*, **28**, 231–9.

72. Bellamy, W. T., Richter, L., Sirjani, D. *et al.* (2001). Vascular endothelial cell growth factor is an autocrine promoter of abnormal localized immature myeloid precursors and leukemia progenitor formation in myelodysplastic syndromes. *Blood*, **97**, 1427–34.

73. Pruneri, G., Bertolini, F., Soligo, D. *et al.* (1999). Angiogenesis in myelodysplastic syndromes. *Br. J. Cancer*, **81**, 1398–401.

74. Aguayo, A., Kantarjian, H., Manshouri, T. *et al.* (2000). Angiogenesis in acute and chronic leukemias and myelodysplastic syndromes. *Blood*, **96**, 2240–5.

75. Ogata, T., Nakamura, K., Yokose, N. *et al.* (2002). Clinical significance of phenotypic features of blasts in patients with myelodysplastic syndrome. *Blood*, **100**, 3887–96.

76. Wells, D. A., Benesch, M., Loken, M. R. *et al.* (2003). Myeloid and monocytic dyspoiesis as determined by flow cytometric scoring in myelodysplastic syndrome correlates with the IPSS and with outcome after hematopoietic stem cell transplantation. *Blood*, **102**, 394–403.

77. Dunn, D. E., Tanattanacharoen, P., Boccuni, P. *et al.* (1999). Paroxysmal nocturnal hemoglobinuria cells in patients with bone marrow failure syndromes. *Ann. Intern. Med.*, **131**, 401–8.

78. Saunthararajah, Y., Nakamura, R., Nam, J. M. *et al.* (2002). HLA-DR15 (DR2) is over-represented in myelodysplastic syndrome and aplastic anemia and predicts a response to immunosuppression in myelodysplastic syndrome. *Blood*, **100**, 1570–4.

79. Maciejewski, J. P., Follman, D., Nakamura, R. *et al.* (2001). Increased frequency of HLA-DR2 in patients with paroxysmal nocturnal hemoglobinuria and the PNH/aplastic anemia syndrome. *Blood*, **98**, 3513–19.

80. Padua, R. A., Guinn, B., Al-Sabah, A. I. *et al.* (1998). RAS, FMS and *p53* mutations and poor clinical outcome in myelodysplasias: a 10-year follow-up. *Leukemia*, **12**, 887–92.

81. Shih, L. Y., Huang, C., Wang, P. N. *et al.* (2004). Acquisition of *FLT3* or *N-ras* mutations is frequently associated with progression of myelodysplastic syndrome to acute myeloid leukemia. *Leukemia*, **18**, 466–75.

82. Paquette, R. L., Landaw, E., Pierre, R. V. *et al.* (1993). *N-ras* mutations are associated with poor prognosis and increased risk of leukemia in myelodysplastic syndrome. *Blood*, **82**, 590–9.

83. Neubauer, A., Greenberg, P., Negrin, R. *et al.* (1994). Mutations in the *ras* proto-oncogenes in patients with myelodysplastic syndromes. *Leukemia*, **8**, 638.

84. Ridge, S. A., Worwood, M., Oscier, D. *et al.* (1990). *FMS* mutations in myelodysplastic, leukemic, and normal subjects. *Proc. Natl Acad. Sci. U.S.A.*, **87**, 1377.

85. Tobal, K., Pagliuca, A., Bhatt, B. *et al.* (1990). Mutation of the human *FMS* gene (M-CSF receptor) in myelodysplastic syndromes and acute myeloid leukemia. *Leukemia*, **4**, 486.

86. Fidler, C., Watkins, F., Bowen, D. T. *et al.* (2004). *N-Ras, Flt3* and *TP53* mutations in patients with myelodysplastic syndrome and a del(5q). *Haematologica*, **89**, 865–6.

87. Sugimoto, K., Hirano, N., Toyoshima, H. *et al.* Mutations of the *p53* gene in myelodysplastic syndrome (MDS) and MDS-derived leukemia. *Blood*, **81**, 3022.

88. Adamson, D. J., Dawson, A., Bennett, B. *et al.* (1995). *p53* mutation in the myelodysplastic syndromes. *Br. J. Haematol.*, **89**, 61.

89. Horiike, S., Kita-Sasai, Y., Nakao, M., and Taniwaki, M. (2003). Configuration of the *TP53* gene as an independent prognostic parameter of myelodysplastic syndrome. *Leuk. Lymphoma*, **44**, 915–22.

90. Tang, J. L., Tien, H., Lin, M. T. *et al.* (1998). *p53* mutation in advanced stage of primary myelodysplastic syndrome. *Anticancer Res.*, **18**, 3757.

91. Mori, N., Hidai, H., Yokota, J. *et al.* (1995). Mutations of the *p53* gene in myelodysplastic syndrome and overt leukemia. *Leuk. Res.*, **19**, 869.

92. Horiike, S., Misawa, S., Kaneko, H. *et al.* (1999). Distinct genetic involvement of the *TP53* gene in therapy-related leukemia and myelodysplasia with chromosomal losses of nos 5 and/or 7 and its possible relationship to replication error phenotype. *Leukemia*, **13**, 1235.

93. Wattel, E., Preudhomme, C., Hecquet, B. *et al.* (1994). *p53* mutations are associated with resistance to chemotherapy and short survival in hematologic malignancies. *Blood*, **84**, 3148.

94. Ben-Yehuda, D., Krichevsky, S., Caspi, O. *et al.* (1996). Microsatellite instability and *p53* mutations in therapy-related leukemia suggest mutator phenotype. *Blood*, **88**, 4296.

95. Kita-Sasai, Y., Horiike, S., Misawa, S. *et al.* (2001). International prognostic scoring system and *TP53* mutations are independent prognostic indicators for patients with myelodysplastic syndrome. *Br. J. Haematol.*, **115**, 309–12.

96. Lai, J. L., Preudhomme, C., Zandecki, M. *et al.* (1995). Myelodysplastic syndromes and acute myeloid leukemia with 17p deletion. An entity characterized by specific dysgranulopoiesis and a high incidence of *p53* mutations. *Leukemia*, **9**, 370.

97. Cilloni, D., Gottardi, E., Messa, F. *et al.* (2003). Significant correlation between the degree of *WT1* expression and the International Prognostic Scoring System Score in patients with myelodysplastic syndromes. *J. Clin. Oncol.*, **21**, 1988–95.

98. Boudard, D., Vasselon, C., Bertheas, M. F. *et al.* (2002). Expression and prognostic significance of Bcl-2 family proteins in myelodysplastic syndromes. *Am. J. Hematol.*, **70**, 115–25.

99. Rajapaksa, R., Ginzton, N., Rott, L. (1996). Altered oncogene expression and apoptosis in myelodysplastic syndrome marrow cells. *Blood*, **88**, 4275–87.

100. Parker, J. E., Mufti, G., Rasool, F. *et al.* (2000). The role of apoptosis, proliferation, and the Bcl-2-related proteins in the myelodysplastic syndromes and acute myeloid leukemia secondary to MDS. *Blood*, **96**, 3932–8.

101. Davis, R. E. and Greenberg, P. L. (1998). Bcl-2 expression by myeloid precursors in myelodysplastic syndromes: impact on disease progression. *Leuk. Res.*, **22**, 767–77.

102. Quesnel, B., Guillerm, G., Vereecque, R. *et al.* (1998). Methylation of the *p15(INK4b)* gene in myelodysplastic syndromes is frequent and acquired during disease progression. *Blood*, **91**, 2985–90.

103. Nakao, M., Horiike, S., Fukushima-Nakase, Y. *et al.* (2004). Novel loss-of-function mutations of the haematopoiesis-related transcription factor, acute myeloid leukaemia 1/runt-related transcription factor 1, detected in acute myeloblastic leukaemia and myelodysplastic syndrome. *Br. J. Haematol.*, **125**, 709–19.

104. Harada, H., Harada, Y., Niimi, H. *et al.* (2004). High incidence of somatic mutations in the *AML1/RUNX1* gene in myelodysplastic syndrome and low blast percentage myeloid leukemia with myelodysplasia. *Blood*, **103**, 2316–24.

105. Shih, L. Y., Lin, T., Wang, P. N. *et al.* (2004). Internal tandem duplication of *fms*-like tyrosine kinase 3 is associated with poor outcome in patients with myelodysplastic syndrome. *Cancer*, **101**, 989–98.

106. Ohyashiki, J. H., Iwama, H., Yahata, N. *et al.* (1999). Telomere stability is frequently impaired in high-risk groups of patients with myelodysplastic syndromes. *Clin. Cancer Res.*, **5**, 1155–60.

2

Morphologic classifications of myelodysplastic syndromes: French–American–British (FAB) and World Health Organization (WHO)

Richard D. Brunning

University of Minnesota, Minneapolis, MN, USA

In 1976, a French–American–British (FAB) cooperative group introduced a morphologic, cytochemical classification of acute leukemia.[1] In the same publication, they also introduced the concept of dysmyelopoietic syndrome which they defined as "disorders associated with bone marrow hyper-cellularity in which confusion with acute myeloid leukemia is possible." Two major groups of dysmyelopoietic syndrome were delineated: refractory anemia with excess of blasts (RAEB) and chronic myelomonocytic leukemia (CMML). Subsequently, in 1982, the FAB group proposed a more complete classification for this group of disorders which they then referred to as myelodysplastic syndromes (MDS).[2] This proposed classification included five types of MDS: (1) refractory anemia (RA); (2) RA with ringed sider-oblasts (RARS); (3) RAEB; (4) RAEB in transformation (RAEB-T); and (5) CMML. Defining criteria for two types of blasts, type I or agranular blasts, and type II blasts with a few azurophilic granules, were also presented. A summary of the characteristics of the five types of MDS in the FAB classification is presented in Table 2.1.[2]

As with all classifications, there were some problems inherent in this proposal; there was particularly some ambiguity regarding the RA and CMML categories. In addition, unrelated to the classification per se, there was some variability in the application of definitional criteria for myelodys-plasia by different observers. Nevertheless, the FAB classification has served

Myelodysplastic Syndromes: Clinical and Biological Advances, ed. Peter L. Greenberg. Published by Cambridge University Press. © Cambridge University Press 2006.

Table 2.1 French–American–British classification of myelodysplastic syndromes[2]

Refractory anemia (RA)

Anemia

Usually no blasts in peripheral blood; if present, < 1%

Marrow myeloblasts (types I and II) < 5%

Erythroid hyperplasia and/or dyserythropoiesis

Granulocytes and megakaryocytes almost always normal

Rarely patients with isolated neutropenia and/or thrombocytopenia but no anemia may be included in this category

Refractory anemia with ringed sideroblasts (RARS)

Findings similar to refractory anemia with the addition of ≥ 15% ringed sideroblasts in the marrow

Possible dimorphic erythrocytes in blood

Refractory anemia with excess of blasts (RAEB)

Always some degree of cytopenia involving two or more myeloid cell lineages

Peripheral blood shows conspicuous abnormalities in all three myeloid cell lineages

Circulating myeloblasts < 5%

Marrow myeloblasts (types I and II) 5–20%

Varying degrees of either granulocytic or erythroid hyperplasia

Always evidence of dysgranulopoiesis, dyserythropoiesis, and/or dysmegakaryocytopoeisis

Refractory anemia with excess of blasts in transformation (RAEB-T)

Cytopenias in patients, generally with an indolent course

Hematologic features similar to RAEB with addition of one or more of the following:

(1) 5–30% myeloblasts (types I and II) in the peripheral blood

(2) Marrow myeloblasts (types I and II) 20–30%

(3) Presence of Auer rods in granulocytic precursors in patients with < 30% blasts in blood and/or marrow

Chronic myelomonocytic leukemia

Defining criterion presence of monocytosis (> 1×10^9/l)

Often associated with increase in mature granulocytes

< 5% myeloblasts in peripheral blood

Bone marrow shows significant increase in monocyte precursors

Percent of marrow myeloblasts 1–20%

---

as a valuable tool for classifying patients with myelodysplastic disorders and as the classification system of MDS in several clinical trials.

In 1997, as part of a World Health Organization (WHO) project on classification of tumors of the hematopoietic system, an international committee composed of hematologists and hematopathologists was charged with developing a new classification for the acute leukemias and MDS. The proposed classifications were published in final form by the WHO in 2001.[3] The WHO classification retained much of the terminology of the FAB classification. However, significant conceptual changes were proposed in an attempt to reflect biologic behavior more accurately. The changes relate principally to four categories: (1) RA; (2) RAEB; (3) RAEB-T; and (4) CMML.

The WHO classification of the MDS includes eight entities; CMML has been placed in a new category of diseases, myelodysplastic/myeloproliferative disorders, which will be discussed (Table 2.2).[3] The relationship of the FAB MDS categories to the WHO categories is shown in Figure 2.1.

Because both the FAB and WHO classifications are morphology-based, it is important to recognize the morphologic features that result in the diagnosis of MDS and the specific categorization of a process.[3–5] In assessing dysplasia, it is critical to evaluate carefully all of the major myeloid cell lines.[3,4] This can only be optimally accomplished on very well-prepared and stained smear preparations. Poorly prepared and stained slides may result in artifactual changes in both the nucleus and cytoplasm which may mimic dysplasia or conceal subtle dysplastic changes. This same cautionary note also applies to marrow biopsy specimens.

The peripheral blood findings vary substantially in different cases. The most frequent abnormalities are increased red blood cell anisopoikilocytosis and macrocytosis. The red blood cells may manifest anisochromasia with a dimorphic population in sideroblastic anemia (Plate 1). The granulocyte abnormalities include nuclear hyposegmentation, pseudo Pelger–Huët changes and hypogranularity. Hypergranularity and abnormal granules may be present.

Morphologically, dyserythropoiesis manifests principally as abnormalities in nuclear structure, including nuclear budding, karyorrhexis, multinuclearity, internuclear bridging, and megaloblastoid changes; cytoplasmic alterations include ringed sideroblasts, vacuolization, and periodic acid–Schiff

Table 2.2 World Health Organization classification of myelodysplastic syndromes[3]

Disease	Blood findings	Bone marrow findings
Refractory anemia (RA)	Anemia No or rare blasts	Erythroid dysplasia only[a] < 5% blasts < 15% ringed sideroblasts
Refractory anemia with ringed sideroblasts (RARS)	Anemia No blasts	≥ 15% ringed sideroblasts in erythroid population Erythroid dysplasia only < 5% blasts
Refractory cytopenia with multilineage dysplasia (RCMD)	Cytopenias (bicytopenia or pancytopenia) No or rare blasts No Auer rods < 1 × 10^9/l monocytes	Dysplasia in ≥ 10% of the cells in ≥ 2 hemopoietic cell lines < 5% blasts No Auer rods < 15% ringed sideroblasts
Refractory cytopenia with multilineage dysplasia and ringed sideroblasts (RCMD-RS)	Cytopenias (bicytopenia or pancytopenia) No or rare blasts No Auer rods < 1 × 10^9/l monocytes	Dysplasia in ≥ 10% of the cells in ≥ 2 hematopoietic cell lines ≥ 15% ringed sideroblasts < 5% blasts No Auer rods
Refractory anemia with excess blasts-1 (RAEB-1)	Cytopenias < 5% blasts No Auer rods < 1 × 10^9/l monocytes	Unilineage or multilineage dysplasia 5–9% blasts No Auer rods
Refractory anemia with excess blasts-2 (RAEB-2)	Cytopenias 5–19% blasts Auer rods ± < 1 × 10^9/l monocytes	Unilineage or multilineage dysplasia 10–19% blasts Auer rods ±
Myelodysplastic syndrome – unclassified (MDS-U)	Neutropenia or thrombocytopenia No or rare blasts No Auer rods	Unilineage dysplasia[a] < 5% blasts No Auer rods ± specific cytogenetic anomalies
MDS associated with isolated del(5q)	Anemia Usually normal or increased platelet count < 5% blasts	Normal to increased megakaryocytes with hypolobulated nuclei < 5% blasts Isolated del(5q) cytogenetic abnormality No Auer rods

[a]Unilineage dysplasia must be present for ≥ 6 months with no other etiology found.

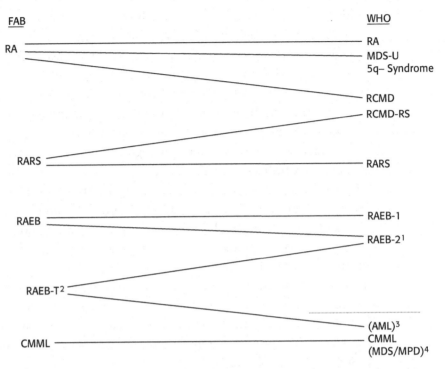

Fig. 2.1   Relation of French–American–British (FAB) and World Health Organization (WHO) classifications of myelodysplastic syndromes.

[1] RAEB-2 includes patients with one or more of the following: (1) 10–19% blasts in marrow; (2) 5–19% blasts in blood; (3) Auer rods in blasts in patients with < 20% blasts in marrow and/or blood.

[2,3] RAEB-T is not included in the WHO classification; patients with > 20% blasts in marrow and/or blood are classified as acute myeloid leukaemia (AML). See 1 for patients with other criteria for RAEB-T.

[4] Chronic myelomonocytic leukemia (CMML) is classified in a newly designated category of myeloid disorders, myelodysplastic/myeloproliferative diseases (MDS/MPD), which includes CMML, atypical chronic myeloid leukemia (aCML), and juvenile myelomonocytic leukaemia (JMML).

RA, refractory anemia; RARS, RA with ringed sideroblasts; RAEB, RA with excess blasts; RAEB-T, RAEB in transformation; MDS-U, myelodysplastic syndrome, unclassified; RCMD, refractory cytopenia with multilineage dysplasia; RCMD-RS, RCMD and ringed sideroblasts; AML, acute myeloid leukemia; MDS/MPD, MDS/myeloproliferative disease.

positivity (Plates 2 and 3). Gigantic erythroblasts with multiple nuclei may uncommonly be present, usually in low numbers.

Dysgranulopoiesis is manifest principally as nuclear hypolobulation (pseudo Pelger-Huët nuclei) and cytoplasmic hypogranularity (Plate 4). The degree of nuclear hypolobulation varies from non-lobulated hyperchromatic nuclei to hyperchromatic bilobed nuclei. Hypogranular neutrophils have a pale, somewhat gray cytoplasm. Other manifestations of dysgranulopoiesis include small size, bizarre nuclear hypersegmentation, nuclear twinning, and giant pseudo Chédiak–Higashi granules.

Dysplastic changes in the developing neutrophils are primarily characterized by nuclear cytoplasmic dyssynchrony and abnormalities of the granules. The nuclear cytoplasmic dyssynchrony manifests more frequently as hypogranularity. Occasionally the granules are larger than normal. Uncommonly, the azurophilic and secondary granules fuse and resemble Chédiak–Higashi granules. Auer rods may be present in promyelocytes and myelocytes in addition to blasts in RAEB-2. Large areas of cytoplasmic basophilia may persist into the myelocyte and later stages. Promyelocytes may lack azurophilic (primary) granules and myelocytes may show diminished secondary granules (Plate 5).

Megakaryocytic dysplasia usually includes hypolobulated nuclei, multiple widely placed small nuclei, nuclear cytoplasmic dyssynchrony, and marked variation in size (Plate 6). Biopsy sections may be more advantageous then marrow smears in evaluating dysmegakaryocytopoiesis (Plate 7).

The blast percentage in the blood and marrow and the characteristics of the dysplasia are the basis for the morphologic classification of the myelodysplastic syndromes in both the FAB and WHO classifications. In the WHO classifications, unilineage dysplasia in the erythroid cells is the only morphologic abnormality characterizing RA. An increase in blasts but less than 20% in the marrow or blood is the hallmark of RAEB-1 and RAEB-2.[3] Multilineage dysplasia without an increase in blasts (< 5%) is a feature of refactory cytopenia with multilineage dysplasia (RCMD).[3,6–8] The presence of ≥ 15% ringed sideroblasts in the marrow characterizes RARS. The combination of multilineage dysplasia and ≥ 15% ringed sideroblasts denotes RCMD with ringed sideroblasts.[3] Macrocytic erythrocytes in conjunction with small or normal-sized hypolobulated megakaryocytes and $< 5\%$ blasts in the marrow suggest the possibility of an isolated 5q– syndrome.[9]

One of the most critical aspects in the diagnosis and morphologic classification of the MDS is the recognition that evidence of myelodysplasia per se is not diagnostic of a myelodysplastic syndrome. This is particularly relevant to those MDS in which the blasts are not increased. Remarkable degrees of dysplasia, particularly in the erythroid cells, may be related to vitamin deficiencies, congenital disorders, and exposure to drugs or chemicals.[3,10–13] Congenital dyserythropoiesis may be characterized by marked dyserythropoiesis; in these disorders the dysplasia is restricted to the erythroid series. Exposure to heavy metals, particularly arsenic, may lead to marked dysplasia, primarily in the erythroid cells (Plate 8). Vitamin B_{12} and/or folate deficiency causes panmyeloid dysplasia; in severe deficiency there may be an extraordinary degree of dysplasia more marked than usually encountered in MDS. The folic acid antagonists can, because of their mechanism of action on folate metabolism, give the same morphologic features as folate deficiency; when several of these drugs are used in combination, extraordinary dysplasia may occur. Parvovirus B_{19} infection has a stage of erythroblastopenia with giant erythroblasts.[14] This stage may be followed by marked erythroid hyperplasia with some erythroid dysplasia.

The administration of granulocyte colony-stimulating factor may result in marked dysplastic changes in the neutrophils with pseudo Pelger–Huët nuclei, marked hypergranularity, and Döhle bodies.[15] Myeloblasts may be observed in the peripheral blood and reach levels of 9–10%. Dysplasia has frequently been observed in patients with human immunodeficiency virus (HIV) infections.[16,17] Paroxysmal nocturnal hemoglobinuria may present with hematologic features suggestive of a myelodysplastic syndrome, particularly if associated with concurrent folic acid deficiency. Megakaryocytic abnormalities occur in vitamin B_{12} and folate deficiency and in HIV-infected patients.

Because of these possible non-clonal etiologies of myelodysplasia, it is imperative to have an accurate and current medical history, particularly of drug therapy, for a patient before establishing a diagnosis of a myelodysplastic syndrome; all possibilities of a non-clonal disorder must be excluded. As previously noted, the presence of morphologic evidence of myelodysplasia is not per se diagnostic of a myelodysplastic syndrome.

WHO classification

Refractory anemia

The term "refractory anemia" in the WHO classification is restricted to those MDS with dysplasia and hematologic findings involving only the erythroid lineage. The presenting symptoms are related to anemia.[3] The erythrocytes in the blood are usually normochromic, normocytic or normochromic, macrocytic. Unusually the red blood cells are slightly hypochromic. There may be no or marked anisopoikilocytosis. Blasts are rarely present in the blood and are always fewer than 1 per 100 leukocytes. The neutrophils and platelets are normal. Erythroid precursors in the marrow vary from decreased to markedly increased and dyserythropoiesis varies from slight to marked. Ringed sideroblasts may be present but are less than 15% of the erythroid precursors. The granulocytic and megakaryocytic series are normal or show minimal dysplasia, always fewer than 10% of the cells. Auer rods are not present and blasts are not increased in the marrow. The marrow biopsy is usually hypercellular, primarily related to erythroid hyperplasia.[18] Occasional patients present with a hypoplastic marrow.

If a case of MDS satisfies the criteria for RA but has hypolobated megakaryocytes and an associated isolated 5q− chromosome abnormality, it is classified as a 5q− syndrome.[3,9]

The diagnosis of RA should only be established after all other possibilities for the erythroid abnormalities have been excluded, including exposure to drugs and toxins, viral illnesses, immunologic disorders, congenital abnormalities, vitamin deficiencies, and paroxysmal nocturnal hemoglobulinuria.

Refractory cytopenias with multilineage dysplasia

The category of RA in the FAB classification has been associated with some imprecision because of the application of somewhat different diagnostic criteria by different observers. As defined by the FAB group, the dysplastic changes in RA are essentially limited to the erythroid series. However, because of a statement in the original defining criteria that allows for granulocytic and megakaryocytic abnormalities, the term understandably has been used by some observers for cases of MDS involving the granulocytes and megakaryocytes, i.e., cases with multilineage dysplasia but no increase in blasts. Because MDS by definition may involve a multilineage stem cell, some observers have proposed that a unilineage dysplasia MDS does not exist. However, involvement of a multilineage stem cell does not necessarily exclude unilineage morphologic manifestation. This variability in approach to the use of the term has led to somewhat imprecise diagnostic criteria by different observers and variability in survival statistics. Because of the ambiguity relating to the entity RA in the FAB classification, the WHO classification recognized a recently described entity, RCMD, for those cases of MDS that present with cytopenias of varying degree, multilineage dysplasia, and no increase in blasts or Auer rods.[3,6–8] Definitionally, dysplastic changes are present in $\geq$ 10% of the cells in two or more myeloid lineages in RCMD. RCMD may present with or without a significant number (> 15%) of ringed sideroblasts. If there are $\geq$ 15% ringed sideroblasts the process is categorized as RCMD with ringed sideroblasts (RCMD-RS).

Refractory anemia with ringed sideroblasts

Several studies of RARS have suggested two prognostic groups, one with prolonged survival with low or no evolution to acute leukemia or a higher-grade MDS in which the dysplasia is restricted to the erythroid series and characterized by anemia and $\geq$ 15% ringed sideroblasts in the marrow.[19] There is generally an erythroid hyperplasia. In many, if not most, of these cases, it is not possible to demonstrate a clonal abnormality and probably they are the result of a metabolic dysfunction unrelated to neoplasia. In other cases of RARS, dysplastic features are present in the granulocytes and/or the megakaryocytes in addition to the erythroid cells. This latter group is recognized in the WHO classification as a variant of refractory cytopenia with multilineage dysplasia, RCMD and $\geq$ 15% ringed sideroblasts (RCMD-RS).[3] The distinction of the two types of RARS is analogous to the distinction of RA and RCMD.

Refractory anemia with excess blasts

In the FAB classification, RAEB is defined by 5–20% blasts in the marrow and < 5% in the blood.[1,2,5] Based on data cited by the International Workshop on Prognostic Factors in MDS which indicated that patients with RAEB with 10–20% blasts in the marrow had a shorter survival and higher rate of evolution to acute leukemia than patients with 5–10% blasts, the WHO proposal stratifies RAEB into two categories: (1) RAEB-1, which has 5–9% blasts in the marrow, and less than 5% in the blood; and (2) RAEB-2, which has 10–19% blasts, in the marrow.[3,20]

RAEB in transformation (RAEB-T) in the FAB classification is defined by one or more of three criteria: (1) 20–30% blasts in the marrow; (2) 5–30% blasts in the blood; and (3) the presence of Auer rods with blast counts of < 30% in the marrow or blood.[2] Because of survival data in the literature showing similarities between patients with 20–30% blasts in the marrow and patients with > 30% marrow blasts,[21–23] the WHO classification of acute myeloid leukemia recognizes 20% blasts in the marrow or blood as a minimum threshold for diagnosis of acute leukemia. Patients with 5–19% blasts in the blood, 10–19% blasts in the marrow, or Auer rods in blasts, with or without the other two criteria are classified as RAEB-2.[3,24]

MDS – unclassified

Uncommonly, cases present with convincing hematologic, morphologic, or cytogenetic evidence of an MDS which do not satisfy the criteria for a specific type of MDS. These cases may present with an isolated thrombocytopenia or neutropenia.[25,26] There is no increase in blasts in the blood or marrow and the dysplasia is restricted to one or other of these cell lineages. In the FAB classification these cases would probably be classified as RA. In the WHO classification these cases are placed in a category of MDS, unclassified (MDS-U).[3] These cases may be problematic. All possible etiologies for the thrombocytopenia or neutropenia must be excluded, with particular emphasis on immunologic/or drug-related etiologies before a diagnosis of a MDS is made; a careful and detailed drug history along with appropriate laboratory studies, including vitamin B_{12}, folic acid, and paroxysmal nocturnal hemoglobinuria-related tests must be performed.[25] Marginal morphologic evidence of dysplasia must be viewed with considerable caution and, if there is any doubt, a diagnosis should be deferred until there is additional morphologic or genetic evidence.

In addition to the cases of MDS with unilineage dysplasia involving the megakaryocyte-platelet or granulocyte lineages, cases of MDS established only on the basis of appropriate cytogenetic findings may be placed in this category if there are no qualifying morphologic features.[27]

As noted, the major differences between the FAB and WHO classifications relate to RA, RAEB, RAEB-T, and CMML.

Myelodysplastic syndromes associated with specific recurring cytogenetic abnormalities

Cytogenetic abnormalities in the MDS are an important factor in the prognostic stratification. The incidence of detectable abnormalities is augmented with the addition of interphase and molecular techniques.[28,29] Although several different cytogenetic patterns may be observed with an MDS, only a small number have been shown to correlate with relatively specific morphologic findings. The most notable example of a morphologic cytogenetic correlation is the 5q− syndrome, which is characterized by an isolated del(5q), including bands of 31–33 and RA, frequently macrocytic, normal to elevated platelet count, < 5% blasts in the blood or marrow, and increased megakaryocytes, frequently with hypolobulated nuclei (Plates 6 and 7).[9,30–32] Dyserythropoiesis of variable degree is usually present. The 5q− syndrome predominantly occurs in middle-aged females, but is not exclusive to that group. It is generally accompanied by a favorable prognosis. Cytogenetic evolution usually heralds a change to acute myeloid leukemia or a higher-grade MDS. The diagnosis of 5q− syndrome should be reserved for patients with the findings described; cases with additional cytogenetic abnormalities or > 5% blasts in the marrow or blood should be classified in the appropriate morphologic classification without the designation 5q− syndrome.[30,31]

Other cytogenetic abnormalities have also been associated with some morphologic correlates. These include del(17), which is associated with acute myeloid leukemia or MDS, and neutrophils with pseudo Pelger–Huët nuclei, small vacuolated neutrophils, *TP53* mutation and an unfavorable prognosis and isolated del(12p) and 20q− which are associated with erythroid and megakaryocyte abnormalities.[33–35] However, at the time of the classification there appeared to be insufficient evidence to recognize these entities as specific clinical, morphologic, cytogenetic correlates.

Therapy-related myelodysplastic syndrome

The therapy-related myelodysplastic syndromes (t-MDS) and acute myeloid leukemias occur in patients treated with cytotoxic chemotherapy and/or radiation therapy. There are two major types: (1) alkylating agent and/or radiation-related type and (2) topoisomerase II inhibitor-related type.[3,36–45] Some cases appear to be unrelated to these two groups.

The major t-MDS is of the alkylating agent and/or radiation therapy type. This usually arises 5–6 years after exposure to the mutagenic agent but may occur after a shorter or longer period. The risk is related to the total dose of the causative agent and the patient's age; older patients are more susceptible. These cases are primarily associated with unbalanced chromosome translocations and/or deletions involving chromosomes 5 and/or 7, consisting of loss of all or part of the long arm of the chromosome. The loss of the long arm of chromosome 5 usually includes bands q23 to q32. Complex chromosome patterns are common. The presenting hematologic features are pancytopenia or isolated cytopenia. Approximately 40–70% of cases of this type of t-MDS present as refractory cytopenia with multilineage dysplasia; approximately one-third of these cases have ≥ 15% ringed sideroblasts. About 25% of cases can be classified as RAEB-1 or 2.[3,4] Cases of MDS with del(17p) may be therapy-related.[40] Extreme degrees of dysplasia may occur. The patients with the alkylating type of t-MDS may succumb in the MDS phase or evolve to a form of acute leukemia, frequently acute myeloid leukemia with multilineage dysplasia.[41]

The topoisomerase II-related type of MDS has a shorter latency period than the alkylating agent-related type; the reported interval ranges from 12 to 130 months, with a median of 33–34 months. This type has been reported following therapy with epidophyllotoxins,[43,46] etoposide and teniposide, and the anthracyclines, and frequently presents as acute leukemia with monocytic features and associated 11q23 cytogenetic abnormalities or other types of leukemia with recurring cytogenetic abnormalities, including t(8;21) involving band q22 and inv16.[43,45–48] Typical cases of acute promyelocytic leukemia with t(15;17) may also be observed.[47]

Cases of MDS-acute myeloid leukemia associated with a long latency period and cytogenetic abnormalities more characteristic of alkylating agent-related type MDS-acute myeloid leukemia, abnormalities of 5 and/or 7, have been reported in patients with acute promyelocytic leukemia in remission after therapy with or without *all*-trans retinoic acid (ATRA). Several of the reported patients had not received alkylating agents during treatment of acute promyelocytic leukemia.[38,49]

Bone marrow histopathology in myelodysplastic syndromes

The criteria for the classification of the MDS are based primarily on examination of the blood and bone marrow smears. However, the histopathology in marrow biopsies can contribute significantly to the evaluation of these specimens.[18,50–52] This is particularly relevant to cases of MDS with marrow fibrosis or hypocellular marrows.

Marrow fibrosis in the MDS has been the subject of several reports; the majority of these reports have found a higher association of fibrosis with chronic myelomonocytic leukemia than other types of MDS and shorter survival than for patients with MDS without fibrosis.[53–55] There is some difficulty in making comparisons of different studies. Cases reported as acute myelodysplasia with myelofibrosis may more appropriately be classified as acute panmyelosis with myelofibrosis rather than an MDS. Some of these cases also fall in the category of the therapy-related MDS–leukemia syndrome, which is an aggressive process.[56] Whether myelodysplasia with myelofibrosis is a distinct entity is controversial.[55] In the WHO classification it is not treated as a distinct entity. If a case of MDS has significant fibrosis it should be classified according to the criteria applied to blood and marrow smears with the qualifying term "with myelofibrosis."

Similar to cases with myelofibrosis, a low percentage of cases of MDS present with hypocellular marrows; the reported incidence ranges from 8 to 20%.[51,57,58] The major distinction of this finding is aplastic anemia.[59,60] There is insufficient evidence for recognizing hypocellular MDS as a distinct entity at this time. Cases of MDS with hypocellular marrows should be classified according to the usual criteria, with the qualifying term "with hypocellular marrow." Since these cases may be difficult to distinguish from true aplastic anemia, additional studies may be necessary. Immunohistochemical reactions with antibodies to CD34, PCNA, and myeloperoxidase should solve the problem in the vast majority of cases.[60] With careful examination of the blood and marrow smears the correct diagnosis should be apparent.

Some of the patients with MDS and hypocellular marrows appear to have an immune-related process and may respond to immunosuppressive agents.[61]

Myelodysplastic/myeloproliferative diseases

In the discussions of the WHO committee on the classification of the myeloid disorders, a consensus developed that there was a small number of myeloid processes that, by virtue of the initial clinical and hematologic presentation, appear to overlap an MDS and a myeloproliferative disorder. CMML is the most notable example of this group of diseases.[62–66] The two other disorders placed in this category are atypical chronic myeloid leukemia and juvenile myelomonocytic leukemia.[3] Because of the somewhat ambiguous biology of these processes, the decision was made to recognize them in a separate category of myeloid diseases: myelodysplastic/myeloproliferative disease. A fourth disorder, RARS and thrombocytosis, was considered for possible inclusion in this group; however, at present, the relationship of these two findings is too uncertain to be recognized as a specific entity and the process is recognized as a variant of RARS until there is evidence for a more definitive categorization.

The myelodysplastic/myeloproliferative diseases are clonal myeloid disorders that present with a constellation of clinical, laboratory, and morphologic features which may be associated with both a myelodysplastic and a myeloproliferative process; i.e., the features lack specificity for classification exclusively either as a myelodysplastic disorder or a myeloproliferative process.[24,64,66] The marrow is generally hypercellular as a result of an expansion of one or more of the myeloid lineages, granulocytic, monocytic, erythroid, or megakaryocytic. There is usually a combination of effective and ineffective hematopoiesis with concurrent cytopenias and cytosis, e.g., anemia and increased granulocytes. Thrombocytopenia may be found in all three subtypes in this category. The neutrophils may be both increased and dysplastic. Splenomegaly and hepatomegaly may be present or absent.

This category is only intended for patients who present with a de novo process; it excludes cases of recognized chronic myeloproliferative disorders such as chronic myeloid leukemia which may manifest dysplastic features in the accelerated phase of the disease. These latter cases should be classified as the primary disease process with a qualifying term, e.g., accelerated phase or blast transformation.

Chronic myelomonocytic leukemia

CMML is a myeloid disorder with protean clinical and morphologic manifestations.[62–64,67,68] Because it lacks an identifying biologic marker analogous to the *BCR-ABL* fusion gene in chronic myeloid leukemia, the diagnostic term encompasses a somewhat heterogeneous group of diseases.[62–64,67–69] At one end of the diagnostic spectrum some cases present with elevated leukocyte counts and splenomegaly, features suggesting a chronic myeloproliferative process whereas other cases present with cytopenias, prominent dysplasia, and no evidence of organomegaly more suggestive of a MDS. The unifying morphologic feature of this spectrum of patients is a persistent monocytosis $> 1 \times 10^9/l$ in the blood and the demonstrated absence of the *BCR/ABL* fusion gene by cytogenetics, fluorescent in situ hybridization (FISH) or molecular studies, and $< 20\%$ blasts and promonocytes in the blood and marrow.[66,69] All possible etiologies of secondary monocytosis must be excluded. In some instances, it is not possible to establish a morphologic diagnosis of CMML at initial encounter because of ambiguity in the clinical and morphologic findings and a period of clinical and hematologic observation may be necessary.

The heterogenous presentation of disorders which appear to fulfill the diagnostic criteria for CMML as defined in the FAB classification has been well documented in several studies; some cases have more of the features of MDS while others present with findings more consistent with a myeloproliferative disorder.[5,62,64–67,69] The FAB group addressed this issue in 1994 and suggested the magnitude of the presenting leukocyte count as the distinguishing feature between CMML myelodysplastic and CMML myeloproliferative; leukocytosis $\geq 13 \times 10^9/l$ categorized a process as CMML myeloproliferative; the cases presenting with leukocyte counts $< 13 \times 10^9/l$ would be classified as CMML myelodysplastic if the defining criteria are present.[70] However, this distinction did not appear to distinguish subgroups with uniform biologic characteristics.

The WHO diagnostic criteria for CMML are presented in Table 2.3.[24,69] The defining characteristic of CMML, either myelodysplastic or myeloproliferative, is a blood monocytosis $> 1.0 \times 10^9/l$; the count is usually between 2 and $5 \times 10^9/l$ but may exceed $80 \times 10^9/l$. The monocytes are generally mature but may manifest atypical granules and nuclear lobulation. Two categories of CMML are recognized by the WHO based on the percentage of combined blasts and promonocytes in the blood: CMML-1, in which the blasts and promonocytes are $< 5\%$ in the blood and $< 10\%$ in the marrow, and CMML-2, in which one or more of three criteria are present: (1) 5–19% blasts and promonocytes in the blood; (2) 10–19% blasts and promonocytes in the marrow; and (3) Auer rods in blasts with or without criteria 1 and/or 2.[3] If eosinophilia is present, it should be added to the diagnostic terminology.

Table 2.3 World Health Organization diagnostic criteria for chronic myelomonocytic leukemia (CMML)[66]

1. Persistent peripheral blood monocytosis $> 1 \times 10^9/l$
2. No Philadelphia chromosome or other evidence of *BCR/ABL* fusion gene
3. Fewer than 20% blasts[a] in the blood or bone marrow
4. Dysplasia in one or more hemopoietic lineages. If dysplasia is absent or minimal, the diagnosis of CMML may still be made if the other requirements are met, and:
   – an acquired, clonal cytogenetic abnormality is present in the marrow cells, or
   – the monocytosis has persisted for at least 3 months and all other causes of monocytosis have been excluded

[a]Blasts include myeloblasts, monoblasts, and promonocytes. Promonocytes are monocytic precursors with abundant light-gray or slightly basophilic cytoplasm with a few scattered, fine lilac-colored granules, finely distributed, stippled nuclear chromatin, variably prominent nucleoli, and delicate nuclear folding or creasing, and in this classification are equivalent to blasts.

Cases of CMML with eosinophilia may have an associated translocation t(5; 12) resulting in an abnormal fusion gene, *TEL/PDGFBRecepto*.

In the predominantly myelodysplastic form of CMML, there are usually associated cytopenias: neutropenia, thrombocytopenia or anemia. Dysplasia is usually present in monocytes with granulation and/or nuclear abnormalities; one or more of the other major myeloid lineages may show minimal dysplasia; the dysplasia is similar to that in other types of MDS and includes neutrophil nuclear hypolobulation and/or granulation abnormalities and dyserythropoiesis. Dysplasia is a less prominent feature of the more myeloproliferative form of CMML and the only morphologic finding may be monocytosis. The anemia in CMML may be normocytic or macrocytic. Large atypical platelets may be found in the blood.

Approximately 25% of patients who present with CMML with low or normal leukocyte counts, i.e., the dysplastic type of CMML, may evolve into a more proliferative type of CMML with elevated leukocyte counts and organomegaly.[71]

The bone marrow is hypercellular in the majority of cases but may be normocellular and uncommonly is hypocellular. The degree of monocyte proliferation is variable in both the smears and sections. The trephine biopsies may show a focal character of the proliferation, with foci of blasts and promonocytes.[72] This may be accentuated in biopsies with immunohistochemical reactions for CD68 (KP-1 and PGM-1) and lysozyme. Alpha-naphthyl acetate esterase and alpha-naphthyl butyrate esterase may highlight the monocytes in smears.

Atypical chronic myeloid leukemia

Atypical chronic myeloid leukemia (aCML) is a myeloid leukemia that morphologically manifests features that are associated with both myelodysplastic and myeloproliferative processes and is only similar to typical chronic myeloid leukemia in that there is a neutrophilia with immature and mature neutrophils; in contrast to typical chronic myeloid leukemia in which dysplastic features are not present in neutrophils in the chronic phase, the neutrophils in aCML invariably show some degree of dysplasia. Unlike typical cases of *ABL/BCR* chronic myeloid leukemia,[65] the basophil percentage in atypical CML is normal or only slightly increased; some of the neutrophils in atypical CML have dysplastic features such as nuclear hypolobulation and hypogranulation. The number of blasts in the blood and marrow does not exceed 20% and is usually less than 5%. Dysplasia of both the megakaryocyte-platelet and erythroid series may be present and there is usually anemia and thrombocytopenia. There must be no cytogenetic or molecular evidence of the *ABL/BCR* fusion gene.[66,69] aCML is a very uncommon disorder, occurring primarily in older adults. The term "atypical chronic myeloid leukemia" should not be used for cases of chronic myeloid leukemia which appear to be negative for the Philadelphia chromosome by G-banding chromosome study but which are positive for the *ABL/BCR* fusion gene by FISH or molecular analyses. There is no specific cytogenetic correlate of aCML; +8, +13,del(20q), i(17q), and del(12p) have been reported.[66,69] aCML usually has an aggressive clinical course.

aCML is a somewhat unsatisfactory term for several reasons, the major one being an apparent but erroneous association with typical *ABL/BCR*-positive chronic myeloid leukemia. However, because of the historical use of this term and no clearly better term, the term is retained.

Juvenile myelomonocytic leukemia

Juvenile myelomonocytic leukemia is a myeloid leukemia occurring in infancy or early childhood characterized primarily by proliferation of

Table 2.4 Diagnostic criteria for juvenile myelomonocytic leukemia[66]

1. Blood monocyte count $> 1 \times 10^9/l$
2. Blood and marrow blasts less than 20%
3. No t(9;22) or other evidence of *BCR/ABL* fusion gene and two or more of the following:
   (a) elevated hemoglobin F for the age
   (b) leukocytes $> 10 \times 10^9/l$
   (c) immature granulocytes in the blood
   (d) clonal chromosome abnormality (including monosomy 7)
   (e) GM-CSF hypersensitivity of myeloid precursors in vitro

GM-CSF, granulocyte–macrophage colony-stimulating factor.

granulocytes and monocytes (Plate 9). The term "juvenile chronic myelomonocytic leukemia" was previously used for this entity. As defined in the WHO criteria, children with the entity, previously referred to as infantile monosomy 7 syndrome, are subsumed in the juvenile myelomonocytic leukemia category.[66] The disorder has a male predilection.

Children with neurofibromatosis type 1 (NF-1) have a 200–500-fold risk of developing juvenile myelomonocytic leukemia compared to children without NF-1.[73] Approximately 10–14% of children with juvenile myelomonocytic leukemia have a clinical diagnosis of NF-1 and approximately 30% of cases of juvenile myelomonocytic leukemia have NF-1 gene mutations.[73]

The WHO diagnostic criteria for juvenile myelomonocytic leukemia are listed in Table 2.4.[66] These criteria are modified from Niemeyer *et al.*[74] In addition to the criteria listed in Table 2.4, other features may be helpful in the diagnosis, including: spontaneous granulocyte–macrophage colonies in vitro, polyclonal hypergammaglobulinemia, increased serum lysozyme, and clinical features, including macular rash (particularly facial), hepatosplenomegaly, and lymphadenopathy.[66,74,75] Because the clinical and laboratory features of juvenile myelomonocytic leukemia may be mimicked by some infectious diseases, it is recommended that studies to exclude Epstein–Barr virus infection, cytomegalovirus, human herpesvirus 6, *Histoplasma*, *Mycobacterium*, and *Toxoplasma* be performed before a diagnosis of juvenile myelomonocytic leukemia is established.[74]

The presenting laboratory findings of juvenile myelomonocytic leukemia are usually leukocytosis and anemia; thrombocytopenia is common.[63,69,74,75] The median leukocyte count ranges from 25 to 35 $\times 10^9$/l; counts in excess of 100 $\times 10^9$/l occur in a minority of cases. The leukocytes include mature and immature neutrophils, including blasts and promyelocytes; the blasts are usually < 5%. There is a monocytosis and some monocytes have unusual nuclear lobulation. Occasional immature monocytes may be present. Eosinophilia and basophilia may also be present. Normoblasts are usually present in the blood and may be numerous. Occasional immunoblasts may be noted.

The bone marrow is usually hypercellular but may be hypocellular with evidence of interstitial cell depletion in occasional cases. The hypercellularity is principally related to granulocytic proliferation; in some patients there may be an erythroid hyperplasia. Monocytes usually comprise 5–10% of the nucleated cells. Blasts are < 20% and frequently < 5%. Auer rods are not found. Dysplastic changes are generally minimal.

Leukemic infiltration of liver and spleen is usually present; other common sites of involvement include the skin, lymph nodes, and respiratory tract. Juvenile myelomonocytic leukemia usually has an aggressive clinical course. However, evolution to acute leukemia is uncommon.[66]

Pediatric myelodysplastic syndromes

MDS are uncommon in childhood and when they occur they frequently have somewhat unique characteristics.[75,76] Some modifications of the WHO classification of MDS have been proposed for pediatric cases.[75,76] A proposed classification of pediatric MDS conforming with the WHO proposed classification is shown in Table 2.5. The two major entities that have been proposed in the pediatric MDS category are juvenile myelomonocytic leukemia (see section on myelodysplastic/myeloproliferative diseases, above) and the myeloid leukemia associated with Down syndrome.

Myeloid leukemia in Down syndrome

Down-syndrome children have an increased risk of developing acute leukemia during the first years of life compared to non-Down-syndrome children. Approximately 1 in 100–200 children with Down syndrome develop

Table 2.5 Proposed classification of pediatric myelodysplastic syndromes[75,76]

Myelodysplastic/myeloproliferative disease
Juvenile myelomonocytic leukemia
Chronic myelomonocytic leukemia (secondary only)
BCR/ABL-negative chronic myeloid leukemia (atypical
    chronic myeloid leukemia)
Down syndrome myeloid disease
Transient abnormal myelopoiesis
Myeloid leukemia of Down syndrome
Myelodysplastic syndromes
Refractory cytopenia
Refractory anemia with excess blasts
Refractory anemia with excess of blasts in
    transformation

---

acute leukemia, which is 10–20 times more frequent than in non-Down-syndrome children.[77–83] The leukemia is usually myeloid with prominent megakaryocyte involvement. There appears to be a higher incidence of MDS preceding the acute leukemia in Down-syndrome patients than in non-Down-syndrome patients.[78–80]

A transient myeloproliferative process morphologically indistinguishable from acute myeloid leukemia may occur in Down-syndrome patients, most commonly in the neonatal period or first few months of life.[79,83] The transient disorder is estimated to occur in approximately 10% of children with Down syndrome. The process usually undergoes spontaneous remission in a few weeks. Recurrence may occur; the recurrent episode may also undergo spontaneous remission or persist and require antileukemic therapy. It is estimated that approximately 10–20% of children with Down syndrome with a history of the transient myeloproliferative disorder will develop acute megakaryoblastic leukemia within 3 years.[83]

Mutagenesis of GATA-1, a transcription factor regulating growth and maturation of a distinct set of tissues including hematopoietic cells, appears to be an early event in Down-syndrome myeloid disorders.[82,84–86] Acquired mutations of GATA-1 are found in the majority of Down-syndrome patients with acute megakaryoblastic leukemia and nearly all Down-syndrome patients with a transient myeloproliferative disorder.

The other types of MDS are uncommon in children. The diagnostic criteria are similar to those for adult cases.

Summary and future directions

The FAB classification of the MDS was initially introduced in 1976; the revised version was introduced in 1982 and has served as the basis of the morphologic classification for 25 years of this heterogeneous and poorly understood group of diseases.[20,87,88] In 2001, the WHO committee for the classification of the hematopoietic disorders introduced a new classification of the MDS which retained much of the framework of the FAB classification but with significant modifications. Several commentaries in regard to the WHO classification and studies comparing the FAB and WHO classifications have been published.[30,76,88–95] In some of these studies, the WHO classification was more predictive of clinical behavior than the FAB classification. This is particularly relevant to the WHO's distinction of RCMD from RA. In other studies the WHO classification did not appear to be an improvement over the FAB classification.[89,94]

The elimination of the FAB category of RAEB-T and the inclusion of patients with 20–30 blood and/or marrow blasts in the acute myeloid leukemia category in the WHO classification has been the subject of several commentaries and it is recognized that debate exists regarding this issue.[91,95] The rationale for the WHO change has been briefly mentioned earlier in this chapter and is discussed more extensively by Vardiman *et al.*[24] This is a problematic area and blast percentage per se should not dictate therapy. The MDS are diseases not only related to blast percentage but also may manifest differing tempos than de novo acute myeloid leukemia and may be associated with distinctive biologic features. Some of these patients have a higher incidence than de novo acute myeloid leukemia of complex, poor-risk cytogenetic changes, early stem cell phenotype, increased expression of multidrug resistance on the blasts and a more unfavorable response to standard acute myeloid leukemia therapy.[96–99] Some patients with RAEB-T in the FAB classification are more appropriately classified as acute myeloid leukemia with multilineage dysplasia with associated poor risk factors; others have a more indolent course characteristic of an MDS. Further studies are warranted to determine the biology of these processes so that classification accurately reflects clinical course.

A similar comment can be applied to other types of MDS which have an indolent clinical course. Some of the cases of unilineage sideroblastic anemia and RA are more likely related to metabolic dysfunction then to disorders of the hematopoietic stem cell.

Classification of disease processes should not be viewed as endproducts but as beginnings which provide a framework for further studies. To be effective they must evolve as additional data derived from laboratory and clinical studies emerge. Critical evaluation must be ongoing and, when sufficient data become available to indicate the necessity for change, changes should be made. The original FAB classification of the MDS was an excellent starting point for codifying a group of poorly recognized and understood hematologic diseases and most hematologists and hematopathologists developed a certain comfort level in its use. The FAB classification, in establishing diagnostic criteria, improved remarkably the diagnostic discipline for acute leukemia and MDS. The WHO classification of the MDS should be viewed as a stage in the evolution of the FAB classification. It attempts to sharpen definitions and focus on aspects of the FAB classification that were problems for diagnosticians. These have been addressed in this chapter.

REFERENCES

1. Bennett, J. M., Catovsky, D., Daniel, M. T. *et al.* (1976). Proposals for the classification of the acute leukaemias. *Br. J. Haematol.*, **33**, 451–8.
2. Bennett, J. M., Catovsky, D., Daniel, M. T. *et al.* (1982). Proposals for the classification of the myelodysplastic syndromes. *Br. J. Haematol.*, **51**, 189–99.
3. Brunning, R. D., Bennett, J. M., Flandrin, G. *et al.* (2001). Myelodysplastic syndromes and acute myeloid leukaemias. In *World Health Organization Classification of Tumours. Pathology and Genetics of Tumours of Haematopoietic and Lymphoid Tissues*, ed. E. S. Jaffe, N. L. Harris, H. Stein and J. W. Vardiman. Lyon: IARC Press, pp. 61–106.

4. Brunning, R. D. and McKenna, R. W. (1994). Myelodysplastic syndromes. In *Tumors of the Bone Marrow, Atlas of Tumor Pathology*, third series, fascicle 9, ed. J. Rosai. Washington, DC: Armed Forces Institute of Pathology, pp. 143–94.

5. Phelan, J. T. II, Kouides, P. A., and Bennett, J. M. (2002). Myelodysplastic syndromes: historical aspects and classification. New York: Marcel Dekker, pp. 1–14.

6. Balduini, C. L., Guarnone, R., Pecci, A., Centenara, E., and Ascari, E. (1998). Multilineage dysplasia without increased blasts identifies a poor prognosis subset of myelodysplastic syndromes. *Leukemia*, **12**, 1655–6 (letter).

7. Michels, S., Chan, W., Jakubowski, D., and Vogler, R. (1990). Unclassifiable myelodysplastic syndrome: a study of sixteen cases with a proposal for a new subtype. *Lab. Invest.*, **62**, 67 (abstract).

8. Rosati, S., Mick, R., Xu, F. *et al.* (1996). Refractory cytopenia with multilineage dysplasia: further characterization of an "unclassifiable" myelodysplastic syndrome. *Leukemia*, **10**, 20–6.

9. Boultwood, J., Lewis, S., and Wainscoat, J. S. (1994). The 5q– syndrome. *Blood*, **84**, 3253–60.

10. Gregg, X. T., Reddy, V., and Prchal, J. T. (2002) Copper deficiency masquerading as myelodysplastic syndrome. *Blood*, **100**, 1493–5.

11. Irving, J. A., Mattman, A., Lockitch, G., and Farrell, K. (2003). Element of caution: a case of reversible cytopenias associated with excessive zinc supplementation. *C.M.A.J.*, **169**, 129–31.

12. Rosati, S., Anastasi, J., and Vardiman, J. (1996). Recurring diagnostic problems in the pathology of the myelodysplastic syndromes. *Semin. Hematol.*, **33**, 111–26.

13. Westhoff, D. D., Samaha, R. J., and Barnes, A. Jr. (1975). Arsenic intoxication as a cause of megaloblastic anemia. *Blood*, **45**, 241–6.

14. Baurmann, H., Schwatz, T. F., Oertel, J. *et al.* (1992). Acute parvovirus infection mimicking myelodysplastic syndrome of the bone marrow. *Ann. Hematol.*, **64**, 43–5.

15. Schmitz, L. L., McClure, J. S., Litz, C. E. *et al.* (1994). Morphologic and quantitative changes in blood and marrow cells following growth factor therapy. *Am. J. Clin. Pathol.*, **101**, 67–75.

16. Katoutsi, V., Kohlmeyer, U., Maschek, H. *et al.* (1994). Comparison of bone marrow and hematologic findings in patients with human immunodeficiency virus infection and those with myelodysplastic syndromes and infectious disease. *Am. J. Clin. Pathol.*, **101**, 123.

17. Treacy, M., Lai, L., Costello, C., and Clark, A. (1987). Peripheral blood and bone marrow abnormalities in patients with HIV related disease. *Br. J. Haematol.*, **65**, 289–94.

18. Delacetaz, F., Schmidt, P. M., Piguet, D. *et al.* (1987). Histopathology of myelodysplastic syndromes. *Am. J. Clin. Pathol.*, **87**, 180–6.

19. Germing, U., Gattermann, N., Aivado, M. *et al.* (2000). Two types of acquired idiopathic sideroblastic anaemia (AISA): a time-tested distinction. *Br. J. Haematol.*, **108**, 724–8.

20. Greenberg, P., Cox, C., Le Beau, M. M. *et al.* (1997). International scoring system for evaluating prognosis in myelodysplastic syndromes. *Blood*, **89**, 2079–88.

21. Bernstein, S. H., Brunetto, V. L., and Davey, F. R. (1996). Acute myeloid leukemia-type chemotherapy for newly diagnosed patients without antecedent cytopenias having myelodysplastic syndromes as defined by French–American–British criteria: a Cancer and Leukemia Group B study. *J. Clin. Oncol.*, **14**, 2486–94.

22. Estey, E., Pierce, S., Kantarjian, H. *et al.* (1993). Treatment of myelodysplastic syndromes with AML-type chemotherapy. *Leuk. Lymphoma*, **11** (suppl. 2), 59–63.

23. Estey, E., Thall, P., Beran, M. *et al.* (1997). Effects of diagnosis (refractory anemia with excess blasts, refractory anemia with excess blasts in transformation or acute myeloid leukemia [AML]) on outcome of AML-type chemotherapy. *Blood*, **90**, 2969–77.

24. Vardiman, J. W., Harris, N. L., and Brunning, R. D. (2002). The World Health Organization (WHO) classification of myeloid neoplasms. *Blood*, **100**, 2292–302.

25. Menke, D. M., Colon-Otero, G., Cockerill, K. J. *et al.* (1992). Refractory thrombocytopenia: a myelodysplastic syndrome that may mimic immune thrombocytopenic purpura. *Am. J. Clin. Pathol.*, **98**, 502–10.

26. Tricot, G., Criel, A., and Verwilghen, R. L. (1982). Thrombocytopenia as presenting symptom of preleukaemia in three patients. *Scand. J. Haematol.*, **28**, 243–50.

27. Steensma, D. P., DeWald, G. W., Hodnefield, J. M. *et al.* (2003). Clonal cytogenetic abnormalities in bone marrow specimens without clear morphologic evidence of dysplasia: a form fruste of myelodysplasia? *Leuk. Res.*, **27**, 235–42.

28. Olney, H. J. and Le Beau, M. M. (2002). Cytogenetics and molecular biology of myelodysplastic syndromes. In *The Myelodysplastic Syndromes, Pathobiology and Clinical Management*, ed. J. M. Bennett. New York: Marcel Dekker, pp. 89–119.

29. Rigolin, G. M., Bigoni, R., Milani, R. *et al.* (2001). Clinical importance of interphase cytogenetics detecting occult chromosome lesions in myelodysplastic syndromes with normal karyotype. *Leukemia*, **15**, 1841–7.

30. Cermak, J., Michalova, K., Brezinova, J. *et al.* (2003). A prognostic impact of separation of refractory cytopenia with multilineage dysplasia and 5q− syndrome from refractory anemia in primary myelodysplastic syndrome. *Leuk. Res.*, **27**, 221–9.

31. Giagounidis, A. N. N., Germing, U., Haase, S. *et al.* (2004). Clinical, morphological, and prognostic features of patients with myelodysplastic syndromes and del(5q) including band q31. *Leukemia*, **18**, 113–19.

32. Lai, F., Godley, L. A., Joslin, J. *et al.* (2001). Transcript map and comparative analysis of the 1.5 Mb commonly deleted segment of human 5q31 in malignant myeloid diseases with a del (5q). *Genomics*, **71**, 235–45.

33. Kurtin, P. J., Dewald, G. W., Shields, D. J., and Hanson, C. A. (1996). Hematologic disorders associated with deletions of chromosome 20q: a clinicopathologic study of 107 patients. *Am. J. Clin. Pathol.*, **106**, 680–8.

34. Lai, J. L., Preudhomme, C., Zandecki, M. *et al.* (1995). Myelodysplastic syndromes and acute myeloid leukemia with 17p deletion. An entity characterized by specific dysgranulopoiesis and a high incidence of P53 mutations. *Leukemia*, **9**, 370–81.

35. Sankar, M., Tanaka, K., Kumaravel, T. S. *et al.* (1998). Identification of a commonly deleted region at 17p13.3 in leukemia and lymphoma associated with 17p abnormality. *Leukemia*, **12**, 510–16.

36. Ellis, M., Ravid, M., and Lishner, M. (1993). A comparative analysis of alkylating agent and epipodophyllotoxin-related leukemias. *Leuk. Lymphoma*, **11**, 9–13.

37. Godley, L. A. and Larson, R. A. (2002). The syndrome of therapy related myelodysplasia and myeloid leukemia. In *The Myelodysplastic Syndromes, Pathobiology and Clinical Management*, ed. J. M. Bennett. New York: Marcel Dekker, pp. 139–76.

38. Latagliata, R., Petti, M. C., Fenu, S. *et al.* (2002). Therapy-related myelodysplastic syndrome–acute myelogenous leukemia in patients treated for acute promyelocytic leukemia: an emerging problem. *Blood*, **99**, 822–4.

39. Le Beau, M. M., Albain, K. S., Larson, R. A. *et al.* (1986). Clinical and cytogenetic correlations in 63 patients with therapy-related myelodysplastic syndromes and acute nonlymphocytic leukemia: further evidence for characteristic abnormalities of chromosomes no. 5 and 7. *J. Clin. Oncol.*, **4**, 325–45.

40. Merlat, A., Lai, J. L., Sterkers, Y. *et al.* (1999). Therapy-related myelodysplastic syndrome and acute myeloid leukemia with 17p deletion. A report on 25 cases. *Leukemia*, **13**, 250–7.

41. Michels, S. D., McKenna, R. W., Arthur, D. C., and Brunning, R. D. (1985). Therapy-related acute myeloid leukemia and myelodysplastic syndrome: a clinical and morphologic study of 65 cases. *Blood*, **65**, 1364–72.

42. Pedersen-Bjergaard, J., Andersen, M. K., Christiansen, D. H., and Nerlov, C. (2002). Genetic pathways in therapy-related myelodysplasia and acute myeloid leukemia. *Blood*, **99**, 1909–12.

43. Pedersen-Bjergaard, J., Phillip, P., Larsen, S. O. *et al.* (1993). Therapy-related myelodysplasia and acute myeloid leukemia. Cytogenic characteristics of 115 consecutive cases and risk in seven cohorts of patients treated intensively for malignant disease in the Copenhagen series. *Leukemia*, **7**, 1975–86.

44. Pedersen-Bjergaard, J. (2005). Insights into leukemogenesis from therapy-related leukemia. *N. Engl. J. Med.*, **352**, 1591–4.

45. Quesnel, B., Kantarjian, H., Pedersen-Bjergaard, J. *et al.* (1993). Therapy-related acute myeloid leukemia with t(8;21), Inv(16) and t(8;16): a report on 25 cases and review of the literature. *J. Clin. Oncol.*, **11**, 2370–9.

46. Pui, C. H., Relling, M. V., Rivera, G. K. *et al.* (1995). Epipodophyllotoxin-related acute myeloid leukemia; a study of 35 cases. *Leukemia*, **9**, 1990–6.

47. Rowley, J. D. and Olney, H. J. (2002). International workshop on the relationship of prior therapy to balanced chromosome aberrations in therapy-related leukemia and myelodysplastic syndromes and acute leukemia: overview report. *Genes Chromosomes Cancer*, **33**, 331–45.

48. Secker-Walker, L. M., Moorman, A. V., Bain, B. J., and Mehta, A. B. (1998). Secondary acute leukemia and myelodysplastic syndrome with 11q23 abnormalities: EU concerted action 11q23 workshop. *Leukemia*, **12**, 840–4.

49. Lobe, I., Rigal-Huguet, F., Vekhoff, A. *et al.* (2003). Myelodysplastic syndrome after acute promyelocytic leukemia: the European APL group experience. *Leukemia*, **17**, 1600–4.

50. Rios, A., Canizo, M. C., Sanz, A. *et al.* (1990). Bone marrow biopsy in myelodysplastic syndromes: morphologic characteristics and contribution to the study of prognostic factors. *Br. J. Haematol.*, **75**, 26–33.

51. Tomonga, M. and Nagai, K. (2002). Hypocellular myelodysplastic syndromes and acute myeloid leukemia: relationship to aplastic anemia. In *The Myelodysplastic Syndromes, Pathobiology and Clinical Management*, ed. J. M. Bennett. New York: Marcel Dekker, pp. 121–38.

52. Tricot, G., DeWolf-Peeters, C., Vlietinck, R., and Verwilghen, R. L. (1984). Bone marrow histology in myelodysplastic syndromes II. Prognostic value of abnormal localization of immature precursors in MDS. *Br. J. Haematol.*, **58**, 217–25.

53. Lambertenghi-Deliliers, G., Annaloro, C., Oriani, A., and Soligo, D. (1992). Myelodysplastic syndrome associated with bone marrow fibrosis. *Leuk. Lymphoma*, **8**, 51–5.

54. Maschek, H., Georgii, A., Kaloutsi, V. *et al.* (1992). Myelofibrosis in primary myelodysplastic syndromes: a retrospective analysis of 352 patients. *Eur. J. Haematol.*, **48**, 208–14.

55. Steensma, D. P., Hanson, C. A., Letendre, L., and Tefferi, A. (2001). Myelodysplasia with fibrosis: a distinct entity? *Leuk. Res.*, **25**, 829–38.

56. Sultan, C., Sigaux, F., Imbert, M., and Reyes, F. (1981). Acute myelodysplasia with myelofibrosis: a report of eight cases. *Br. J. Haematol.*, **49**, 11–16.

57. Tuzuner, N., Cox, C., Rowe, J. M. *et al.* (1995). Hypocellular myelodysplastic syndromes (MDS): new proposals. *Br. J. Haematol.*, **91**, 612–17.

58. Yoshida, Y., Oguma, S., Uchino, H., and Maekawa, T. (1988). Refractory myelodysplastic anaemias with hypocellular bone marrow. *J. Clin. Pathol.*, **41**, 763.

59. Maschek, H., Kaloutsi, V., Rodriguez-Kaiser, M. *et al.* (1993). Hypoplastic myelodysplastic syndrome: incidence, morphology, cytogenetics and prognosis. *Ann. Hematol.*, **66**, 117–22.

60. Orazi, A., Albiter, M., Heerema, N. A. *et al.* (1997). Hypoplastic myelodysplastic syndrome can be distinguished from acquired aplastic anemia by CD34 and PCNA immunostaining of bone marrow biopsy specimens. *Am. J. Clin. Pathol.*, **107**, 268–74.

61. Barrett, J., Saunthararajah, Y., and Molldrem, J. (2000). Myelodysplastic syndrome and aplastic anemia: distinct entities or diseases linked by a common pathophysiology? *Semin. Hematol.*, **37**, 15–29.

62. Group Français de Cytogénetique Hématologique (1991). Chronic myelomonocytic leukemia: single entity or heterogeneous disorder? A prospective multicenter study of 100 patients. *Cancer Genet. Cytogenet*, **55**, 57–65.

63. Krsnik, I., Srivastava, P. C., and Galton, D. A. G. (1992). Chronic myelomonocytic leukaemia and atypical chronic myeloid leukaemia. In *Myelodysplastic Syndromes*, ed. F. Schmalzl and G. J. Multi. New York: Springer-Verlag, pp. 131–9.

64. Nossinger, T., Reisner, R., Gruner, H. *et al.* (2000). Dysplastic versus proliferative CMML – a retrospective analysis of 91 patient from a single institution. *Leuk. Res.*, **25**, 741–7.

65. Shepherd, P. C., Ganesan, T. S., and Galton, D. A. (1987). Haematological classification of the chronic myeloid leukaemias. *Baillière's Clin. Haematol.*, **1**, 887–906.

66. Vardiman, J. W. (2001). Myelodysplastic/myeloproliferative disease: introduction. In *World Health Organization Classification of Tumours. Pathology and Genetics of Tumours of Haematopoietic and Lymphoid Tissues*, ed. E. S. Jaffe, N. L. Harris, H. Stein, and J. W. Vardiman. Lyon: IARC Press, pp. 47–48.

67. Germing, U., Gattermann, N., Minning, H. *et al.* (1998). Problems in the classification of CMML – dysplastic versus proliferative type. *Leuk. Res.*, **22**, 871–8.

68. Steensma, D. P., Tefferi, A., and Li, C. Y. (2003). Splenic histopathological variants in chronic myelomonocytic leukemia: reinforcement of the heterogeneity of the syndrome. *Leuk. Res.*, **27**, 775–82.

69. Vardiman, J. W. (2003). Myelodysplastic syndromes, chronic myeloproliferative diseases, and myelodysplastic/myeloproliferative diseases. *Semin. Diag. Pathol.*, **20**, 154–79.

70. Bennett, J. M., Catovsky, D., Daniel, M. T. *et al.* (1994). The chronic myeloid leukemias: guidelines for distinguishing the chronic granulocytic, atypical chronic myeloid and chronic myelomonocytic leukaemias. *Br. J. Haematol.*, **87**, 746–54.

71. Greenberg, P., Anderson, J., de Witte, T. *et al.* (2000). Problematic WHO reclassification of myelodysplastic syndromes. *J. Clin. Oncol.*, **18**, 3447–9.

72. Chen, T.-C., Chou, J.-M., Ketterling, R. P. *et al.* (2003). Histologic and immunohistochemical study of bone marrow monocytic nodules in 21 cases with myelodysplasia. *Am. J. Clin. Pathol.*, **120**, 874–81.

73. Side, L. E., Emanuel, P. D., Taylor, B. *et al.* (1998). Mutations of the NF1 gene in children with juvenile myelomonocytic leukemia without clinical evidence of neurofibromatosis, type 1. *Blood*, **92**, 267–72.

74. Niemeyer, C. M., Fenu, S., Hasle, H. *et al.* (1998). Differentiating juvenile myelomonocytic leukemia from infectious disease. *Blood*, **91**, 365–7.

75. Hasle, H. and Niemeyer, C. (2002). Myelodysplastic syndrome and juvenile myelomonocytic leukemia in children. In *The Myelodysplastic Syndromes, Pathobiology and Clinical Management*, ed. J. M. Bennett. New York: Marcel Dekker, pp. 299–344.

76. Hasle, H., Niemeyer, C. M., Chessells, J. M. *et al.* (2003). A pediatric approach to the WHO classification of myelodysplastic and myeloproliferative diseases. *Leukemia*, **17**, 277–82.

77. Gurbuxani, S., Vyas, P., and Crispino, J. D. (2004). Recent insights into the mechanisms of myeloid leukemogenesis in Down syndrome. *Blood*, **103**, 399–406.

78. Hasle, H., Clemmensen, I. H., and Mikkelsen, M. (2000). Risks of leukaemia and solid tumours in individuals with Down's syndrome. *Lancet*, **355**, 165–9.

79. Lange, B. J., Kobrinsky, N., Barnard, D. R. *et al.* (1998). Distinct demography, biology, and outcome of acute myeloid leukemia and myelodysplastic syndrome in children with Down syndrome: Children's Cancer Study Group Studies 2861 and 2891. *Blood*, **91**, 608–15.

80. Lange, B. (2000). The management of neoplastic disorders of haematopoiesis in children with Down's syndrome. *Br. J. Haematol.*, **110**, 512–24.

81. Ma, S. K., Wan, T. S. K., Chan, G. C. F. *et al.* (2001). Relationship between transient abnormal myelopoiesis and acute megakaryoblastic leukaemia in Down's syndrome. *Br. J. Haematol.*, **112**, 824–5.

82. Mundschau, G., Gurbuxani, S., Gamis, A. S. *et al.* (2003). Mutagenesis of GATA1 is an initiating event in Down syndrome leukemogenesis. *Blood*, **101**, 4298–300.

83. Zipursky, A. (2003). Transient leukaemia – a benign form of leukaemia in newborn infants. *Br. J. Haematol.*, **120**, 930–8.

84. Hitzler, J. K., Cheung, J., Li, Y. *et al.* (2003). GATA1 mutations in transient leukemia and acute megakaryoblastic leukemia of Down syndrome. *Blood*, **101**, 4301–4.

85. Rainis, L., Bercovich, D., Strehl, S. *et al.* (2003). Mutations in exon 2 of GATA1 are early events in megakaryocytic malignancies associated with trisomy 21. *Blood*, **102**, 981–6.

86. Wechsler, J., Greene, M., McDevitt, M. *et al.* (2002). Acquired mutations in GATA1 in the megakaryoblastic leukemia of Down syndrome. *Nat. Genet.*, **32**, 148–52.

87. Heaney, M. L. and Golde, D. W. (1999). Myelodysplasia. *N. Engl. J. Med.*, **340**, 1649–60.

88. Steensma, D. P. and Tefferi, A. (2003). The myelodysplastic syndrome(s): a perspective and review highlighting current controversies. *Leuk. Res.*, **27**, 95–120.

89. Brunning, R. D. (2003). MDS – new classification, new problem? *Leuk. Res.*, **27**, 567–9.

90. Cobo, F., Quinto, L. L., Rozman, M. *et al.* (2003). Analysis of 178 myelodysplastic syndrome patients: validation of the World Health Organization classification and the International Prognostic Scoring System. *Leuk. Res.*, **27**, S18–19.

91. Germing, U., Gattermann, N., Strupp, C. *et al.* (2000). Validation of the WHO proposals for a new classification of primary myelodysplastic syndromes: a retrospective analysis of 1600 patients. *Leuk. Res.*, **24**, 983–92.

92. Howe, R., Porwit-MacDonald, A., Wanat, R. *et al.* (2004). The WHO classification of MDS does make a difference. *Blood*, **103**, 3265–70.

93. Lee, J. H., Lee, J. H., Shin, Y. R. *et al.* (2003). Application of different prognostic scoring systems and comparison of the FAB and WHO classifications in Korean patients with myelodysplastic syndrome. *Leukemia*, **17**, 305–13.

94. Nosslinger, T., Reisner, R., Koller, E. *et al.* (2002). Myelodysplastic syndromes from French–American–British to World Health Organization: comparison of classifications on 431 unselected patients from a single institution. *Blood*, **98**, 2935–41.

95. Strupp, C., Gattermann, N., Giagounidis, A. *et al.* (2003). Refractory anemia with excess of blasts in transformation: analysis of reclassification according to the WHO proposals. *Leuk. Res.*, **27**, 397–404.

96. Head, D. R. (1996). Revised classification of acute myeloid leukemia. *Leukemia*, **10**, 1826–31.

97. Willman, C. L. (1998). Molecular genetic features of myelodysplastic syndromes. *Leukemia*, **12**, S2–6.

98. Wattel, E., DeBotton, S., Luc Lai, J. *et al.* (1997). Long-term follow-up of de novo myelodysplastic syndromes treated with intensive chemotherapy: incidence of long-term survivors and outcome of partial responders. *Br. J. Haematol.*, **98**, 983–91.

99. DeWitte, T., Sucio, S., Peetermans, M. *et al.* (1995). Intensive chemotherapy for poor prognosis myelodysplasia (MDS) and secondary acute myeloid leukemia following MDS of more than 8 months duration. A pilot study by the Leukemia Committee of the EORTC. *Leukemia*, **9**, 1805.

3

Pathogenetic mechanisms underlying myelodysplastic syndromes

Peter L. Greenberg

Stanford University Medical Center, Stanford, and VA Palo Alto Health Care System, Palo Alto, CA, USA

The clonal myeloid hemopathies, including myelodysplastic syndromes (MDS), comprise a group of disorders in which abnormal hemopoietic regulation plus inherent hemopoietic stem cell (HSC) anomalies underlie its biologic and clinical expression. Targets of this dysregulation include cellular programs for stem cell survival, proliferation, differentiation, and inhibition. An apparent paradox in MDS relates to the finding of generally increased marrow hemopoietic cellularity associated with peripheral blood cytopenias. These features indicate the occurrence of ineffective hematopoiesis with intramedullary destruction of a substantial portion of developing hematopoietic cells.

Factors associated with the biologic nature of MDS need to incorporate the two major discerning features of the disease – the defective differentiation of the patients' hemopoietic cells resulting in marrow failure, and expansion of the abnormal clone in those patients who undergo evolution to or toward acute myeloid leukemia (AML). The pathogenesis of these clinical and biological features of marrow dysfunction in MDS is multifactorial and involves both aberrant microenvironmental marrow stromal influences on hemopoietic cells as well as intrinsic abnormalities within the HSCs and their progeny.[1]

Microenvironmental marrow stromal abnormalities

Hematopoietic regulatory interactions

Accumulating evidence has demonstrated the significant role of the marrow microenvironment in the developmental regulation of normal and neoplastic

Myelodysplastic Syndromes: Clinical and Biological Advances, ed. Peter L. Greenberg. Published by Cambridge University Press. © Cambridge University Press 2006.

Table 3.1 Growth factor regulation of hemopoiesis[a]

	HGF production			HGF responsiveness		
	Proliferative	Differentiative	Inhibitory	Proliferative	Differentiative	Inhibitory
Normal	++	++	++	++	++	++
AML	++	+/−	++++	++++	−	−
MDS	++	+	+++	+	+	+

[a] Proliferative factors: *c-kit* ligand, interleukin-3, granulocyte–macrophage colony-stimulating factor, *c-mpl* ligand.

Differentiative factors: granulocyte colony-stimulating factor, erythropoietin, macrophage colony-stimulating factor.

Inhibitory factors: transforming growth factor-ß, interferons-α, β, γ; tumor necrosis factor-α, Fas ligand, vascular endothelial cell growth factor (VEGF), interleukin-1β, TRAIL (tumor necrosis factor-related apoptosis-inducing ligand) prostaglandin E, macrophage inflammatory protein-1α, interleukin-8.

HGF, hemopoietic growth factor; AML, acute myeloid leukemia, MDS, myelodysplastic syndrome.

cells. MDS shares with other neoplasms characteristics of defective proliferation and loss of cellular organization. This is a process whereby reciprocal signaling between the altered stroma, inflammatory mediators, and stem cells occurs. Hemopoietic growth factors (HGFs) are produced within the marrow microenvironment, regulating blood cell production. These factors have stimulatory, differentiative, or inhibitory activity. Imbalances in the production of and responsiveness to these factors contribute to the marrow dysfunction and cytopenias in MDS.[2–4]

Marrow stromal derangements within MDS marrow which enhance hemopoetic cell apoptosis include suboptimal production of stimulatory factors (granulocyte colony-stimulating factor (G-CSF), granulocyte–macrophage colony-stimulating factor (GM-CSF), *c-kit* ligand (stem cell factor), interleukin-3 (IL-3), erythropoietin, *c-mpl* ligand) and increased paracrine (intramedullary) production of inhibitory cytokines along with enhanced angiogenesis[1–3,5–11] (Table 3.1, Fig. 3.1). Treatment of MDS patients with either G-CSF or erythropoietin may increase their neutrophil counts or hemoglobin levels.[12] Thus, the defective production of a variety of HGFs, in addition to decreased precursor cell responsiveness to some of these factors, appears to contribute to the hemopoietic derangements extant

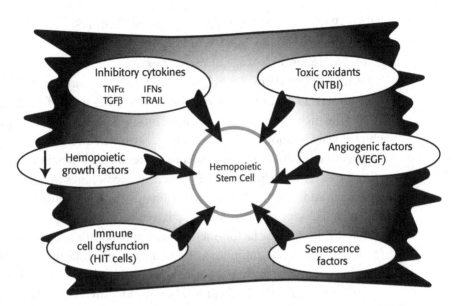

Fig. 3.1   Myelodysplastic syndrome (MDS) pathogenesis. Marrow microenvironmental factors regulating hemopoiesis and impacting on MDS and normal hemopoietic cells are depicted. TNF-α, tumor necrosis factor-α; TGF-β, transforming growth factor-β; IFNs, interferons-α, -β, -γ; TRAIL, TNF-related apoptosis-inducing ligand; NTBI, non-transferrin-bound iron; VEGF, vascular endothelial growth factor; HIT cells, hemopoietic-inhibitory T cells.

in MDS (Table 3.1). In MDS, GM-CSF and IL-3 have greater myeloid proliferative effects in vitro than G-CSF, whereas G-CSF has greater myeloid differentiative effects.[13] This is particularly evident for refractory anemia with excess blasts (RAEB)/RAEB in transformation (RAEB-T) patients and those with normal cytogenetics. The relative impact and production of these factors in AML are also indicated in Table 3.1.

Also contributing to the inhospitable marrow microenvironment in MDS are the increased endogenous marrow levels of the inhibitory and inflammatory cytokines. These factors cause the marrow suppression and enhanced hemopoietic cell apoptosis in MDS. Such cytokines include tumor necrosis factor-α (TNF-α), Fas ligand, transforming growth factor-β (TGF-β), interferons-α, β, and γ, vascular endothelial growth factor (VEGF), IL-1β, intercrine chemokines, and TRAIL (TNF-related apoptosis-inducing ligand)[1,8–11,14–20] (Table 3.1). In addition, increased levels of the cognate receptors are present in MDS compared to normal marrow cells, for TNFR-1,

TRAIL-R1, 2, *fas*, VEGFR-1, 2 and occur within the HSC and progenitor cell compartment (CD34+ cells)[11,19,20] (Fig. 3.1).

TNF-α enhances leakage of reactive oxygen species from the mitochondrial respiratory chain, leading to oxidative DNA damage.[21] Exposure of CD34+ cells to TNF-α or interferon-γ upregulates the surface receptor Fas (CD95), which in turn generates apoptotic signals.[21–25] TGF-ß, produced ubiquitously by monocytic, neutrophilic, stromal, and lymphoid cells and by platelets, inhibits early normal and leukemic multipotent HSC proliferation in vitro.[26,27] The family of intercrine chemokines includes members which, in addition to their proinflammatory and chemotactic effects for leukocytes, also possess inhibitory activity for early hemopoietic precursors and stem cells.[28] These factors include macrophage inflammatory protein-1α (MIP-1α, stem cell inhibitor), IL-8, and platelet factor 4. MIP-1α is inhibitory for normal early stem cells, but with lesser effects on leukemic precursors.[28] The effects of stimulatory/proliferative HGFs block many of these hemopoietic inhibitory effects.[4,29,30]

The supportive function of marrow stromal cells from patients has been assessed using long-term bone marrow culture systems to stimulate CD34-positive hemopoietic cell proliferation and differentiation. Compared to normal stroma, MDS marrow stroma generally demonstrated poor support, although a portion were normal.[31–34] In the former group, the cultured hemopoietic cells were associated with frequent apoptotic change and induced expression of fas/CD95.[31] Childhood MDS marrow stromal cell monolayers showed poor myelosupportive properties and were composed of myofibroblasts, collagen IV, laminin, and fibronectin.[35] Consistent with the generally suboptimal hemopoietic support has been the demonstration in MDS stromal cultures of increased levels of TGF-β, macrophage-CSF, IL-6, IL-7, angiogenic factors, and leukemia-inhibitory factor.[33–37] These findings support the hypothesis that alterations in the marrow stromal environment contribute to the abnormal hemopoiesis in MDS (Fig. 3.1).

Angiogenesis

Angiogenesis helps support the growth of hematologic malignancies as well as solid tumors.[38] The major angiogenic peptide, VEGF, stimulates angiogenesis directly by binding to VEGF receptors, which are present on endothelial and hemopoietic cells. Angiogenic molecules generated by malignant myelomonocytic precursors are diffusable stimuli which enhance leukemia progenitor self-renewal while promoting the generation of proapoptotic cytokines and intramedullary angiogenic responses.[39,40] VEGF is expressed by AML cells and acts as a paracrine growth factor in the development of AML. Elevated intracellular VEGF levels in AML patients are an independent prognostic factor of shortened survival.[40,41] Autocrine production of VEGF has been demonstrated to enhance leukemia colony formation and atypical localization of immature myeloid precursors (ALIP) in chronic myelomonocytic leukemia (CMML) and other types of MDS.[39] Microvascular density (MVD) is significantly increased in marrow biopsies of MDS patients compared with normal controls, but lower than in AML or myeloproliferative disorder (MPD).[11,42] Among MDS French–American–British (FAB) subtypes, MVD is higher in RAEB-T and CMML subsets compared with refractory anemia (RA), RA with ringed sideroblasts (RARS), or RAEB, suggesting a link in MDS between angiogenesis and progressive disease.

p38 kinase signaling cascade

Regulatory cascades exist whereby these inhibitory cytokines stimulate members of the mitogen-activated protein kinases (MAPK) superfamily.[43] The three major groups of MAPKs are the *p38*, extracellular signal-regulated kinase (*ERK*), and *JNK* kinase families. The *ERK* family mediates mitogenic and antiapoptotic signals, whereas the *p38* and *JNK* families regulate apoptosis, cell cycle, cell differentiation, and cytokine production. In vitro studies with p38 inhibitors established that the *p38* MAPK pathway is a common effector for hemopoietic inhibitors such as interferons (IFNs), TNF-α, and TGF-β. Thus, *p38* is central for downstream signaling in human hemopoietic progenitors and plays a critical role in the induction of the suppressive effects of these cytokines on normal hemopoiesis[43,44] (Fig. 3.2). Recent investigations using inhibitors of *p38* indicate that aplastic anemia marrow cell inhibition may be mediated through effects of this kinase.[45] Further studies are needed to clarify the role of this molecular signaling cascade in MDS.

Secondarily acquired inhibitory features

Toxic oxidants

Plasma and intramedullary molecular markers of oxidative stress are present in MDS and possess an increased concentration of the lipid peroxidation

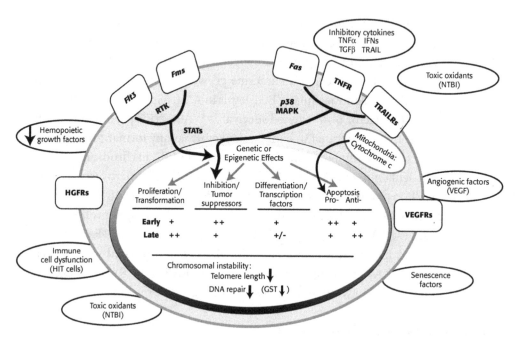

Fig. 3.2   Multifactorial myelodysplastic syndrome (MDS) pathogenesis. Selected factors implicated in MDS pathogenesis and involved with regulating hemopoietic stem cells are
depicted. A number of hemopoietic regulatory cell surface receptors activated by stromal
factors (e.g., hemopoietic growth factors (HGFs), inhibitory or angiogenic cytokines, toxic
oxidants) trigger specific signaling pathways (signal transducers and activators of transcription (STATs), p38 mitogen-activated protein kinases (MAPKs)) which act on nuclear
programs.

Functional nuclear categories may be separated into proliferation/transformation,
inhibition/tumor suppressor, differentiation/transcription factor, or apoptotic programs.
Apoptotic programs are pro- or antiapoptotic, with mitochondrial release of cytochrome
c being proapoptotic. In addition to specific gene transcription effects, epigenetic translational effects may have a major impact on gene expression.

"Early" indicates, early-stage MDS (e.g., International Progostic Scoring System (IPSS)
low, intermediate 1); "late" indicates later MDS stages (e.g., IPSS intermediate 2, high),
with their associated differing levels of responsiveness for the depicted functional
programs. Alteration of chromosomal stability relates to decreased telomere length and
DNA repair mechanisms in MDS.

Stromal influences: HGFRs (HGF receptors (e.g., granulocyte–macrophage colony-
stimulating factor receptor (GM-CSFR), granulocyte colony-stimulating factor receptor
(G-CSFR), interleukin-3 receptor (IL-3R), c-kit, c-mpl) generate proliferative signals on
specific ligand activation. fms and flt3, receptor tyrosine kinases (RTKs), are constitutively activated by mutations or activated by their specific ligands to trigger STATs

product malondialdehyde and the presence of oxidized bases in marrow CD34+ cells.[21–23,46] Mechanisms of oxidative stress include mitochondrial dysfunction via iron overload (non-transferrin-bound iron, NTBI) and mitochondrial DNA mutation, systemic inflammation, and bone marrow stromal defects.[23] A mechanism by which the increased TNF-α levels in MDS promote apoptosis is via intracellular oxygen free radical production, with its subsequent oxidation of DNA and proteins.[22] A direct relationship exists between plasma TNF-α concentrations and DNA oxidation and glutathione depletion in CD34+ progenitors. Oxidized pyrimidine nucleotides are present in the progenitor-enriched bone marrow CD34+ cell compartment from MDS patients, but are absent in both CD34− MDS cells and CD34+ cells from normal subjects[22] (Figs. 3.1 and 3.2).

As mentioned above, in vitro studies of the integrity of the hematopoietic microenvironment in MDS have indicated alterations in the function of MDS marrow adherent cell layers, including increased levels of TNF-α. Abnormalities of both the macrophage and fibroblast stromal components include an increased apoptotic index and enhanced production of TNF-α and IL-6.[31–34] MDS stromal supernatant contains a higher superoxide concentration than normal stromal supernatant.[37] As TNF-α increases oxygen free radical production and *fas* expression, these data suggest a role for these mechanisms contributing to the ineffective hemopoiesis and increased apoptosis in MDS (Figs. 3.1 and 3.2).

Recent gene expression data indicate downregulation of many stress-response proteins in CD34+ cells from MDS patients, consistent with a

---

effecting genetic changes. *fas*, tumor necrosis factor receptor-1 (TNFR-1) TNF-related apoptosis inducing ligand receptors-1, 2 (TRAILRs) are stimulated by inflammatory cytokines (e.g., *fas* ligand, TNF-α, TRAIL) and trigger (along with interferons and TGF-β) hemopoietic inhibitory signals through the *p38* family of MAPKs. Vascular endothelial growth factor receptors-1 and 2 (VEGFRs), activated by VEGF, generate proapoptotic cytokines as well as positive stimuli for (pre)leukemic cells. Toxic oxidant generated by TNF or by non-transferrin-bound iron (NTBI) may lead to genomic instability and decreased DNA repair, particularly in the presence of low levels of glutathione S-transferase (GST). (The GST gene mediates protection against oxidative stress.) In a proportion of MDS patients, hemopoietic-inhibitory T (HIT) cells cause marrow suppression.

relative failure of stress defense mechanisms in this cellular compartment.[47] These data have been extended by showing markedly upregulated expression of antioxidant defense enzymes in MDS neutrophils, but only modest upregulation of these molecules in the hemopoietic precursor compartment (CD34+ cells).[48]

Additive to these innate marrow microenvironmental derangements in MDS is the acquired intramedullary microenvironmental damage due to the toxic oxidant effects of iron overload. This cause of oxidant stress is consequent to both ineffective utilization of iron by the defective erythroid cells and by the tissue iron accumulation caused by excessive red blood cell (RBC) transfusions. Studies in patients with transfusional siderosis have demonstrated the adverse effects of such iron toxicity on hepatic, cardiac, endocrine, and marrow function.[49–51] Increased NTBI, generated when plasma iron exceeds transferrin's binding capacity, combines with oxygen to form intramedullary oxygen and hydroxyl radicals.[49] These toxic elements cause lipid peroxidation and cell membrane, protein, DNA, and organ damage.

Potential consequences of oxidative stress via iron overload include mitochondrial dysfunction, genotoxic effects causing mitochondrial and nuclear DNA mutations, and bone marrow stromal defects. Enhanced release of cytochrome c from the damaged mitochondria causes apoptosis through caspase activation.[20,23] MDS is a prominent RBC transfusion state, and as such the marrow in this disorder shows a number of abnormalities similar to those in thalassemia major,[49] which relate in part to the presence of high levels of oxidant-damaging substances such as NTBI. Both disorders have ineffective erythropoiesis with intramedullary hemolysis, and enhanced apoptosis of the marrow progeny with dysfunctional mitochondria. However, in contrast to thalassemia, the oxidant damaging effects in MDS have genotoxic effects on the marrow cells from these patients, due to the aberrant nature of their stem cells (multipotent, clonal, often with multiple cytogenetic abnormalities) plus the afore-mentioned plethora of stromal anomalies in MDS. Data have indicated the improvement of marrow function with effective iron chelation therapy in both MDS and thalassemia.[51,52]

Immunologic cell dysfunction has also been demonstrated in MDS patients. In these individuals, T cells, natural killer (NK) cells and B cells are generally defective in incidence and function.[53] Decrements have been documented in the T-helper cell population and the mitogenic response of

T cells.[54,55] These abnormalities also contribute to the decreased HGF production in MDS. In contrast, a portion of patients with immune-related MDS have an increase of hemopoietic inhibitory T cells.[56]

Together, this mixture of anomalous biologic features provides an abnormal intramedullary microenvironmental milieu in MDS and diminishes the survival and differentiation of normal hemopoietic precursors relative to their (pre)leukemic counterparts (Figs. 3.1 and 3.2). Such paracrine anomalies enhance intracellular activation of apoptosis-generating proteases (caspases), which underlie much of the pathogenesis of this disorder. These features provide a growth advantage for abnormal (pre)leukemic hemopoiesis compared to normal cells.

Inherent hemopoietic stem cell abnormalities

As two or more hemopoietic lineages are generally affected in MDS, the basic lesions initiating this disorder occur as a neoplastic process at the pluripotent HSC level. Biologic data, including clonal analysis evaluating restriction fragment length polymorphisms (RFLP), marrow cytogenetics, and in vitro hemopoietic cell clonogenic growth characteristics, indicate that the marrow stem cells of MDS patients generally derive from a myeloid malignant clone despite not yet clinically demonstrating overt leukemia.[57–60] Lymphoid cells are part of the abnormal clone in some but not all cases of MDS, as clonal T cells and both clonal and polyclonal B cells have been demonstrated.[61–63]

Despite the more indolent nature of MDS than AML, many in vitro myeloid clonogenic abnormalities evident in AML are also present in MDS.[64] The colony-forming capacities of all of the marrow hemopoietic precursor cells (colony-forming unit (CFU)-granulocyte, erythroid, monocyte, megakaryocyte (GEMM), burst-forming unit-erythroid (BFU-E), CFU-E (erythroid), CFU-GM (granulocyte, monocyte, CFU-Meg (megakaryocyte)) (CFU-GEMM, BFU-E, CFU-E, CFU-GM, CFU-Meg) are quite low or absent in the majority of MDS patients,[64] as found in most AML patients. Also similar to leukemic patients, an increased proportion of CFU-GMs are of light buoyant density, and abortive myeloid cluster formation and defective cellular maturation occur within the colonies.[64] Suboptimal responses of MDS erythroid precursors to erythropoietin has been demonstrated.[65]

In addition to the relatively low serum erythropoietin levels in most MDS patients,[5] the anemia in MDS is mainly influenced by the size of the BFU-E population, whose severe deficiency results in insufficient influx of erythropoietin-responsive cells.[65] G-CSF synergistically augments the in vitro and in vivo erythropoietin responsiveness of BFU-E in normal and MDS marrow.[6,11]

Apoptosis

The predominant final common pathway underlying the inherent marrow derangement causing ineffective hematopoiesis in MDS has been varying degrees of apoptosis of the hemopoietic precursors and their progeny.[66–70] The potential progression of MDS to/toward AML relates to altered expression of tumor-related genes within the patients' HSCs. The abnormal marrow stromal influences described above impact strongly and negatively on both of these processes (Fig. 3.2).

Histological study of MDS bone marrow biopsies revealed a significant increase of morphologically recognizable apoptosis in erythroid and myeloid precursors, compared to that in normal biopsies.[66] Analysis of cell kinetics and apoptosis in MDS bone marrow cells revealed a high rate of cellular proliferation, coinciding with increased apoptosis,[68] consistent with the ineffective hemopoiesis occurring in MDS.

Buttressing these morphologic and kinetic studies, increased levels of apoptosis in MDS marrow cells have been demonstrated by flow cytometric, cytochemical, and DNA laddering techniques.[17,67,69,70–72] Most investigators have found this process predominantly within the CD34+ hemopoietic precursor cell population, whereas others have found it evident within more differentiated cells and in stromal cells. Treatment of MDS patients with the cytokines G-CSF and erythropoietin, alone or in combination, enhanced effective hemopoiesis in vivo associated with decreased apoptosis.[29,30]

Increased levels of several of the proapoptotic caspases (caspase-1, caspase-3, caspase-9) occur in marrow cells of MDS patients and correlate inversely with blast counts and Bcl-2+ cells.[73,74] CFU-E number was particularly decreased in early MDS and associated with high marrow cell levels of caspase-3. Approximately half of the erythroid progenitor cells derived from patients with MDS (particularly those with RARS) exhibited spontaneous release of cytochrome c from mitochondria, with ensuing activation of caspase-9 and apoptosis.[74] Exposure of these MDS marrow cells to inhibitors of these caspases significantly increased the erythropoietic colonies obtained in vitro from MDS patients, whereas no changes occurred in normal marrow progenitors.[74] These data indicate that sequential activation of these caspases and constitutive activation of the mitochondrial axis of the apoptotic signaling pathway form an important biochemical pathway of marrow cell death in MDS patients.

Hemopoietic cell apoptosis is markedly increased early in MDS (i.e., during the RA, RARS, and RAEB-1 stages), whereas this process decreases later in disease progression (i.e., during RAEB-2, RAEB-T).[69,75] RAEB-T patients had higher apoptotic levels than did those with AML, suggesting biologic differences between these entities.[72] The enhanced apoptosis of the hemopoietic cells in MDS patients relates to intracellular alteration of proapoptotic (e.g., c-myc) versus antiapoptotic (bcl-2) oncoprotein levels, deranged telomere dynamics/genetic instability, abnormal apoptotic signaling, and enhanced oxidant stress susceptibility (Fig. 3.2).

Several of the genes responsible for the regulation of apoptosis have been identified (Fig. 3.3). Bcl-2 and certain members of the Bcl-2 gene family (Bcl-2, bcl-x_L and Mcl-1) are antiapoptotic, whereas other members (Bax, Bcl-x_S, Bad), c-myc, and p53 act as potent inducers of apoptosis for hemopoietic cells.[76,77] The intracellular ratio of c-myc to Bcl-2 oncoproteins is increased in MDS CD34+ cells compared to those from normal and AML CD34+ cells.[69] The increased ratio of proapoptotic (Bax, Bad) to antiapoptotic (Bcl-2, Bcl-x, c-myc) oncoproteins occurs in the CD34+ cells of patients with early MDS, and with reversal of this ratio in more advanced stages of the disease.[69,75] Similar, but less prominent relative degrees of protein expression were found for these oncogenes in the CD34− population. Enhanced apoptotic signaling occurs in MDS hemopoietic cells through their increased receptors for fas ligand, TRAIL, and VEGF.[10,19,20,40] Bcl-2 expression within early myeloid precursors in MDS marrow biopsies (in both proportion and absolute number) correlated with initial MDS stage (i.e., higher levels in later-stage patients), progressed over time, and was associated with evolution to AML.[78,79] These findings are consistent with the hypothesis that an altered balance between cell-death and cell-survival programs is associated with the increased degrees of apoptosis present in MDS hematopoietic precursors and contributes to the ineffective hemopoiesis in this disorder. In

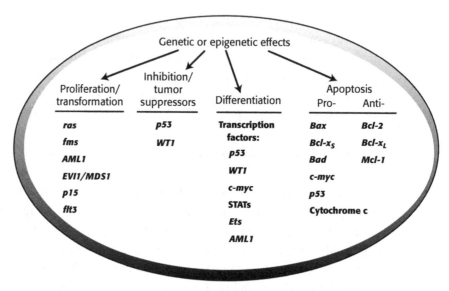

Fig. 3.3   Altered gene expression in myelodysplastic syndrome (MDS). Four categories (prolif-
eration/transformation, inhibition/tumor suppressor, differentiation/transcription factor,
or apoptosis) are listed, depicting the functional programs of genes which have been
demonstrated to be mutated or to have altered degrees of expression in a portion of
MDS patients. In addition to specific gene transcription effects of the mutated genes, epigenetic translational effects may have a major impact on gene expression. STATs, signal
transducer and activator of transcription.

contrast, decreased apoptosis relates to the enhanced leukemic cell survival
as MDS progresses toward AML.

Cytogenetic abnormalities

Chromosomal abnormalities identify areas of the genome which are susceptible to damage and which may be important in the pathogenesis of disease.
The incidence of non-random cytogenetic abnormalities in de novo MDS
is approximately 40–60% at diagnosis, whereas more than 80% of cases
with secondary MDS show abnormal karyotypes.[80,81] Evolutionary changes
may occur during the course of the disorder.[82] These genetic derangements
reflect the multistep process believed to underlie the evolution of MDS. Generally, the more aggressive stage of the disorder, in terms of rapidity of clinical
course and high number of marrow blasts, the more abnormal the karyotype.

Although both structural and numerical changes may be found in MDS, in contrast to AML, MDS is most often associated with chromosome deletions as a primary karyotypic anomaly. Deletions leading to gene loss suggest a recessive mechanism in the origin of leukemic transformation and that as-yet unidentified deletions of tumor-suppressor genes have important roles in the molecular mechanisms of MDS.

A detailed analysis of chromosome aberrations shows apparent similarities between those present in MDS and in other myeloid clonal hemopathies, such as AML and MPD.[83] The frequent occurrence of the 5q chromosomal region abnormality implicates the involvement of one or more genes residing in this region for the development and maintenance of abnormal hemopoiesis. Recent investigations have also shown that a group of patients with MDS/MPD, most with eosinophilia but some of whom have CMML, have 5q33–35 cytogenetic abnormalities which may be associated with rearrangement of the platelet-derived growth factor-β receptor (PDGFRβ) gene.[84] The diseases in such patients may be responsive to imatinib mesylate (Glivec) therapy.[85] These observations suggest that segmental genetic differences detectable by molecular but not standard cytogenetic methods exist in MDS, MPD, and AML HSCs which contribute to the phenotypic heterogeneity of the myeloid clonal hemopathies.

Molecular abnormalities

Altered levels of a number of major signal transduction molecules regulating hemopoiesis have been identified and their genetic alterations have been extensively analyzed in both MDS and AML. These features include receptors for growth factors, *ras*-signaling molecules, cell cycle regulators, and transcription factors. The disruption of the normal flow of the signal transduction pathways involving these molecules in MDS contributes to ineffective multilineage hemopoiesis, bone marrow failure, and AML evolution. Hemopoietic cells from MDS patients have been investigated for abnormalities in expression of genes regulating hemopoiesis (Fig. 3.3). These genes have been placed into at least four categories based on their functional roles: proliferation/transformation, inhibition/tumor suppressors, differentiation, and apoptosis (Figs. 3.2 and 3.3). Some genes have multiple functional roles (e.g., *p53* is proapoptotic as well as being a tumor suppressor and a transcription factor).

The family of *Ras* proto-oncogenes encodes guanosine triphosphate-binding proteins which function as molecular switches regulating diverse signaling pathways involved in cell growth, differentiation, and apoptosis.[86] Oncogenic *N-Ras* mutations are frequently found in hematologic malignancies. In several series of patients with MDS, the frequency of *Ras* mutations ranged from 3 to 33%, most commonly in CMML.[86–91] Most studies of MDS patients have indicated that *Ras* mutations were associated with poor survival or progression to AML.[87,89,90] These mutations are less common in therapy-related (t)-MDS/t-AML than in de novo AML. The dyserythropoiesis was also linked to an increase in the *ras*-expressing cells undergoing apoptosis during their differentiation program. Three major pathways are abnormally activated by oncogenic *ras*: *Raf/ERK*, phosphatidyl inositol 3 (PI3)-kinase/*Akt*, and *RalGEF/RalA*. However, recent studies demonstrated that only constitutive activation of the MEK (MAPK/ERK kinase)/ERK pathway alone recapitulated all of the effects of oncogenic *H-ras* or *N-ras* expression in blocking erythroid differentiation and inducing erythropoietin-independent proliferation.[92] Taken together, these data suggest that mutational activation of *ras* and constitutive MEK/ERK signaling are potentially involved in the dyserythropoiesis and pathogenesis of MDS.

The *fms* proto-oncogene encodes the tyrosine kinase receptor for macrophage colony-stimulating factor (M-CSF receptor) and point mutations within the gene can confer transforming activity to the gene.[87] *Fms* mutations occur in < 20% of MDS patients, and, similar to *ras* mutations, are preferentially observed in CMML.[87,93,94] The *fms* gene maps to chromosome 5q33, a critical region containing genes for numerous HGFs and HGF receptors, which are commonly deleted in the 5q− syndrome.[9]

The mutation status for *ras* and *fms* was related to the patients' clinical prognostic subgroups (i.e., International Prognostic Scoring System (IPSS) categories[95]), increasing in incidence with poor-risk disease.[87,93,94] The highest incidence of these mutations was in the CMML subgroup. In contrast, these lesions were not present in patients with 5q− cytogenetic abnormalities who had a low potential for AML evolution.[96]

p53 is a tumor-suppressor gene and also induces regulatory adherence of HSCs to stromal integrins.[97] The frequency of mutations of this gene in de novo MDS cases has been in the 5–20% range, with higher rates observed in t-MDS/AML patients.[87,98–107] These mutations of *p53* correlated with resistance to chemotherapy, evolution to leukemia, advanced IPSS scores, and shorter survival. Patients with *p53* mutations are more frequently found in advanced MDS categories and had poorer outcomes within the IPSS subgroups. In studies of t-MDS/AML, *p53* mutations were associated with complex karyotypes, and microsatellite instability, suggesting a mutator phenotype.[105–107]

The Wilms tumor-suppressor gene (*WT1*) is a transcription factor involved in a number of developmental processes. The degree of *WT1* expression was highly correlated with the FAB and IPSS categories of MDS, was higher in RAEB and t-AML compared with RA, and increased further during disease progression.[108] Moreover, a significant correlation was found between *WT1* expression levels, blast cell percentage, the presence of cytogenetic abnormalities, and IPSS category.

An enhanced incidence of somatically acquired point mutations in the *AML1* gene has been reported in MDS, AML, and t-MDS or t-AML.[109,110] *AML1* point mutations were predominantly found in high-risk MDS patients and AML following MDS. The MDS/AML patients with an *AML1* mutation had significantly worse prognoses than those without such mutations.

The fusion gene *MDS1/EVI1* is a strong activator of specific hemopoietic promoters, whereas *EVI1* by itself is a repressor of these genes. Although *EVI1* represses activation by the GATA-1 erythroid factor, *MDS1/EVI1* does not, and is itself repressed by *EVI1*.[111] Recent results indicate that the gene rearrangements at 3q26 affect expression of *EVI1*, but not of *MDS1/EVI1*.[111,112] The leukemia-associated fusion gene *AML1/MDS1/EVI1* (AME) encodes a chimeric transcription factor that results from the (3;21)(q26;q22) translocation. AME is a transcriptional repressor that induces leukemia in murine models. This translocation is observed in patients with t-MDS and with post-MDS AML.[113] Data suggest that rearrangements at 3q26 involving *EVI1* could result in leukemia by a two-step process involving first, transcriptional disruption of *MDS1/EVI1*, and next, by inappropriately activating expression of *EVI1*.

Analysis of the *flt3*-receptor tyrosine kinase mutations showed that this mutation was associated with a high risk of transformation to AML and poor survival in MDS patients.[88,107,114] Approximately one-third of MDS patients acquired mutations of *flt3* or *N-ras* gene during AML evolution, which further predicted poor clinical outcomes.[115]

Transcription factors

Cellular responses to environmental stimuli are controlled by a series of signaling cascades, including DNA-binding transcription factors, that transduce extracellular signals from ligand-activated cell surface receptors to the nucleus. Although most pathways were initially thought to be linear, data indicate that there is a dynamic interplay between signaling pathways that result in the complex pattern of cell-type specific responses required for proliferation, differentiation, and survival.[116,117] A number of transcription factors such as *AML1*, retinoic acid receptor-α, *MZF-1*, *Hox*, *c-myb* and the STAT (signal transducer and activator of transcription) and *Ets* families play important roles in myeloid cell maintenance and differentiation.[117]

The *Ets* family of transcription factors directs cytoplasmic signals to the control of gene expression.[118] This family is defined by a highly conserved DNA-binding domain which binds the core consensus sequence GGAA/T. As mentioned above regarding stromal influences, signaling pathways such as the MAPK, *Erk*1 and 2, *p38* and *JNK*, the PI3 kinases, and Ca^{2+}-specific signals activated by growth factors, inhibitory cytokines, or cellular stresses, converge on the *Ets* family of factors, controlling their activity, protein partnerships, and specification of downstream target genes[118] (Figs. 3.2 and 3.3). *Ets* family members can act as both upstream and downstream effectors, of signaling pathways. As such, they may coordinate interactions between stem and stromal cells. As downstream effectors, their activities are directly controlled by specific phosphorylations, resulting in their ability to activate or repress specific target genes, including those involved in myeloid cell development, HSC maintenance, and expansion and tumor progression.[118–121] As upstream effectors they are responsible for the spatial and temporal expression of numerous growth factor receptors.[118,120] This family of transcription factors is regulated through cellular signaling by *Ras*-responsive elements, the MAP Ks (*Erks*, *p38*, and *JNK*) and Ca^{2+}-specific pathways. Activation of *Ets* and *Ets*-like genes have been implicated in myeloid malignancies, including MDS.[122,123] Their role in the pathogenesis of these diseases needs further evaluation.

These aberrant molecular findings in MDS thus often relate to the patients' cytogenetics, clinical status, prognostic scores, survival, and potential for transformation to acute leukemia. Such studies demonstrate that cytogenetic and gene mutations, indicative of chromosomal and genetic instability, are associated with disease progression and poor survival in a proportion of MDS patients. However, as these anomalies are not consistently found in all (or even most) MDS patients, other features need to be discerned to understand better the molecular framework underlying this disease.

Multistep/multigenic model

These molecular findings are consistent with a multistep model in which the MDS and AML phenotype requires at least two cooperating mutations in the hemopoietic progenitor cells: one promoting proliferation/tranformation and enhanced cell survival (such as oncogenic *ras* or a constitutively activated receptor tyrosine kinase – *fms, flt3*) and one associated with impaired differentiation and enhanced immortalization (such as mutations in or abnormal activation of hemopoietic transcription factors).[124] Constitutively and abnormally active receptors generate quantitatively and qualitatively different signals compared to wild-type receptors, and mediate the oncogenic phenotype characterized by abnormal proliferation and differentiation.

The activated kinase enzymes phosphorylate STAT factors, which translocate to the cell nucleus and regulate the expression of genes, are associated with survival and proliferation. Anomalous phosphorylation and activation of STAT family members occur in MDS and various leukemias.[125] Signal transduction of *flt3* involves activation of several conserved pathways, including the *ras*/MAPK and the PI3-kinase/*Akt* signaling cascades. Transforming versions of *flt3* exhibit altered signaling, with pronounced activation of STAT5, ultimately resulting in alternate profiles of gene expression.[126] The *Ets* family of transcription factors also plays a central role in hemopoietic regulation. Together, these cooperating lesions appear to be relevant candidates which may contribute to leukemic and preleukemic cells becoming capable of proliferation and expansion but with poor differentiation (Figs. 3.2 and 3.3).

Telomere dynamics

Telomeres, the terminal components of chromosomes providing genetic stability, and telomerase, the enzyme permitting telomeric renewal, have been analyzed in MDS. Metaphases from most MDS patients showed homogeneous telomere shortening.[127,128] In contrast, marrow metaphases from normal individuals demonstrated a relatively wide range of telomere length in each metaphase. These findings indicate dysregulation of telomere-shortening mechanisms within MDS cells. Most MDS patients had normal-to-low levels of telomerase activity, suggesting that changes in telomere length rather than telomerase activity more accurately reflects the abnormal biology of MDS.[129] Replicative senescence, the aging characteristic of somatic cells, is caused by short dysfunctional telomeres, which arise when DNA is replicated in the absence of adequate telomerase activity. Data indicate that the senescence response to telomere dysfunction is reversible and is primarily maintained by intact *p53*.[130] Thus, abnormal telomere maintenance in MDS patients, particularly those with *p53* mutations, appears to be an early indication of genomic instability (Fig. 3.2).

Epigenetic hypermethylation

Methylation of cytosine residues in CpG dinucleotide islands by DNA methyltransferase leads to transcriptional silencing of genes during normal hemopoiesis and has emerged as an important epigenetic mechanism contributing to loss of tumor-suppressor gene expression in MDS (Figs. 3.2 and 3.3). The potential for leukemia evolution is enhanced by epigenetic events, including methylation silencing of proto-oncogenes or activating *ras* point mutations.[131] Transformed cells undergo a dramatic change in their DNA methylation patterns. The profile of gene hypermethylation in hematologic malignancies is an epigenetic signature that is unique for subtypes of neoplasms. This phenomenon occurs in an overall genomic environment of DNA hypomethylation.

Several genes have been shown to be hypermethylated in MDS and leukemias. The most widely studied genes are the cyclin-dependent kinase cell-cycle inhibitors $p15^{INK4B}$ and $p16^{INK4A}$, although the list of methylation-repressed genes in these neoplasms is expanding.[131–133] The $p15^{INK4B}$ and $p16^{INK4A}$ genes are important negative cell cycle regulators often inactivated by deletions, mutations, or hypermethylation in malignancy, whose expression is induced by TGF-β. Reports indicate frequent hypermethylation of the $p15^{INK4B}$ gene promoter in MDS and leukemias.[132,133] Methylation silencing of *p15* is believed either to override or worsen genetic aberrations, increasing the risk for leukemia transformation in MDS (Fig. 3.2). This silencing of *p15* is rare in patients with low-risk MDS, but is detected in the majority of marrow cells of patients with excess blasts, with increased incidence upon progression to AML, implicating this mechanism of epigenetic gene-silencing in the control of disease progression.[132,133] Methylation of *p15* is associated with deletion or loss of chromosome arm 7q. As an independent prognostic factor in t-MDS and t-AML, the *p15* methylation frequency and density both increased significantly with advanced disease stage.[134] Thus, hypermethylation may be used as a marker of progression in MDS. These data suggest that proliferation of leukemic cells may require an escape from cell cycle regulation through specific gene hypermethylation, with loss of the TGF-β-inhibitory effect. Of interest, the therapeutic hypomethylating agent decitabine has shown good correlation with clinical hematologic improvement and effective hypomethylation of *p15*.[135,136]

Aging

MDS and a number of other hematologic malignancies occur predominantly in relatively elderly individuals, with the incidence rising exponentially with age.[137] Approximately 75% of MDS patients are > 60 years, with median ages being 65–70 years old. The reasons underlying the vulnerability of more elderly patients to develop MDS (or other cancers) or the role of aging in this process are not known. However, recent studies have suggested possible mechanisms whereby this may occur.

As indicated above, for MDS (and leukemia) to develop, at least two critical changes are essential: an accumulation of oncogenic mutations within hemopoietic stem cells and a permissive tissue environment in which mutant cells can survive, proliferate, and express their neoplastic phenotype. Increasing evidence suggests that the rise in cancer incidence with age results from a synergy between the accumulation of mutations and age-related, pro-oncogenic changes in the tissue milieu.[138,139] An age-related change occurring in hemopoietic tissues is the accumulation of senescent cells. Cellular senescence is a potent tumor-suppressive mechanism that irreversibly arrests proliferation in response to damage or stimuli which put cells at risk for neoplastic transformation.[140] Senescent cells, particularly senescent stromal fibroblasts, secrete factors which disrupt tissue architecture and/or stimulate neighboring cells to proliferate. Data suggest that senescent cells may create a tissue environment which synergizes with oncogenic mutations to promote the progression of age-related cancers.[141] As indicated above, such abnormal stroma is evident in marrow of MDS patients (Fig. 3.1).

A possible basis underlying oxidative stress as contributing to the aging process is the age-related loss of physiological function which results from the progressive and irreversible accumulation of oxidative cellular and tissue damage.[23,142] Oxidative stress increases mutations and impacts on the genomic integrity of hemopoietic cells during senescence and immortalization.[23,142] Age-related increments in the levels of the specific oxidized bases, which are known oxidative DNA damage products, have been reported in various cells and tissues, including mutations in *p53* and *ras*.[130,141] Age-associated decline in DNA repair mechanisms follows treatment with ultraviolet radiation or hydrogen peroxide. The glutathione S-transferase (GST) gene mediates protection against oxidative stress by conjugating glutathione to toxic peroxide products of alkylating agents (Fig. 3.2). The polymorphic *GSTT1* null and *GSTM1/GSTT1* genotypes were found to be overrepresented in patients with either MDS or aplastic anemia who had an increased frequency of chromosomal abnormalities.[143] Polymorphisms in the *GSTP1* gene are associated with an increased susceptibility for developing AML.[144,145] These findings provide a framework for further evaluating the impact of aging on the development of MDS and leukemia.

Summary and future directions

The multifactorial and multistep pathogenetic features underlying MDS relate to the aberrant intramedullary microenvironmental milieux and secondary toxic iron radical damage, combined with primary disease-specific inherent HSC lesions (Figs. 3.1–3.3). Such effects are enhanced by processes fundamental to aging in these predominantly elderly individuals. These findings demonstrate that cytogenetic and oncogene mutations, indicative of chromosomal and genetic instability, as well as epigenetic changes, are associated with disease progression in MDS. The data presented herein provide a framework for further studies to better assess the biologic nature of MDS. Although single gene anomalies have provided valuable clues to potential molecular lesions in MDS, these lesions are not specific for MDS and current evidence suggests that this disease, and most cancers, are multigenic. Thus, evaluation of more comprehensive sets of differential gene expression profiles using microarray techniques in MDS marrow cells will likely provide the next generation of critical markers underlying the pathogenesis of this disease.

REFERENCES

1. Greenberg, P. L. (2000). The myelodysplastic syndromes. In *Hematology: Basic Principles and Practice*, 3rd edn, ed. R. Hoffman, E. Benz, S. Shattil, and H. Cohen. New York: Churchill Livingstone, pp. 1106–29.

2. Metcalf, D. (1986). The molecular biology and functions of the granulocyte-macrophage colony stimulating factors. *Blood*, **67**, 257–67.

3. Verbeek, W., Vehmeyer, K., Wormann, B. *et al.* (1995). The effect of stem-cell factor, interleukin-3 and erythropoietin on in vitro erythropoiesis in myelodysplastic syndromes. *J. Cancer Res. Clin. Oncol.*, **121**, 338–42.

4. Williams, G. T., Smith, C., Spooncer, E., Dexter, T. M., and Taylor, D. R. (1990). Haemopoietic colony stimulating factors promote cell survival by suppressing apoptosis. *Nature*, **343**, 76.

5. Jacobs, A., Janowska, A., Caro, J. *et al.* (1989). Circulating erythropoietin in patients with myelodysplastic syndrome. *Br. J. Haematol.*, **73**, 36.

6. Greenberg, P. L., MacKichan, M., Negrin, R., Renick, M., and Ginzton, N. (1990). Production of granulocyte colony stimulating factor by normal and myelodysplastic syndrome peripheral blood cells. *Blood*, **76** (suppl. 1), 146.

7. Verhoef, G. E., DeSchouwer, P., Ceuppens, J. L. *et al.* (1992). Measurement of serum cytokine levels in patients with myelodysplastic syndromes. *Leukemia*, **6**, 1268.

8. Axelrad, A. (1990). Some hemopoietic negative regulators. *Exp. Hematol.*, **18**, 143–50.

9. Deeg, H. J., Beckham, C., Loken, M. R. *et al.* (2000). Negative regulators of hemopoiesis and stroma function in patients with myelodysplastic syndrome. *Leuk. Lymphoma*, **37**, 405–14.

10. Gersuk, G. M., Lee, J., Beckham, C. A., Anderson, J., and Deeg, J. H. (1996). Fas (CD95) receptor and *Fas*-ligand expression in bone marrow cells from patients with myelodysplastic syndrome. *Blood*, **88**, 1122.

11. Pruneri, G., Bertolini, F., Soligo, D. *et al.* (1999). Angiogenesis in myelodysplastic syndromes. *Br. J. Cancer*, **81**, 1398–401.

12. Greenberg, P. L. (1992). Treatment of MDS with hemopoietic growth factors. *Semin. Oncol.*, **19**, 106.

13. Nagler, A., Ginzton, N., Bangs, C. *et al.* (1990). In vitro differentiative and proliferative effects of human recombinant colony-stimulating factors on marrow hemopoiesis in myelodysplastic syndromes. *Leukemia*, **4**, 193–202.

14. Broxmeyer, H. E., Lu, L., Platzer, E. *et al.* (1983). Comparative analysis of the influence of human gamma, alpha, and beta interferons on human multipotential, erythroid and granulocyte-macrophage progenitor cells. *J. Immunol.*, **131**, 1300–5.

15. Peetre, C., Gullberg, U., Nilsson, E. *et al.* (1986). Effects of recombinant tumor necrosis factor on proliferation and differentiation of leukemic and normal hemopoietic cells in vitro: relationship to cell surface receptor. *J. Clin. Invest.*, **78**, 1694–700.

16. Murase, T., Hofta, T., Saito, H. *et al.* (1987). Effect of recombinant human tumor necrosis factor on the colony growth of human leukemia progenitor cells and normal hematopoietic progenitor cells. *Blood*, **69**, 467–72.

17. Shetty, V., Mundle, S., Alvi, S. *et al.* (1996). Measurement of apoptosis, proliferation and three cytokines in 46 patients with myelodysplastic syndromes. *Leuk. Res.*, **20**, 891–900.

18. Budel, L. M., Dong, F., Lowenberg, B. *et al.* (1995). Hematopoietic growth factor receptors: structure variations and alternatives of receptor complex formation in normal hematopoiesis and in hematopoietic disorders. *Leukemia*, **9**, 553–61.

19. Bouscary, D., De Vos, J., Guesnu, M. *et al.* (1997). *Fas/Apo-1* (CD95) expression and apoptosis in patients with myelodysplastic syndromes. *Leukemia*, **11**, 839–45.

20. Zang, D. Y., Goodwin, R., Loken, M. R., Bryant, E., and Deeg, H. J. (2001). Expression of tumor necrosis factor-related apoptosis-inducing ligand, *Apo2L*, and its receptors in myelodysplastic syndrome: effects on in vitro hemopoiesis. *Blood*, **98**, 3058–65.

21. Goossens, V., Grooten, J., De Vos, K., and Fiers, W. (1995). Direct evidence for tumor necrosis factor-induced mitochondrial reactive oxygen intermediates and their involvement in cytotoxicity. *Proc. Natl Acad. Sci. U.S.A.*, **92**, 8115.

22. Peddie, C., Wolf, R., McLellan, L., Collins, A. R., and Bowen, T. (1997). Oxidative DNA damage in CD34+ myelodysplastic cells is associated with intracellular redox changes and elevated plasma tumour necrosis factor-α concentration. *Br. J. Haematol.*, **99**, 625.

23. Farquhar, M. J. and Bowen, D. (2003). Oxidative stress and the myelodysplastic syndromes. *Int. J. Hematol.*, **77**, 342–50.

24. Maciejewski, J. P., Selleri, C., Anderson, S., and Young, N. (1995). Fas antigen expression in CD34+ human marrow cells is induced by interferon-α and tumor necrosis factor-α and potentiates cytokine-mediated hematopoietic suppression in vitro. *Blood*, **85**, 3183.

25. Gersuk, G., Beckham, C., Loken, M. *et al.* (1998). A role for TNF-α, *Fas* and *Fas* ligand in marrow failure associated with myelodysplastic syndrome. *Br. J. Haematol.*, **103**, 176–88.

26. Massague, J. (1987). The TGF-beta family of growth and differentiation factors. *Cell*, **49**, 437–8.

27. Sing, G. K., Keller, J., Ellingsworth, J. R. *et al.* (1988). Transforming growth factor beta selectively inhibits normal and leukemic human bone marrow cell growth in vitro. *Blood*, **72**, 1504–11.

28. Broxmeyer, H. E., Sherry, B., Cooper, S., Lu, L. *et al.* (1993). Comparative analysis of the human macrophage inflammatory protein family of cytokines (chemokines) on proliferation of human myeloid progenitor cells. *J. Immunol.*, **150**, 3448–58.

29. Schmidt-Mende, J., Tehranchi, R., Forsblom, A. M., Joseph, B. *et al.* (2001). Granulocyte colony-stimulating factor inhibits Fas-triggered apoptosis in bone marrow cells isolated from patients with refractory anemia with ringed sideroblasts. *Leukemia*, **15**, 742–51.

30. Tehranchi, R., Fadeel, B., Forsblom, A. M. *et al.* (2003). Granulocyte colony-stimulating factor inhibits spontaneous cytochrome c release and mitochondria-dependent apoptosis of myelodysplastic syndrome hematopoietic progenitors. *Blood*, **101**, 1080–6.

31. Aizawa, S., Nakano, M., Iwase, O. *et al.* (1999). Bone marrow stroma from refractory anemia of myelodysplastic syndrome is defective in its ability to support normal CD34-positive cell proliferation and differentiation in vitro. *Leuk. Res.*, **23**, 239–46.

32. Tennant, G. B., Walsh, V., Truran, L. N. *et al.* (2000). Abnormalities of adherent layers grown from bone marrow of patients with myelodysplasia. *Br. J. Haematol.*, **111**, 853–62.

33. Coutinho, L. H., Geary, C., Chang, J., Harrison, C., and Testa, N. G. (1990). Functional studies of bone marrow haemopoietic and stromal cells in the myelodysplastic syndrome (MDS). *Br. J. Haematol.*, **75**, 16–25.

34. Tauro, S., Hepburn, M., Peddie, C. M., Bowen, D. T., and Pippard, M. J. (2002). Functional disturbance of marrow stromal microenvironment in the myelodysplastic syndromes. *Leukemia*, **16**, 785–90.

35. Borojevic, R., Roela, R., Rodarte, R. S. *et al.* (2004). Bone marrow stroma in childhood myelodysplastic syndrome: composition, ability to sustain hematopoiesis in vitro, and altered gene expression. *Leuk. Res.*, **28**, 831–44.

36. Duhrsen, U., Martinez, T., Vohwinkel, G. *et al.* (2001). Effects of vascular endothelial and platelet-derived growth factor receptor inhibitors on long-term cultures from normal human bone marrow. *Growth Factors*, **19**, 1–17.

37. Carvalho, M. A., Arcanjo, K., Silva, L. C., and Borojevic, R. (2000). The capacity of connective tissue stromas to sustain myelopoiesis depends both upon the growth factors and the local intercellular environment. *Biol. Cell*, **92**, 605–14.

38. Ferrara, N. and Alitalo, K. (1999). Clinical applications of angiogeneic growth factors and their inhibitors. *Nat. Med.*, **5**, 1359–64.

39. Bellamy, W. T., Richer, L., Sirjani, D. *et al.* (2001). Vascular endothelial cell growth factor is an autocrine promoter of abnormal localized immature myeloid precursors

and leukemia progenitor formation in myelodysplastic syndromes. *Blood*, **97**, 1427–34.

40. List, A. F. (2001). Vascular endothelial growth factor signaling pathway as an emerging target in hematologic malignancies. *Oncologist*, **6** (suppl. 5), 24–31.

41. Zhang, L., Eastmond, D., and Smith, M. T. (2002). The nature of chromosomal aberrations detected in humans exposed to benzene. *Crit. Rev. Toxicol.*, **32**, 1–42.

42. Aguayo, A., Kantarjian, H., Manshouri, T. *et al.* (2000). Angiogenesis in acute and chronic leukemias and myelodysplastic syndromes. *Blood*, **96**, 2240–5.

43. Platanias, L. C. (2003). Map kinase signaling pathways and hematologic malignancies. *Blood*, **101**, 4667–79.

44. Verma, A., Deb, D., Sassano, A. *et al.* (2002). Activation of the p38 mitogen-activated protein kinase mediates the suppressive effects of type I interferons and transforming growth factor-beta on normal hematopoiesis. *J. Biol. Chem.*, **277**, 7726–35.

45. Verma, A., Deb, D., Sassano, A. *et al.* (2002). Cutting edge: activation of the *p38* mitogen-activated protein kinase signaling pathway mediates cytokine-induced hemopoietic suppression in aplastic anemia. *J. Immunol.*, **168**, 5984–8.

46. Cortelezzi, A., Cattaneo, C., Cristiani, S. *et al.* (2000). Non-transferrin-bound iron in myelodysplastic syndromes: a marker of ineffective erythropoiesis? *Hematol. J.*, **1**, 153–8.

47. Hofmann, W. K., De Vos, S., Komor, M. *et al.* (2002). Characterization of gene expression of CD34+ cells from normal and myelodysplastic bone marrow. *Blood*, **100**, 3553–60.

48. Bowen, D., Wang, L., Frew, M., Kerr, R., and Groves, M. (2003). Antioxidant enzyme expression in myelodysplastic and acute myeloid leukemia bone marrow: further evidence of a pathogenetic role for oxidative stress? *Haematologica*, **88**, 1070–2.

49. Hershko, C., Link, G., and Cabantchik, I. (1996). Pathophysiology of iron overload. *Ann. N.Y. Acad. Sci.*, **850**, 191.

50. Olivieri, N. and Brittenham, G. (1997). Iron-chelating therapy and the treatment of thalassemia. *Blood*, **89**, 739.

51. Jensen, P. D., Heickendorff, L., Pedersen, B. *et al.* (1996). The effect of iron chelation on haemopoiesis in MDS patients with transfusional iron overload. *Br. J. Haematol.*, **94**, 288–99.

52. Pootrakul, P., Sinrankapracha, P., Sankote, J., Kachintorn, U. *et al.* (2003). Clinical trial of deferiprone iron chelation therapy in beta-thalassaemia/haemoglobin E patients in Thailand. *Br. J. Haematol.*, **122**, 305–10.

53. Hamblin, T. (1992). Immunologic abnormalities in myelodysplastic syndromes. *Hematol. Oncol. Clin. North Am.*, **6**, 571.

54. Bynoe, A. G., Scott, C., Ford, P. *et al.* (1983). Decreased T helper cells in the myelodysplastic syndromes. *Br. J. Haematol.* **54**, 97.

55. Knox, S. J., Greenberg, P., Anderson, R. W. *et al.* (1983). Studies of T lymphocytes in preleukemic disorders and acute nonlymphocytic leukemia: in vitro radiosensitivity, mitogenic responsiveness, colony formation, and enumeration of lymphocytic subpopulations. *Blood*, **61**, 449.

56. Richert-Boe, K. E. and Bagby, G. J. (1992). In vitro hematopoiesis in myelodysplasia: liquid and soft-gel culture studies. *Hematol. Oncol. Clin. North Am.*, **6**, 543–56.

57. Janssen, J. W. G., Buschle, M., Layton, M. *et al.* (1989). Clonal analysis of myelodysplastic syndromes: evidence of multipotent stem cell origin. *Blood*, **73**, 248.

58. Abrahamson, G., Boultwood, J., Madden, J. *et al.* (1991). Clonality of cell populations in refractory anaemia using combined approach of gene loss and X linked restriction fragment length polymorphism methylation analysis. *Br. J. Haematol.*, **79**, 550.

59. Anastasi, J., Feng, J., Le Beau, M. M. *et al.* (1993). Cytogenetic clonality in myelodysplastic syndromes studied with fluorescence in situ hybridization: lineage, response to growth factor therapy and clonal expansion. *Blood*, **81**, 1580.

60. Tsukamot, N., Morita, K., Maehara, T. *et al.* (1993). Clonality in MDS: demonstration of pluripotent stem cell origin using X linked restriction fragment length polymorphisms. *Br. J. Haematol.*, **83**, 589.

61. van Kamp, H., Fibbe, W., Jansen, R. P. M. *et al.* (1992). Clonal involvement of granulocytes and monocytes, but not of T and B lymphocytes and natural killer cells in patients with myelodysplasia: analysis by X linked restriction fragment length polymorphisms and polymerase chain reaction of the phosphoglycerate kinase gene. *Blood*, **80**, 1774.

62. Culligan, D. J., Cachai, P., Whittaker, J. *et al.* (1992). Clonal lymphocytes are detectable in only some cases of MDS. *Br. J. Haematol.*, **81**, 346.

63. Kroef, M. J. P. L., Fibbe, W., Mout, R. *et al.* (1993). Myeloid but not lymphoid cells carry the 5q deletion: polymerase chain reaction analysis of loss of heterozygosity using mini repeat sequences on highly purified cell fractions. *Blood*, **81**, 1849.

64. Greenberg, P. L. (1996). Biologic and clinical implications of marrow culture studies in the myelodysplastic syndromes. *Semin. Hematol.*, **33**, 163–75.

65. Merchav, S., Nielson, O., Rosenbaum, H. *et al.* (1990). In vitro studies of erythropoietin-dependent regulation of erythropoiesis in myelodysplastic syndromes. *Leukemia*, **4**, 771–4.

66. Clark, D. M. and Lambert, I. (1990). Apoptosis is a common histopathological finding in myelodysplasia: the correlate of ineffective haematopoiesis. *Leuk. Lymphoma*, **2**, 415.

67. Raza, A., Gezer, S., Mundle, S. *et al.* (1995). Apoptosis in bone marrow biopsy samples involving stromal and hematopoietic cells in 50 patients with myelodysplastic syndromes. *Blood*, **86**, 268.

68. Raza, A., Mundle, S., Iftikhar, A. *et al.* (1995). Simultaneous assessment of cell kinetics and programmed cell death in bone marrow biopsies of myelodysplastics reveals extensive apoptosis as the probable basis for ineffective hematopoiesis. *Am. J. Hematol.*, **48**, 143.

69. Rajapaksa, R., Ginzton, N., Rott, L., and Greenberg, P. L. (1996). Altered oncogene expression and apoptosis in myelodysplastic syndrome marrow cells. *Blood*, **88**, 4275–87.

70. Greenberg, P. L. (1998). Apoptosis and its role in MDS: implications for disease natural history and treatment. *Leukemia Res.*, **22**, 1123–36.

71. Shimazaki, K., Ohshima, K., Suzumiya, J., Kawasaki, C., and Kikuchi, M. (2000). Evaluation of apoptosis as a prognostic factor in myelodysplastic syndromes. *Br. J. Haematol.*, **110**, 584–90.

72. Huh, Y. O., Jilani, I., Estey, E. *et al.* (2002). More cell death in refractory anemia with excess blasts in transformation than in acute myeloid leukemia. *Leukemia*, **16**, 2249–52.

73. Ali, A., Mundle, S., Ragasa, D. *et al.* (1999). Sequential activation of caspase-1 and caspase-3-like proteases during apoptosis in myelodysplastic syndromes. *J. Hematother. Stem Cell Res.*, **8**, 343–56.

74. Hellstrom-Lindberg, E., Schmidt-Mende, J., Forsblom, A. M. *et al.* (2001). Apoptosis in refractory anaemia with ringed sideroblasts is initiated at the stem cell level and associated with increased activation of caspases. *Br. J. Haematol.*, **112**, 714–26.

75. Parker, J., Mufti, G., Rasool, F. *et al.* (2000). The role of apoptosis, proliferation and the Bcl2-related proteins in the myelodysplastic syndromes and acute myeloid leukemia secondary to MDS. *Blood*, **96**, 3932–8.

76. Korsmeyer, S. (1995). Regulators of cell death. *Trends Genet.*, **11**, 101.

77. Reed, J. C. (1997). Bcl-2 family proteins: regulators of apoptosis and chemoresistance in hematologic malignancies. *Semin. Hematol.*, **34**, 9.

78. Davis, R. E. and Greenberg, P. (1998). *Bcl-2* expression by myeloid precursors in myelodysplastic syndromes: impact on disease progression. *Leuk. Res.*, **22**, 767–77.

79. Boudard, D., Vasselon, C., Bertheas, M. F. *et al.* (2002). Expression and prognostic significance of Bcl-2 family proteins in myelodysplastic syndromes. *Am. J. Hematol.*, **70**, 115–25.

80. Jacobs, R. A., Cornbleet, M., Vardiman, J. *et al.* (1986). Prognostic implications of morphology and karyotype in primary myelodysplastic syndromes. *Blood*, **67**, 1765.

81. Pedersen-Bjergaard, J., Philip, P., Larsen, S. O. *et al.* (1990). Chromosome aberrations and prognostic factors in therapy-related myelodysplasia and acute non-lymphocytic leukemia. *Blood*, **76**, 1083.

82. Horiike, S., Taniwaki, M., Misawa, S. *et al.* (1988). Chromosome abnormalities and karyotypic evolution in 83 patients with myelodysplastic syndrome and predictive value for prognosis. *Cancer*, **62**, 1129.

83. Rossi, G., Pelizzari, A., Bellotti, D., Tonelli, M., and Barlati, S. (2000). Cytogenetic analogy between myelodysplastic syndrome and acute myeloid leukemia of elderly patients. *Leukemia*, **14**, 636–41.

84. Carroll, M., Tomasson, M., Barker, G. F., Golub, T. R., and Gilliland, D. G. (1996). The TEL/platelet-derived growth factor beta receptor (PDGF beta R) fusion in chronic myelomonocytic leukemia is a transforming protein that self-associates and activates PDGF beta R kinase-dependent signaling pathways. *Proc. Natl Acad. Sci. U.S.A.*, **93**, 14845–50.

85. Magnusson, M. K., Meade, K., Nakamura, R., Barrett, J., and Dunbar, C. E. (2002). Activity of STI571 in chronic myelomonocytic leukemia with a platelet-derived growth factor beta receptor fusion oncogene. *Blood*, **100**, 1088–91.

86. Yunis, J. J., Boot, A. J. M., Mayer, M. G., and Bos, J. L. (1989). Mechanisms of *ras* mutation in myelodysplastic syndrome. *Oncogene*, **4**, 609.

87. Padua, R. A., Gunn, B., Al-Sabah, A. I. *et al.* (1998). *RAS, FMS* and *p53* mutations and poor clinical outcome in myelodysplasias: a 10-year follow-up. *Leukemia*, **12**, 887–92.

88. Shih, L. Y., Huang, C., Wang, P. N. *et al.* (2004). Acquisition of *FLT3* or *N-ras* mutations is frequently associated with progression of myelodysplastic syndrome to acute myeloid leukemia. *Leukemia*, **18**, 466–75.

89. Paquette, R. L., Landow, E., Pierre, R. V. *et al.* (1993). *N-ras* mutations are associated with poor prognosis and increased risk of leukaemia in myelodysplastic syndrome. *Blood*, **82**, 590–9.

90. Parker, J. and Mufti, G. (1996). *Ras* and myelodysplasia: lessons from the last decade. *Semin. Hematol.*, **33**, 206.

91. Neubauer, A., Greenberg, P., Negrin, R. *et al.* (1994). Mutations in the *ras* proto-oncogenes in patients with myelodysplastic syndromes. *Leukemia*, **8**, 638.

92. Zhang, J. and Lodish, H. (2004). Constitutive activation of the MEK/ERK pathway mediates all effects of oncogenic *H-ras* expression in primary erythroid progenitors. *Blood*, **104**, 1679–87.

93. Greenberg, P., Cox, C., Le Beau, M. M. *et al.* (1997). International scoring system for evaluating prognosis in myelodysplastic syndromes. *Blood*, **89**, 2079–88.

94. Ridge, S. A., Worwood, M., Oscier, D. *et al.* (1990). *FMS* mutations in myelodysplastic, leukemic, and normal subjects. *Proc. Natl Acad. Sci. U.S.A.*, **87**, 1377.

95. Tobal, K., Pagliuca, A., Bhatt, B. *et al.* (1990). Mutation of the human *FMS* gene (M-CSF receptor) in myelodysplastic syndromes and acute myeloid leukemia. *Leukemia*, **4**, 486.

96. Fidler, C., Watkins, F., Bowen, D. T. *et al.* (2004). *NRAS, FLT3* and *TP53* mutations in patients with myelodysplastic syndrome and a del(5q). *Haematologica*, **89**, 865–6.

97. Hollstein, M., Sidransky, D., Vogelstein, B., and Harris, C. C. (1991). *p53* mutations in human cancers. *Science*, **253**, 49.

98. Jonveaux, P., Fenaux, P., Quiquandon, I. *et al.* (1991). Mutations in the *p53* gene in myelodysplastic syndromes. *Oncogene*, **6**, 2243.

99. Wattel, E., Preudhomme, C., Hecquet, B. *et al.* (1994). *P53* mutations are associated with resistance to chemotherapy and short survival in hematologic malignancies. *Blood*, **84**, 3148.

100. Mori, N., Hidai, H., Yokota, J. *et al.* (1995). Mutations of the *p53* gene in myelodysplastic syndrome and overt leukemia. *Leuk. Res.*, **19**, 869.

101. Sugimoto, K., Hirano, N., Toyoshima, H. *et al.* (1993). Mutations of the *p53* gene in myelodysplastic syndrome (MDS) and MDS-derived leukemia. *Blood*, **81**, 3022.

102. Kaneko, H., Misawa, S., Horiike, S. *et al.* (1995). *TP53* mutations emerge at early phase of myelodysplastic syndrome and are associated with complex chromosomal abnormalities. *Blood*, **85**, 2189.

103. Kita-Sasai, Y., Horiike, S., Misawa, S. *et al.* (2001). International prognostic scoring system and *TP53* mutations are independent prognostic indicators for patients with myelodysplastic syndrome. *Br. J. Haematol.*, **115**, 301–12.

104. Horiike, S., Kita-Sasai, Y., Nakao, M., and Taniwaki, M. (2003). Configuration of the *TP53* gene as an independent prognostic parameter of myelodysplastic syndrome. *Leuk. Lymphoma*, **44**, 915–22.

105. Ben-Yehuda, D., Krichevsky, S., Caspi, O. *et al.* (1996). Microsatellite instability and *p53* mutations in therapy-related leukemia suggest mutator phenotype. *Blood*, **88**, 4296.

106. Horiike, S., Misawa, S., Kaneko, H. *et al.* (1999). Distinct genetic involvement of the *TP53* gene in therapy-related leukemia and myelodysplasia with chromosomal losses of nos 5 and/or 7 and its possible relationship to replication error phenotype. *Leukemia*, **13**, 1235.

107. Side, L. E., Curtiss, N., Teel, K., Kratz, C. *et al.* (2004). *RAS, FLT3*, and *TP53* mutations in therapy-related myeloid malignancies with abnormalities of chromosomes 5 and 7. *Genes Chromosomes Cancer*, **39**, 217–22.

108. Cilloni, D., Gottardi, E., Messa, F., Fava, M. *et al.* (2003). Significant correlation between the degree of *WT1* expression and the International Prognostic Scoring System Score in patients with myelodysplastic syndromes. *J. Clin. Oncol.*, **21**, 1988–95.

109. Nakao, M., Horiike, S., Fukushima-Nakase, Y., Nishimura, M. *et al.* (2004). Novel loss-of-function mutations of the haematopoiesis-related transcription factor, acute myeloid leukaemia 1/runt-related transcription factor 1, detected in acute

myeloblastic leukaemia and myelodysplastic syndrome. *Br. J. Haematol.*, **125**, 709–19.

110. Harada, H., Haroda, Y., Niimi, H. *et al.* (2004). High incidence of somatic mutations in the *AML1/RUNX1* gene in myelodysplastic syndrome and low blast percentage myeloid leukemia with myelodysplasia. *Blood*, **103**, 2316–24.

111. Soderholm, J., Kobayashi, H., Mathieu, C., Rowley, J. D., and Nucifora, G. (1997). The leukemia-associated gene *MDS1/EVI1* is a new type of GATA-binding transactivator. *Leukemia*, **11**, 352–8.

112. Barjesteh van Waalwijk van Doorn-Khosrovani, S., Erpelinck, C., Lowenberg, B., and Delwel, R. (2003). Low expression of *MDS1-EVI1*-like-1 (*MEL1*) and *EVI1*-like-1 (*EL1*) genes in favorable-risk acute myeloid leukemia. *Exp. Hematol.*, **31**, 1066–72.

113. Xu, K., Wang, L., Hao, Y. *et al.* (1999). *Evi-1* and *MDS1-Evi-1* genes in pathogenesis of myelodysplastic syndromes and post-MDS acute myeloid leukemia. *Chin. Med. J. (Engl.)*, **112**, 1112–18.

114. Shih, L. Y., Lin, T., Wang, P. N. *et al.* (2004). Internal tandem duplication of fms-like tyrosine kinase 3 is associated with poor outcome in patients with myelodysplastic syndrome. *Cancer*, **101**, 989–98.

115. Horiike, S., Yokota, S., Nakao, M., Iwai, T. *et al.* (1997). Tandem duplications of the *FLT3* receptor gene are associated with leukemic transformation of myelodysplasia. *Leukemia*, **11**, 1442–6.

116. Gomes, I., Sharma, T., Edassery, S. *et al.* (2002). Novel transcription factors in human CD34 antigen-positive hematopoietic cells. *Blood*, **100**, 107–19.

117. Nagamura-Inoue, T., Tamura, T. T., and Ozato, K. (2001). Transcription factors that regulate growth and differentiation of myeloid cells. *Int. Rev. Immunol.*, **20**, 83–105.

118. Yordy, J. S. and Muise-Helmericks, R. (2000). Signal transduction and the *Ets* family of transcription factors. *Oncogene*, **19**, 6503–13.

119. Hsu, T., Trojanowska, M., and Watson, D. K. (2004). Ets proteins in biological control and cancer. *J. Cell Biochem.*, **91**, 896–903.

120. Kopp, J. L., Wilder, P., Desler, M. *et al.* (2004). Unique and selective effects of five Ets family members, *Elf3*, *Ets1*, *Ets2*, *PEA3*, and *PU.1*, on the promoter of the type II transforming growth factor-beta receptor gene. *J. Biol. Chem.*, **279**, 19407–20.

121. Kim, H. G., De Guzman, C., Swindle, C. S. *et al.* (2004). The ETS-family transcription factor, PU.1, is necessary for the maintenance of fetal liver hematopoietic stem cells. [Epub ahead of print]. *Blood*, **104**, 3894–900.

122. Kerckaert, J. P., Duterque-Coquillaud, M., Collyn-d'Hooghe, M. *et al.* (1990). Polymorphism of the proto-oncogene *ETS-1* in hematological malignancies. *Leukemia*, **4**, 16–19.

123. Wlodarska, I., Mecucci, C., Marynen, P. *et al.* (1995). *TEL* gene is involved in myelodysplastic syndromes with either the typical t(5;12)(q33;p13) translocation or its variant t(10;12)(q24;p13). *Blood,* **85,** 2848–52.

124. Gilliland, D. G. (2002). Molecular genetics of human leukemias: new insights into therapy. *Semin. Hematol.,* **39** (suppl. 3), 6–11.

125. Sternberg, D. W. and Gilliland, D. (2004). The role of signal transducer and activator of transcription factors in leukemogenesis. *J. Clin. Oncol.,* **22,** 361–71.

126. Hoefsloot, L. H., van Amelsvoort, M., Broeders, L. C. *et al.* (1997). Erythropoietin-induced activation of *STAT5* is impaired in the myelodysplastic syndrome. *Blood,* **89,** 1690–700.

127. Ohyashiki, J. H., Iwama, H., Yahata, N. *et al.* (1999). Telomere stability is frequently impaired in high-risk groups of patients with myelodysplastic syndromes. *Clin. Cancer Res.,* **5,** 1155–60.

128. Sashida, G., Ohyashiki, J., Nakajima, A. *et al.* (2003). Telomere dynamics in myelodysplastic syndrome determined by telomere measurement of marrow metaphases. *Clin. Cancer Res.,* **9,** 1489–96.

129. Ohshima, K., Karube, K., Shimazaki, K. *et al.* (2003). Imbalance between apoptosis and telomerase activity in myelodysplastic syndromes: possible role in ineffective hemopoiesis. *Leuk. Lymphoma,* **44,** 1339–46.

130. Beausejour, C. M., Krtolica, A., Galimi, F. *et al.* (2003). Reversal of human cellular senescence: roles of the *p53* and *p16* pathways. *Embo. J.,* **22,** 4212–22.

131. Esteller, M. (2003). Profiling aberrant DNA methylation in hematologic neoplasms: a view from the tip of the iceberg. *Clin. Immunol.,* **109,** 80–8.

132. Quesnel, B., Guillerm, G., Vereecque, R. *et al.* (1998). Methylation of the *p15(INK4b)* gene in myelodysplastic syndromes is frequent and acquired during disease progression. *Blood,* **91,** 2985–90.

133. Lubbert, M. (2003). Gene silencing of the *p15/INK4B* cell-cycle inhibitor by hypermethylation: an early or later epigenetic alteration in myelodysplastic syndromes? *Leukemia,* **17,** 1762–4.

134. Christiansen, D. H., Andersen, M., and Pedersen-Bjergaard, J. (2003). Methylation of *p15INK4B* is common, is associated with deletion of genes on chromosome arm 7q and predicts a poor prognosis in therapy-related myelodysplasia and acute myeloid leukemia. *Leukemia,* **17,** 1813–19.

135. Claus, R. and Lubbert, M. (2003). Epigenetic targets in hematopoietic malignancies. *Oncogene,* **22,** 6489–96.

136. Daskalakis, M., Nguyen, T., Nguyen, C. *et al.* (2002). Demethylation of a hypermethylated *P15/INK4B* gene in patients with myelodysplastic syndrome by 5-Aza-2'-deoxycytidine (decitabine) treatment. *Blood,* **100,** 2957–64.

137. Lichtman, M. A. and Rowe, J. (2004). The relationship of patient age to the pathobiology of the clonal myeloid diseases. *Semin. Oncol.,* **31,** 185–97.

138. Krtolica, A. and Campisi, J. (2003). Integrating epithelial cancer, aging stroma and cellular senescence. *Adv. Gerontol.*, **11**, 109–16.

139. Busuttil, R. A., Rubio, M., Campisi, J., and Vijga, J. (2004). Genomic instability, aging, and cellular senescence. *Ann. N. Y. Acad. Sci.*, **1019**, 245–55.

140. Campisi, J. (2003). Cellular senescence and apoptosis: how cellular responses might influence aging phenotypes. l. *Exp. Gerontol.*, **38**, 5–11.

141. Krtolica, A. and Campisi, J. (2002). Cancer and aging: a model for the cancer promoting effects of the aging stroma. *Int. J. Biochem. Cell Biol.*, **34**, 1401–14.

142. Busuttil, R. A., Rubio, M., Dolle, M. E., Campisi, J., and Vijg, J. (2003). Oxygen accelerates the accumulation of mutations during the senescence and immortalization of murine cells in culture. *Aging Cell*, **2**, 287–94.

143. Sutton, J. F., Stacey, M., Kearns, W. G. *et al.* (2004). Increased risk for aplastic anemia and myelodysplastic syndrome in individuals lacking glutathione S-transferase genes. *Pediatr. Blood Cancer*, **42**, 122–6.

144. Allan, J. M., Wild, C., Rollinson, S. *et al.* (2001). Polymorphism in glutathione S-transferase P1 is associated with susceptibility to chemotherapy-induced leukemia. *Proc. Natl Acad. Sci. U.S.A.*, **98**, 11592–7.

145. Morgan, G. J. and Smith, M. (2002). Metabolic enzyme polymorphisms and susceptibility to acute leukemia in adults. *Am. J. Pharmacogenomics*, **2**, 79–92.

Cytogenetic abnormalities in myelodysplastic syndromes

Harold J. Olney[1] and Michelle M. Le Beau[2]

[1] Université de Montréal, Montreal, Quebec, Canada
[2] University of Chicago, Chicago, IL, USA

The cytogenetic evaluation of a bone marrow sample from patients with a myelodysplastic syndrome (MDS) has become an integral part of clinical care. This analysis not only confirms the diagnosis but is also invaluable in defining the prognosis and median survival, as well as the risk for progression to an acute myeloid leukemia (AML). On a more fundamental level, cytogenetic analysis has been instrumental in establishing the clonality of these syndromes as well as providing hints into the pathobiology of these entities.

The first widely recognized system of classification for MDS was proposed by the French–American–British (FAB) group in 1982, and distinguished chronic myelomonocytic leukemia (CMML), refractory anemia (RA), refractory anemia with ringed sideroblasts (RARS), refractory anemia with excess blasts (RAEB), and refractory anemia with excess blasts in transformation (RAEB-T).[1] While imperfect, the FAB classification system has allowed clinicians and researchers to advance the understanding of the pathogenesis and prognosis of these diseases as well as to evaluate the utility of therapeutic interventions. The current World Health Organization (WHO) classification requires cytogenetic data for diagnostic purposes; thus, cytogenetic analysis is a mandatory step in the full evaluation of a newly diagnosed patient.[2] The WHO classification includes RA, RARS, refractory cytopenias with multilineage dysplasia (RCMD), RCMD with ringed sideroblasts (RCMD-RS), RAEB-1, 2, unclassified MDS, and MDS with isolated del(5q). See

Myelodysplastic Syndromes: Clinical and Biological Advances, ed. Peter L. Greenberg. Published by Cambridge University Press. © Cambridge University Press 2006.

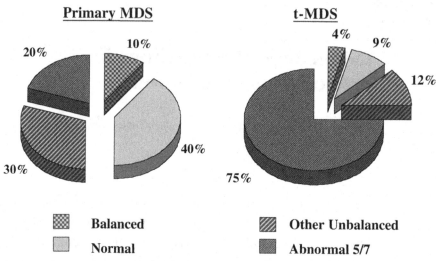

Fig. 4.1   Distribution of karyotypic abnormalities in Primary myelodysplastic syndromes (MDS) and therapy-related MDS (t-MDS).

Chapters 1 and 2 for expanded discussion of the morphologic classification of MDS.

At the time of diagnosis, recurring chromosomal abnormalities are found in 40–70% of patients with primary MDS and in 95% of patients with therapy-related MDS (t-MDS).[3] Numerous authors have reported the value of cytogenetic analysis in predicting survival and risk of leukemic transformation during a patient's clinical course.[4–7] The frequency of cytogenetic abnormalities increases with the severity of disease, as does the risk of leukemic transformation. Clonal chromosome abnormalities can be detected in marrow cells of 40–100% of patients with primary MDS at diagnosis (RA, 25%; RARS, 10%; RCMD, 50%; RAEB-1, 2, 50–70%; MDS with isolated del(5q), 100%).

The most common cytogenetic abnormalities encountered in MDS are del(5q), −7, and +8 (Figs. 4.1 and 4.2), which have been included in prognostic scoring systems of MDS. Clones with unrelated abnormalities, one of which typically has a gain of chromosome 8, are seen at a greater frequency (∼5% versus ∼1%) in patients with MDS than in patients with AML. Among the few independent variables identified that predict clinical

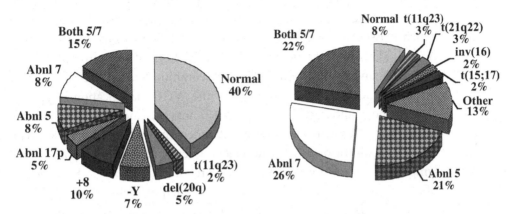

Fig. 4.2   Recurring chromosomal abnormalities in primary myelodsyplastic syndromes (MDS) and therapy-related MDS (t-MDS) and therapy-related acute myeloid leukemia (t-AML).

outcomes in MDS, cytogenetic findings form the cornerstone of successful prognostic scoring systems.[8]

This review will summarize our current understanding of the recurring chromosomal alterations and molecular biological findings in MDS. We emphasize the most current literature, and extend our apologies to the many investigators who contributed earlier to our understanding of MDS but who are not cited here.

Diagnosis

Pathological classification of hematological diseases requires expert evaluation and is crucial for clinical management decisions. The detection of a clonal cytogenetic abnormality may be useful in difficult cases to establish the diagnosis of MDS, distinguishing between a benign reactive lymphoid or myeloid hyperplasia and a malignant monoclonal proliferation.

The most frequent recurring abnormalities found in MDS are unbalanced, namely simple loss or deletions of chromosomes, but unbalanced translocations and more complex derivatives can be found (Figs. 4.1 and 4.2). In rare cases, recurring balanced translocations have been reported. A handful of specific cytogenetic abnormalities are recognized in association with morphologically and clinically distinct subsets of MDS, including the 5q− syndrome,[9] the 17p− syndrome,[10] and the isodicentric X chromosome which is associated with RARS with a high likelihood of transformation to AML.[11] Many findings, including loss or deletions of chromosomes 5 or 7, trisomy 8, and complex karyotypes, are common to both MDS and AML, including the new RCMD subtype of the WHO classification (Fig. 4.2). Other abnormalities, such as the t(15;17), inv(16), and t(8;21), are usually found in acute leukemia without an antecedent myelodysplastic phase.[12] The t(9;22), diagnostic of chronic myelogenous leukemia and a subtype of acute lymphoblastic leukemia, has rarely been reported in MDS[13]. The detection of one of these recurring abnormalities can be quite helpful in establishing the correct diagnosis, and can add information of prognostic importance, permitting tailored treatment planning. Serial evaluations can also be informative, particularly when there is a change in the clinical picture. The identification of new abnormalities in the karyotype often signals a change in the pace of the disease, usually to a more aggressive course, and may herald incipient leukemia.

Prognosis

The initial FAB classification provided the first systematic prognostic classification. The RA and RARS subtypes are generally more favorable (low risk) than CMML (intermediate risk), with RAEB and RAEB-T having the poorest prognosis (high risk). The Spanish,[14] Düsseldorf,[15] Lille,[4] and Bournemouth[16] classification systems attempted to refine prognosis by integrating clinical or laboratory data to the pathologic findings defined by the FAB classification system. More recently, the International MDS Risk Analysis Workshop combined cytogenetic, morphologic, and clinical data from over 800 patients from seven large risk-based studies to describe an International Prognostic Scoring System (IPSS) for MDS (see Chapter 1).[8] The IPSS scores cytogenetic abnormalities (outlined in Table 4.1), percentage of marrow blasts, and number of peripheral cytopenias to define three risk groups: good, intermediate, and poor outcome, with a median survival of 3.8, 2.4, and 0.8 years, respectively. The IPSS has been found to be highly reproducible in predicting survival and risk of leukemic transformation.[7,17−19]

Table 4.1 Cytogenetic abnormalities of the International Prognostic Scoring System

	Cytogenetic abnormalities	25% AML progression (years)	Median survival (years)
Favorable risk	Normal karyotype isolated del(5q) isolated del(20q) isolated −Y	5.6	3.8
Intermediate risk	other abnormalities	1.6	2.4
Poor risk	−7 del(7q) Complex karyotypes	0.9	0.8

AML, acute myeloid leukemia.

Evolution of the karyotype

Cytogenetic evolution is the appearance of an abnormal clone where only normal cells have been seen previously, or the progression from the presence of a single clone (often with a simple karyotype) to multiple related, or occasionally unrelated, abnormal clones. The abnormal clones may evolve, acquiring additional abnormalities with disease progression, and typically resolve with remission of disease following treatment. In published series, most MDS patients die of bone marrow failure, close to half progress to acute leukemia, and a few die of intercurrent illness. The natural history of MDS generally follows one of three patterns: (1) a gradual increase in marrow blast count associated with worsening pancytopenia; (2) a relatively stable clinical course followed by an abrupt change with a clear leukemic transformation; and (3) a stable course over many years without increase in marrow blast counts upon reinvestigation.[20] In the first group, the karyotype typically remains stable, and the progression to leukemia is based on the relatively arbitrary finding of greater than 20% blasts (30% in the FAB classification) in the marrow, making the transition to AML a relatively ill-defined event. In the second group, a change in the karyotype, with the gain of secondary clones, and complex karyotypes, is typical. The karyotype as well as disease

tends to remain stable in the third group. Few series with sequential cytogenetic studies have been published, and most series are small with short
follow-up periods.[21–23] Nonetheless, karyotypic evolution in MDS is associated with transformation to acute leukemia in about 60% of cases, and
reduced survival, particularly for those patients who evolve within a short
period of time (less than 100 days).[22]

Alterations in gene function

A growing body of evidence suggests that mutations of multiple genes mediate the pathogenesis and progression of MDS. A detailed review of these
genes is beyond the scope of this chapter, but is included elsewhere in this
volume. Table 4.2 provides a partial list and overview of some of their salient
features as related to MDS.

The most extensively studied gene family in MDS is the RAS (rat sarcoma
viral oncogene homolog) family. RAS proteins are a critical component of
signaling pathways from cell surface receptors to the nucleus, and result in the
control of cellular proliferation, differentiation, and cell death. These proteins
bind guanine nucleotides, with activation controlled by cycling between the
guanosine triphosphate (GTP)-bound (active) and guanosine diphosphate
(GDP)-bound (inactive) forms.[24] Once activated by a cell surface receptor,
RAS proteins induce a cascade of kinase activity, resulting in the transduction
of the signals to the nucleus. The RAS signaling cascade is downstream of
a number of activated cytokine receptors, including the FLT3 interleukin-3
(IL-3), and granulocyte–macrophage colony-stimulating factor(GM-CSF)
receptors; thus, this signaling pathway plays an important role in hematopoiesis. Mutant RAS proteins retain the active GTP-bound form, promoting constitutive activation. The most frequent mutation is a single base
change at codon 12 of the protein, but codons 13 and 61 are also frequently
mutated. Codons 12 and 13 are located within the pocket that binds GTP,
and mutant proteins have decreased phosphatase activity, reducing inactivation to the GDP form.[25,26] Constitutively activating point mutations of
N-RAS have been detected at high frequency in hematologic malignancies.
In MDS, *N-RAS* mutations have been detected in 10–40% of cases. These
mutations have been associated with a poor prognosis, with higher incidence of transformation to AML and shorter survival. Those patients with

Table 4.2 Partial list of genes altered in myelodysplastic syndrome (MDS)

Gene	Alteration	Associated features	References
BCL 2	Overexpressed in all FAB subtypes	Encodes a protein product that suppresses apoptosis No correlation with survival Highest levels noted in higher-risk entities where apoptosis is reduced	34,35,117
CSF1R/FMS	Mutated in 12–20%, increased with higher-risk MDS	Encodes the macrophage colony-stimulating factor receptor with tyrosine kinase activity Karyotype predominantly normal Increased frequency of transformation to AML and poor survival	28,118
FLT3	Internal tandem duplication (ITD) in ∼ 10% of MDS and AML with trilineage dysplasia	Encodes a class receptor tyrosine kinase playing a role in stem cell differentiation ITD results in constitutive activation of protein Associated with progression to AML and poor prognosis Frequently observed with normal karyotype in AML	119,120
GCSFRG	Point mutations identified	Encodes the G-CSF receptor Severe congenital neutropenia (SCN) patients with G-CSF receptor defects can progress to MDS and/or AML Mutation alone is not sufficient for transformation Progression to leukemia in SCN associated with loss of chromosome 7 and N-RAS/K-RAS1 mutations	121
HLA-DR15 (DR2)	Overrepresented in MDS of RA subtype (36% versus 21% in normal blood donors)	T-cell-mediated autoimmune mechanism implicated in some forms of MDS Correlated with response to immunosuppression of carefully defined MDS	122
KIT	Overexpressed; no mutations found	Encodes the stem cell factor receptor May provide an autocrine growth pathway	123,124
MDR1	Expressed in ∼ 60%	Encodes a transmembrane drug efflux pump May be involved in resistance of MDS to drug therapy Associated with monosomy 7	125

(cont.)

Table 4.2 (cont.)

Gene	Expression/Mutation	Function/Comments	Ref.
MDM2	Overexpressed in ~ 70%	Encodes a protein product (murine double minute-2) which abrogates the function of the p53 tumor suppressor protein via ubiquitination and degradation of p53 Gene amplification not detected Associated with unfavorable cytogenetic abnormalities Shorter remission duration	126,127
MPL	Overexpressed in ~ 45% of CMML, and ~ 40% of RAEB, RAEB-T patients; underexpressed (~ 50% of normal levels) in most MDS patients, especially RA	Encodes the thrombopoietin receptor Higher expression in RAEB and RAEB-T associated with poor prognosis, increased progression to AML correlated with dysmegakaryocytopoiesis	128,129
NF1	Loss and mutations identified, particularly in pediatric MDS/MPS	Encodes neurofibromin, a tumor suppressor gene product, that functions as a GTPase-activating protein (GAP) to downregulate RAS (rat sarcoma viral oncogene homolog) function High incidence of MDS and AML in children with neurofibromatosis type 1 No structural alteration in homologous allele in adults with loss of one chromosome 17	130,131
N-RAS	Mutated in 20–40%; overexpressed in RA, RARS	Encodes a component of various cytokine signal transduction pathways Activating mutations result in constitutive signaling Associated with monocytic component Increased risk of progression to AML Overexpression may represent an early event in the multistep process of transformation	132
CDKN2B/ p15^{INK4B}	Decreased expression via gene-silencing by DNA methylation in 68% of t-MDS/t-AML	Closely associated with deletion or loss of 7q Independently associated with poor survival	133

			Ref.
PTPN11	Somatic missense mutations in 33% of JMML patients	A non-receptor tyrosine phosphatase that relays signals from activated growth factor receptors to RAS proteins Mutations of *N-RAS/K-RAS1*, *NF1*, and *PTPN11* seem to be mutually exclusive	134
Telomerase (including *TERT*, *TR*, and *TP1*)	Increased activity late in disease, particularly *TERT*	Enzyme complex responsible for chromosome telomere maintenance and replication Variable levels of activity Abnormal telomere maintenance may be an early indication of genetic instability Telomeres shortened with disease progression	135–138
TP53	Mutated in 5–25%; higher frequency in t-MDS	Encodes G1, S, and G2 checkpoint protein product which monitors integrity of genome; arrests cell cycle in response to DNA damage Loss of wild-type allele Associated with weak *BCL2* expression Observed as both early and late genetic event in MDS Associated with rapid progression and poor outcome seen with loss of 17p, −5/del(5q), −7/del(7q), suggesting pathogenic exposure to carcinogens Significantly differentiates worse prognosis within each IPSS subgroup	28,139,140
WT1	Associated with overexpression	Overexpressed in 65% of bone marrow specimens and 78% of peripheral blood specimens overexpressed compared to normal cells, including all RAEB and t-AML patient samples Correlated with blast counts and cytogenetic abnormalities Significantly correlated with IPSS score	141

FAB, French–American–British; AML, acute myeloid leukemia; RA, refractory anemia; G-CSF, granulocyte–colony stimulating factor; CMML, chronic myelomonocytic leukemia; RAEB, refractory anemia with excess blasts; RAEB-T, RAEB in transformation; MPS, myeloproliferative syndrome; RARS, RA with ringed sideroblasts; JMML, Juvenile myelomonocytic leukemia; IPSS, International Prognostic Scoring System.

both abnormal karyotypes and *N-RAS* mutations have the highest likelihood of transformation.[25,27–30] Many therapeutic molecules entering clinical trials, including the farnesyl transferease inhibitors and imatinib, interrupt various steps in the RAS signaling pathways.[31,32]

One of the paradoxes associated with the MDSs is the presence of peripheral cytopenias, frequently involving all three lineages (granulocytic, erythroid, and megakaryocytic), with the presence of a hypercellular bone marrow where cells in both the peripheral blood and bone marrow exhibit varying degrees of dysmorphic features. Many genes are involved in the tightly regulated and complex process of cellular death, apoptosis, which plays an important role in maintaining normal homeostasis by removing immature and dysmorphic cells. Although some of the findings are conflicting, there is consensus on a number of points. Measurements of cell cycle kinetics demonstrate an increase in the proliferation of all hematopoietic cell lineages, particularly the myeloid cell line.[33,34] This proliferation is balanced by an increase in apoptosis in MDS. It is well documented that altered cytokine levels play a pivotal role in this process.[35] The proapoptotic tumor necrosis factor-α (TNF-α), transforming growth factor alpha (TGF-α), interferon gamma (IFN-γ), and interleukin-1 beta (IL-1β) are increased in MDS.[36–38] They may function to suppress the growth of hematopoietic progenitors and induce expression of the *FAS* receptor which, when appropriately triggered, can initiate the apoptotic pathways. The prominent role of some cytokines has been examined in clinical studies. Strategies to neutralize TNF-α by decreasing its production with pentoxifylline or thalidomide and with soluble TNF-α receptors (to bind the excess TNF competitively) have resulted in clinical responses in a minority of MDS patients.[39–41]

Molecular models for chromosome abnormalities in MDS

As described earlier, many of the recurring chromosomal abnormalities in MDS lead to the loss of genetic material. Such loss is the hallmark of tumor suppressor genes, which normally function to control cell growth and/or cell death by regulating the cell cycle, the response to DNA damage, and apoptosis. A simple "two-hit" model involving a single target tumor suppressor gene (Knudson's model) predicts that loss of function of both alleles must occur for the malignant phenotype to be expressed.[42] Gene function may be lost by chromosomal deletion or loss, point mutations, or methylation of the control elements of the gene (transcriptional silencing). A clinical example to illustrate this principle is the occurrence of MDS or AML following cytotoxic therapy (t-MDS and t-AML, respectively). Bone marrow dysfunction occurs after a relatively long latency period following cytotoxic exposure. This latency is compatible with a two-step mechanism in which a second mutation of a target gene must occur in a myeloid progenitor cell. Given two normal alleles at the tumor suppressor gene locus initially, one would be mutated as a result of therapy. Subsequent loss of the second allele in a bone marrow stem cell would permit leukemia development. Alternatively, because AML develops in only 5–15% of patients who are treated for a primary tumor, these individuals may have inherited a predisposing mutant allele; subsequent exposure to cytotoxic therapy may induce the second mutation, giving rise to leukemia. In these cases, characterization of the predisposing mutations will be important in identifying individuals who are at risk of developing t-MDS/t-AML, and in the selection of the appropriate therapy for the primary malignant disease.

In an alternative model, loss of only a single copy of a gene may result in a reduction in the level of one or more critical gene products (haploinsufficiency). Several reports implicate haploinsufficiency of the *TP53* and *p27Kip1* genes in the pathogenesis of tumors in mice, where a substantial percentage of tumors developing in heterozygous mice retain a functional copy of *TP53* or *p27Kip1*.[43,44] In humans, haploinsufficiency of the *RUNX1* (runt-related transcription factor 1, also known as *AML1*) gene results in a familial platelet disorder with a predisposition to AML.[45,46] Importantly, the few leukemias available for analysis from affected family members appear to retain one normal *RUNX1* allele. Despite intensive efforts, homozygous deletions have not been detected in myeloid leukemia cells characterized by deletions of 5q, 7q, or 20q in MDS and AML, an observation that is compatible with a haploinsufficiency model in which loss of one allele of the relevant gene (or genes) alters the cell's fate. At present, there is little experimental evidence favoring one or the other of these alternative models in the pathogenesis of MDS.

Cytogenetic findings in MDS

Normal karyotype

Between 30 and 60% of patients with MDS have a normal karyotype. This group of patients is likely to be genetically heterogeneous with alterations responsible for the neoplastic transformation not being detectable by standard cytogenetic methods, or in whom technical factors precluded the detection of chromosomally abnormal cells. Regardless of the heterogeneity, these cases are found as a whole to have a better prognosis than some cases of MDS with cytogenetic abnormalities, and are a standard reference for comparison of outcomes. The median survival for these good-prognosis patients is 3.8 years, and the time to progression to AML of 25% of this cohort was 5.6 years.[8]

−Y

The clinical and biological significance of the loss of the Y chromosome, −Y, is unknown. Loss of the Y chromosome has been observed in a number of malignant diseases, but has also been reported to be a phenomenon associated with aging.[47] A comprehensive analysis of this abnormality by the UK Cytogenetics Group, in both normal and neoplastic bone marrows, found that a −Y could be identified in 7.7% of patients without a malignant hematologic disease and in 10.7% of patients with MDS and thus was not reliable to document a malignant process.[48] The International MDS Risk Analysis Workshop found that, while loss of a Y chromosome may not be diagnostic of MDS, once the disease is identified by clinical and pathologic means, −Y as the sole cytogenetic abnormality conferred a favorable outcome.[8] In a large series of 215 male patients, Wiktor *et al.* found that patients with a hematological disease had a significantly higher percentage of cells with a −Y (52% versus 37%, $P = 0.036$). In this series, the presence of −Y in > 75% of metaphase cells accurately predicted a malignant hematological disease.[49] The authors also noted a neutral or favorable prognosis for an isolated −Y.

del(20q)

A deletion of the long arm of chromosome 20, del(20q), is a common recurring abnormality in malignant myeloid disorders. The abnormality is seen in approximately 5% of MDS cases and 7% of t-MDS cases.[3] Consistent clinical features characterize MDS patients with a del(20q), including low-risk disease (usually RA), low rate of progression to AML, and prolonged survival (median of 45 months versus 28 months for other MDS patients).[50] Morphologically, the presence of a del(20q) is associated with prominent dysplasia in the erythroid and megakaryocytic lineages.[51] The International MDS Risk Analysis Workshop found that patients with a del(20q) observed in association with a complex karyotype identified a poor-risk group with a median survival for the entire poor-risk group of 9.6 months, whereas the prognosis for patients with an isolated del(20q) was favorable.[8] Taken together, these data suggest that the del(20q) in MDS may be associated with a favorable outcome when noted as the sole abnormality, but with a less favorable prognosis in the setting of a complex karyotype. This phenomenon is analogous to that observed for the del(5q) in MDS (discussed below).

Cytogenetic analysis of the deleted chromosome 20 homologs has revealed that the deletions are variable in size; the majority of deletions are large, with loss of most of 20q. By using fluorescence in situ hybridization (FISH) with a panel of probes from 20q, combined with loss of heterozygosity (LOH) studies, investigators have identified an interstitial commonly deleted segment (CDS) of 4 Mb within 20q12 that is flanked by D20S206 proximally and D20S424 distally, containing a number of genes. Despite the availability of detailed physical and transcript maps, the identity of a myeloid tumor suppressor gene on 20q is unknown.[52,53] The functions of candidate genes within the CDS are diverse, and include transcription factors, components of signal transduction pathways, an RNA transcription modulator, and a regulator of apoptosis.[53]

Loss of chromosome 5 or del(5q)

In MDS or AML arising de novo, loss of a whole chromosome 5, or a deletion of its long arm, −5/del(5q), is observed in 10–20% of patients, whereas in t-MDS/t-AML it is identified in 40% of patients (Fig. 4.3).[3,54] A significant occupational exposure to potential carcinogens is present in many patients with AML or MDS de novo and either −5/del(5q) or a −7/del(7q) (discussed below), suggesting that abnormalities of chromosome 5 or 7 may be a marker of mutagen-induced malignant hematologic disease.[55]

In primary MDS, abnormalities of chromosome 5 are observed in the 5q− syndrome (described below) or, more commonly, in RAEB or RAEB-T

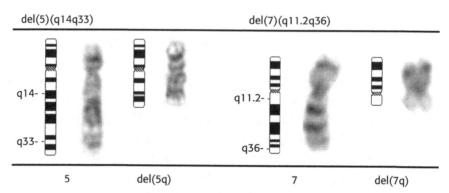

del(5)(q14q33)   del(7)(q11.2q36)

q14-   q11.2-

q33-   q36-

5   del(5q)   7   del(7q)

Fig. 4.3   In this del(5q), breakpoints occur in q14 and q33, resulting in interstitial loss of the intervening chromosomal material. In this del(7q), breakpoints occur in q11.2 and q36. In both cases, the critical commonly deleted segments are lost. Normal chromosome 5 and 7 homologs are shown for comparison.

(RAEB-1 and RAEB-2 in the WHO classification) in association with a complex karyotype. Clinically, the patients with del(5q) coupled with other cytogenetic abnormalities have a poor prognosis, with early progression to leukemia, treatment resistance, and short survival. Abnormalities of 5q are associated with previous exposure to standard and high-dose alkylating agent therapy, including use in immunosuppressive regimens.[56–59] A role for exposure to benzene[60] as well as therapeutic ionizing radiation[61,62] as risks for MDS is emerging.

5q− syndrome

The identification of a del(5q) as the sole karyotypic abnormality is associated with a distinct clinical syndrome.[9,63] Unlike the male predominance in MDS in general, the 5q− syndrome has an overrepresentation of females (2 : 1). The initial laboratory findings are usually a macrocytic anemia with a normal or elevated platelet count. The diagnosis is usually RA (in two-thirds) or RAEB (in one-third). On bone marrow examination, abnormalities in the megakaryocytic lineage (particularly micromegakaryocytes) are prominent. These patients have a favorable outcome − in fact, the best of any MDS subgroup, with low rates of leukemic transformation and a relatively long survival of several years' duration.[8,63]

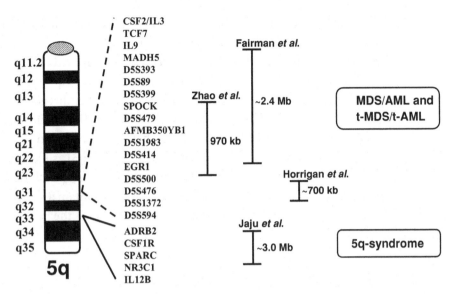

Fig. 4.4   Ideogram of the long arm of chromosome 5 showing chromosome markers and candidate genes within the commonly deleted segments (CDSs) as reported by various investigators. The proximal CDS in 5q31 was identified in myelodysplastic syndrome (MDS), acute myeloid leukemia (AML) and therapy-related MDS/therapy-related AML (t-MDS/t-AML), whereas the distal CDS in 5q33 was identified in the 5q− syndrome.

Molecular analysis of the del(5q)

Several groups of investigators have defined a CDS on the long arm of chromosome 5 predicted to contain a myeloid tumor suppressor gene that is involved in the pathogenesis of MDS and AML (Fig. 4.4).[64–68] By cytogenetic and FISH analysis, Le Beau and colleagues defined a 970-kb CDS within 5q31 flanked by D5S479 and D5S500.[68] The function of the genes within this CDS cover a spectrum of activities including regulation of mitosis and the G2 checkpoint, transcriptional and translational regulators, and cell surface receptors. Analysis of myeloid leukemia cells for inactivating mutations has eliminated 20 genes within the CDS, suggesting that a novel myeloid tumor suppressor gene is located in this interval, or that mechanisms such as haploinsufficiency or transcriptional silencing may be involved in the pathogenesis of these disorders (see[65] and Le Beau et al., unpublished data).

Molecular analysis of bone marrow cells from patients with the 5q− syndrome suggests that a different region is involved. Boultwood and colleagues examined 16 patients with the 5q– syndrome and identified a 1.5-Mb CDS within 5q32 between *D5S413* and *NR3C1* which is also gene-rich.[69] This region is distal to the CDS in 5q31 found in the patients with RAEB, RAEB-T, and AML with del(5q). Whether all patients with the 5q– syndrome have involvement of a gene in this distal region, and whether this gene plays a role in the pathogenesis of other subtypes of MDS or AML, remains uncertain.

In summary, the existing data suggest that there are two non-overlapping CDSs in 5q31 and 5q32. The proximal segment in 5q31 is likely to contain a tumor suppressor gene involved in the pathogenesis of both de novo and therapy-related MDS/AML. Band 5q32 is likely to contain a second myeloid tumor suppressor gene involved in the pathogenesis of the 5q– syndrome.

+8

The incidence of a gain of chromosome 8 in MDS is ~ 10%. This abnormality is observed in all FAB subgroups varying with age, gender, and prior treatment with cytotoxic agents or radiation.[3,4,8,70] It can occur as both a constitutional and an acquired abnormality and can fluctuate throughout the disease course.[71–73] The significance of the gain of chromosome 8 in MDS patients is not fully characterized as a risk factor. The situation is complicated in that +8 is often associated with other recurring abnormalities known to have prognostic significance, and may be seen in isolation as a separate clone unrelated to the primary clone in up to 5% of cases. The International MDS Risk Analysis Workshop ranked this abnormality in the intermediate-risk group.[8] Although only significant in univariate analysis, a large confirmatory study found that +8 as a sole abnormality had a worse behavior than expected for an intermediate IPSS risk group.[7]

Loss of chromosome 7 or del(7q)

A –7/del(7q) is observed as the sole abnormality in approximately 5% of adult patients with de novo MDS,[6,7] but in ~ 50% of children with de novo MDS[74] and in ~ 55% of patients with t-MDS (Fig. 4.2).[54] It can occur in three general contexts (reviewed in[75]): (1) de novo MDS and AML; (2) myeloid leukemia associated with constitutional predisposition; and (3) t-MDS/t-AML. The similar clinical and biological features of the myeloid disorders associated with –7/del(7q) suggest that the same gene(s) is altered in each of these contexts. The IPSS considers the −7/del(7q) a poor prognosis cytogenetic finding.[8]

Monosomy 7 syndrome has been described in young children. It is characterized by a preponderance of males ($\sim$ 4 : 1), hepatosplenomegaly, leukocytosis, thrombocytopenia, and poor prognosis.[76,77] Juvenile myelomonocytic leukemia (JMML, previously known as juvenile chronic myelogenous leukemia) shares many features with this entity, with −7 observed either at diagnosis or as a new cytogenetic finding associated with disease acceleration on marrow examination.[75] An emerging paradigm is that −7 cooperates with deregulated signaling via the RAS pathway in the pathogenesis of JMML. Activation of the RAS pathway occurs as a result of mutations in the *N-RAS* or *K-RAS1* gene, inactivating mutations in the gene encoding NF1, a negative regulator of RAS proteins, or activating mutations in the gene encoding the PTPN11/SHP2 phosphatase, a positive regulator of RAS proteins. In patients constitutionally susceptible to myeloid neoplasms, including Fanconi anemia, neurofibromatosis type 1, and severe congenital neutropenia, a −7/del(7q) is the most frequent bone marrow cytogenetic abnormality detected. As with −5/del(5q), occupational or environmental exposure to mutagens, including chemotherapy, radiotherapy, benzene exposure, and smoking[78] as well as severe aplastic anemia (regularly treated with immunosuppressive agents alone) have been associated with −7/del(7q).

Molecular analysis of the −7/del(7q)

As with the −5/del(5q), investigators have examined the breakpoints and extent of the deletions of 7q in patients to identify a CDS.[79–84] Le Beau *et al.* examined 81 patients with de novo and therapy-related MDS/AML, and identified two distinct CDSs. In 65 patients, the CDS was within q22, whereas in 16 other patients, interstitial deletions of a more distal segment were detected with a CDS of q32–33.[81] By FISH analysis, these investigators identified an $\sim$ 2-Mb CDS in 7q22, a finding that is consistent with most published data.[79,82,85,86] Tosi *et al.*[84] evaluated patients with 7q abnormalities and identified an interesting patient with a complex karyotype and a t(7;7) who had a deletion associated with the translocation breakpoint of 150 kb proximal to the CDS defined by Le Beau *et al.* A number of candidate genes have been identified and evaluated for mutations within the CDS at 7q22, including genes encoding extracellular (or extracellular-like) proteins, replication and transcriptional control elements, a splicing factor kinase and a mitochondrial-processing peptidase[87]; however, no inactivating mutations have been identified in the remaining allele.

Data from cytogenetic, FISH, and LOH studies performed in a number of laboratories paint a complex picture of 7q deletions in myeloid malignancies. There is general agreement that 7q22 is involved in a majority of cases. Defining a consistent CDS has been complicated by: (1) the relatively low frequency of del(7q) versus complete loss of chromosome 7; (2) the use of different techniques to investigate marrow samples, e.g., FISH versus LOH; (3) the wide spectrum of myeloid disorders with alterations in chromosome 7, suggesting genetic heterogeneity; and (4) the existence of multiple and sometimes complex cytogenetic abnormalities in some cases.

17p− syndrome

Loss of the short arm of chromosome 17 (17p−) has been reported in up to 5% of patients with MDS as a result of various abnormalities, including simple deletions, unbalanced translocations, dicentric rearrangements (particularly with chromosome 5), or, less often, −17, or isochromosome formation.[88] A frequent recurring rearrangement is the dic(5;17)(q11.1–13;p11.1–13).[89,90] Approximately one-third of these patients have t-MDS,[91] and most have additional cytogenetic abnormalities. The most common additional changes are unbalanced translocations involving chromosomes 5 or 7.

Morphologically, the 17p− syndrome is associated with a typical form of dysgranulopoiesis combining pseudo Pelger–Huët hypolobulation and the presence of small granules in granulocytes. Clinically, the disease is aggressive, with resistance to treatment and short survival. The *TP53* (*p53*) gene, an important tumor suppressor gene that functions in the cellular response to DNA damage, is located at 17p13.1. One allele of *TP53* is typically lost as a result of the abnormality of 17p in these cases; an inactivating mutation in the second allele on the remaining, normal chromosome 17 occurs in ∼ 70% of cases.[89,90] Sankar *et al.* mapped a CDS in leukemia and lymphoma patients to 17p13.3, suggesting the existence of a novel tumor suppressor gene distal to *TP53*.[92]

11q23

The mixed-lineage leukemia (*MLL*) gene (also known as *ALL1, HTRX, HRX*) is involved in over 50 reciprocal translocations in acute leukemia.[93] In a European workshop of 550 patients with 11q23 abnormalities, 28 cases (5.1%) presented with a MDS, and five others had evolved from t-MDS to t-AML prior to cytogenetic analysis, accounting for up to 6% of all cases examined. A quarter of these cases were t-MDS.[94] Additional abnormalities, including complex karyotypes and a −7/del(7q), often accompany the 11q23 abnormalities in both primary MDS and t-MDS. Whereas RA was overrepresented and RARS underrepresented as compared to most series of MDS patients, no association with an FAB subgroup was identified. The median survival was short (19 months), with leukemic transformation in ∼ 20% of cases. This workshop did not find the classic association of prior exposure to topoisomerase II inhibitors in their 40 cases of t-MDS and t-AML, but this may simply reflect the relatively small number ($n = 23$) of cases with full treatment details.[95]

Just under 12% of the 162 patients with 11q23 involvement included in an international workshop on MDS and leukemia following cytotoxic treatment presented with a t-MDS.[62,96] One-third (6/19) of these patients had progression to an acute leukemia (5 AML, 1 acute lymphoid leukemia (ALL)). No clear association with FAB subtype was identified. The most common translocations were t(9;11)(p22;q23) in 6 cases, t(11;19)(q23;p13.1) in 3 cases, and t(11;16)(q23;p13.3) in 3 cases.

t(11;16)

The t(11;16)(q23;p13.3) occurs primarily in t-MDS, but some cases have presented as t-AML (Fig. 4.5).[97] Among at least 50 recurring translocations of *MLL* in myeloid neoplasms (with AML predominating), the t(11;16) is unique in that most patients have t-MDS. The *MLL* gene on chromosome 11 is fused with the *CBP* (CREB-binding protein) gene on chromosome 16. The MLL protein is a histone methyltransferase that assembles in protein complexes that regulate gene transcription, e.g., *HOX* genes during embryonic development, via chromatin remodeling. CBP is an adapter protein involved in transcription control via histone acetylation, which mediates chromosome decondensation, thereby facilitating transcription. Both genes

t(11;16)(p13.3;q23)

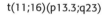

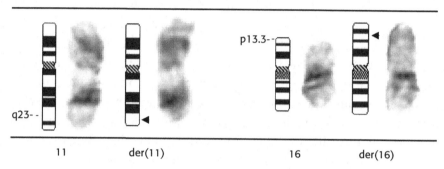

| 11 | der(11) | 16 | der(16) |

Fig. 4.5   In the t(11;16), breakpoints occur in 11q23 and 16p13.3, followed by a reciprocal exchange of chromosomal material. The 5′ end of the *MLL* gene at 11q23 is fused to the 3′ end of the *CBP* gene from 16p13.3 to form the *MLL/CBP* fusion gene on the der(11). Arrowheads indicate the breakpoints. Normal chromosome 11 and 16 homologs are shown for comparison.

have multiple translocation partners in various hematologic disorders; thus, elucidating their function will undoubtedly lead to significant progress in leukemia research.

Complex karyotypes

Complex karyotypes are variably defined, but generally involve the presence of three or more abnormalities. The majority of cases with complex karyotypes involve unbalanced chromosomal abnormalities leading to the loss of genetic material. Complex karyotypes are observed in ∼ 20% of patients with primary MDS, and in as many as 90% of patients with t-MDS.[54,98] Abnormalities involving chromosomes 5, 7, or both are identified in most cases with complex karyotypes. There is general agreement that a complex karyotype carries a poor prognosis.[8,20]

t-MDS

Dose escalation, as well as significantly more toxic agents and combinations of agents, are routinely used in patient care. One of the most serious late consequences of cancer therapy is the development of a second cancer of myeloid origin. In patients treated with high-dose therapy for breast cancer, lymphoma, leukemias and multiple myeloma, the reported incidence of t-MDS/t-AML is 1–24% of treated patients.[58] Increasing numbers of patients with benign disease, particularly rheumatology and dermatology patients, as well as organ transplant recipients, are also being exposed to cytotoxic agents for immunosuppression, placing them at risk for some of the same late complications.

Cytogenetic aberrations are detected in up to 90% of patients with t-MDS.[54,99] Common cytogenetic findings are illustrated in Figure 4.2. The patients exposed to alkylating agents typically have a longer latency period to bone marrow dysfunction (median 5–7 years), and develop t-MDS with trilineage dysplasia, which often progresses to t-AML. Abnormalities of chromosomes 5, and/or 7, and complex karyotypes predominate. Patients exposed to topoisomerase II inhibitors are more likely to present with t-AML, have a shorter latency period, generally within 2 years, and have abnormalities involving *MLL* at 11q23 or *RUNX1* (*AML1*) at 21q22.[62,100,101]

Rare recurring translocations

The identification of genes involved in recurring cytogenetic abnormalities has been extremely useful in gaining insights into their normal functions and their role in leukemogenesis.[93,102] The consequence of the recurring translocations is the deregulation of gene expression with increased production of a normal protein product, or the generation of a novel fusion gene and production of a fusion protein. To date, all of the recurring translocations cloned in malignant myeloid disorders result in fusion proteins. In MDS, several such translocations have been identified and examined by molecular analysis.

The platelet-derived growth factor receptor-β translocations

The t(5;12)(q33;p13) is observed in ~ 1% of patients with CMML. In 1994, the molecular consequences of this translocation were elucidated. The gene encoding the beta chain of the PDGFR (*PDGFRB*) is involved on chromosome 5. A novel erythroblastosis virus transforming sequence (ETS)-like transcription factor, *TEL* (translocated ETS in leukemia, also known as *ETV6*), is the gene affected on chromosome 12. The translocation creates a fusion gene and fusion protein containing the 5' portion of *TEL* and the

3' portion of *PDGFRB*.[103] It is believed that the PDGFRB kinase activity is perturbed, resulting in the transformed phenotype. *TEL* encodes a transcriptional repressor, and is promiscuously involved in translocations with some 40 partner genes in hematologic malignancies.[93] Interest has increased in identifying this translocation which predicts for a clinical response to imatinib, a selective inhibitor of the tyrosine kinase activity of the PDGFRB protein.[32] Similarly, *PDGFRB* participates in other rare translocations involving genes encoding the membrane-associated protein Huntington-interacting protein 1 (HIP1) in the t(5;7)(q33;q11.2),[104] the small GTPase RABPT5 (Rabaptin 5) in the t(5;17)(q33;p13)[105] and H4, a ubiquitous protein of unknown function in the t(5;10)(q33;q21),[106] to produce CMML, and with *CEV14* (clonal evolution-related gene on chromosome 14, also known as *TRIP11*, thyroid hormone receptor interactor 11) in the t(5;14)(q33;q32) in a case of AML.[107] A unifying feature of these various translocations is the presence of eosinophilia.

Translocations of 3q

The t(3;21)(q26.2;q22.1) has been linked to acute leukemia arising after cytotoxic therapy. This abnormality was first recognized in chronic myelogenous leukemia in blast crisis[108] and later in t-MDS/t-AML.[109] The *EAP* gene (Epstein–Barr small RNAs associated protein) at 3q26.2 encodes a highly expressed small nuclear protein associated with Epstein–Barr small RNA (EBER1). *EAP* was found to be fused with the *RUNX1* gene at 21q22, retaining the DNA binding sequences of *EAP*. The fusion is out of frame; thus, the *RUNX1* gene is truncated and loses its functional activity. Further work has identified two additional genes 400–750 kb centromeric to *EAP*, also at 3q26.2, namely *MDS1/EVI1* (MDS-associated sequences) and *EVI1* (ecotropic virus insertion site).[110] Both genes encode nuclear transcription factors containing DNA-binding zinc finger domains, which are identical other than an N-terminal extension of 12 amino acids in the MDS1/EVI1 protein, representing a splicing variant. Each gene has independent and tightly controlled expression during differentiation.[111] The MDS1/EVI1 and EVI1 proteins have opposite functions. EVI1 inhibits granulocyte colony-stimulated factor (G-CSF)-mediated differentiation and TGF-β1 growth-inhibitory effect, whereas MDS1/EVI1 has no effect on G-CSF and enhances TGF-β1 growth inhibition.[111] *RUNX1* fuses with *MDS1/EVI1*, in-frame, resulting in the loss of the first 12 amino acids, producing a novel EVI1 protein, and a phenotype of arrested differentiation, which leads to apoptosis in vitro.[112] MDS1/EVI1 serves as a translocation partner with the ribosome binding protein RPN1 (ribophorin 1)[113] and/or the poorly characterized protein in fetal development GR6[114] in the inv(3)(q21q26.2) or the t(3;3)(q21;q26.2) associated with normal or increased platelet counts as well as TEL[115] (discussed above) in the t(3;12)(q26.2;p13). Common features of myeloid diseases associated with abnormalities of 3q are a previous history of cytotoxic exposure, prominent bone marrow dysplasia, and a poor prognosis. In an international workshop on therapy-related hematologic disease, inv(3)/t(3;3) abnormalities were the most frequent of the 3q abnormalities.[116]

Summary and future directions

As explored in this chapter, the role of cytogenetic analysis clinically in the diagnosis, prognosis, and follow-up of patients with MDS has growing importance to physicians treating these disorders. The information on prognosis is of particular benefit and assists in elaborating an appropriate treatment strategy for the individual patient. The most frequently encountered presentations and abnormalities have been highlighted. On a fundamental level, the classic cytogenetic alterations have been subject to intensive scrutiny and the molecular basis of disease pathogenesis is being increasingly understood. Several particularly well-characterized alterations have been reviewed. Other molecular methods within the domain of the cytogeneticist, such as FISH and spectral karyotyping, have been shown to be complementary, without replacing the information that is obtained with conventional cytogenetic analysis. Further observations and investigations with all of these techniques will undoubtedly contribute to improved understanding and management of patients with MDS.

REFERENCES

1. Bennett, J. M., Catovsky, D., Daniel, M. T. *et al.* (1982). Proposals for the classification of the myelodysplastic syndromes. *Br. J. Haematol.*, **51**, 189–99.

2. Jaffe, E. S., Harris, N. L., Stein, G., and Vardiman, J. W. (ed.) (2001). *World Health Organization Classification of Tumours: Pathology and Genetics of Tumours of Haematopoietic and Lymphoid Tissues.* Lyons, France: IARC Press.

3. Vallespi, T., Imbert, M., Mecucci, C., Preudhomme, C., and Fenaux, P. (1998). Diagnosis, classification, and cytogenetics of myelodysplastic syndromes. *Haematologica*, **83**, 258–75.

4. Morel, P., Hebbar, M., Lai, J. L. *et al.* (1993). Cytogenetic analysis has strong independent prognostic value in de novo myelodysplastic syndromes and can be incorporated in a new scoring system: a report on 408 cases. *Leukemia*, **7**, 1315–23.

5. Jotterand, M. and Parlier, V. (1996). Diagnostic and prognostic significance of cytogenetics in adult primary myelodysplastic syndromes. *Leuk. Lymphoma*, **23**, 253–66.

6. Toyama, K., Ohyashiki, K., Yoshida, Y. *et al.* (1993). Clinical implications of chromosomal abnormalities in 401 patients with myelodysplastic syndromes: a multicentric study in Japan. *Leukemia*, **7**, 499–508.

7. Sole, F., Espinet, B., Sanz, G. F. *et al.* (2000). Incidence, characterization and prognostic significance of chromosomal abnormalities in 640 patients with primary myelodysplastic syndromes. Grupo Cooperativo Español de Citogenética Hematológica. *Br. J. Haematol.*, **108**, 346–56.

8. Greenberg, P., Cox, C., Le Beau, M. M. *et al.* (1997). International scoring system for evaluating prognosis in myelodysplastic syndromes. *Blood*, **89**, 2079–88.

9. Van den Berghe, H. and Michaux, L. (1997). 5q–, twenty-five years later: a synopsis. *Cancer Genet. Cytogenet.*, **94**, 1–7.

10. Jary, L., Mossafa, H., Fourcade, C. *et al.* (1997). The 17p– syndrome: a distinct myelodysplastic syndrome entity? *Leuk. Lymphoma*, **25**, 163–8.

11. Dewald, G. W., Pierre, R. V., and Phyliky, R. L. (1982). Three patients with structurally abnormal chromosomes, each with Xq13 breakpoints and a history of idiopathic acquired sideroblastic anemia. *Blood*, **59**, 100–5.

12. Rowley, J. D. (1999). The role of chromosome translocations in leukemogenesis. *Semin. Hematol.*, **36** (suppl. 7), 59–72.

13. Smadja, N., Krulik, M., Hagemeijer, A. *et al.* (1989). Cytogenetic and molecular studies of the Philadelphia translocation t(9;22) observed in a patient with myelodysplastic syndrome. *Leukemia*, **3**, 236–8.

14. Sanz, G. F., Sanz, M. A., Vallespi, T. *et al.* (1989). Two regression models and a scoring system for predicting survival and planning treatment in myelodysplastic

syndromes: a multivariate analysis of prognostic factors in 370 patients. *Blood*, **74**, 395–408.

15. Aul, C., Gattermann, N., Germing, U. *et al.* (1994). Risk assessment in primary myelodysplastic syndromes: validation of the Dusseldorf score. *Leukemia*, **8**, 1906–13.

16. Parlier, V., van Melle, G., Beris, P. *et al.* (1995). Prediction of 18-month survival in patients with primary myelodysplastic syndrome. A regression model and scoring system based on the combination of chromosome findings and the Bournemouth score. *Cancer Genet. Cytogenet.*, **81**, 158–65.

17. Sanz, G. F., Sanz, M. A., and Greenberg, P. L. (1998). Prognostic factors and scoring systems in myelodysplastic syndromes. *Haematologica*, **83**, 358–68.

18. Nevill, T. J., Fung, H. C., Shepherd, J. D. *et al.* (1998). Cytogenetic abnormalities in primary myelodysplastic syndrome are highly predictive of outcome after allogeneic bone marrow transplantation. *Blood*, **92**, 1910–17.

19. Belli, C., Acevedo, S., Bengio, R. *et al.* (2002). Detection of risk groups in myelodysplastic syndromes. A multicenter study. *Haematologica*, **87**, 9–16.

20. Hamblin, T. J. and Oscier, D. G. (1987). The myelodysplastic syndromes – a practical guide. *Hematol. Oncol.*, **5**, 19–34.

21. Horiike, S., Taniwaki, M., Misawa, S., and Abe, T. (1988). Chromosome abnormalities and karyotypic evolution in 83 patients with myelodysplastic syndrome and predictive value for prognosis. *Cancer*, **62**, 1129–38.

22. Geddes, A. A., Bowen, D. T., and Jacobs, A. (1990). Clonal karyotype abnormalities and clinical progress in the myelodysplastic syndrome. *Br. J. Haematol.*, **76**, 194–202.

23. de Souza Fernandez, T., Ornellas, M. H., Otero de Carvalho, L., Tabak, D., and Abdelhay, E. (2000). Chromosomal alterations associated with evolution from myelodysplastic syndrome to acute myeloid leukemia. *Leuk. Res.*, **24**, 839–48.

24. Rebollo, A. and Martinez, A. C. (1999). *RAS* proteins: recent advances and new functions. *Blood*, **94**, 2971–80.

25. Neubauer, A., Dodge, R. K., George, S. L. *et al.* (1994). Prognostic importance of mutations in the ras proto-oncogenes in de novo acute myeloid leukemia. *Blood*, **83**, 1603–11.

26. Gallagher, A., Darley, R., and Padua, R. A. (1997). *RAS* and the myelodysplastic syndromes. *Pathol. Biol. (Paris)*, **45**, 561–8.

27. Beaupre, D. M. and Kurzrock, R. (1999). *RAS* and leukemia: from basic mechanisms to gene-directed therapy. *J. Clin. Oncol.*, **17**, 1071–9.

28. Padua, R. A., Guinn, B. A., Al-Sabah, A. I. *et al.* (1998). *RAS*, *FMS* and *p53* mutations and poor clinical outcome in myelodysplasias: a 10-year follow-up. *Leukemia*, **12**, 887–92.

29. de Souza Fernandez, T., Menezes de Souza, J., Macedo Silva, M. L., Tabak, D., and Abdelhay, E. (1998). Correlation of *N-RAS* point mutations with specific chromosomal abnormalities in primary myelodysplastic syndrome. *Leuk. Res.*, **22**, 125–34.

30. Tien, H. F., Wang, C. H., Chuang, S. M. *et al.* (1994). Cytogenetic studies, *RAS* mutation, and clinical characteristics in primary myelodysplastic syndrome. A study on 68 Chinese patients in Taiwan. *Cancer Genet. Cytogenet.*, **74**, 40–9.

31. Kurzrock, R., Kantarjian, H. M., Cortes, J. E. *et al.* (2003). Farnesyltransferase inhibitor R115777 in myelodysplastic syndrome: clinical and biologic activities in phase I setting. *Blood*, **102**, 4527–34.

32. Apperley, J. F., Gardembas, M., Melo, J. V. *et al.* (2002). Response to imatinib mesylate in patients with chronic myeloproliferative disease with rearrangements of the platelet-derived growth factor receptor beta. *N. Engl. J. Med.*, **347**, 481–7.

33. Raza, A., Mundle, S., Iftikhar, A. *et al.* (1995). Simultaneous assessment of cell kinetics and programmed cell death in bone marrow biopsies of myelodysplastics reveals extensive apoptosis as the probable basis for ineffective hematopoiesis. *Am. J. Hematol.*, **48**, 143–54.

34. Parker, J. E., Mufti, G. J., Rassool, F. *et al.* (2000). The role of apoptosis, proliferation, and the *BCL-2*-related proteins in the myelodysplastic syndromes and acute myeloid leukemia secondary to MDS. *Blood*, **96**, 3932–8.

35. Westwood, N. B. and Mufi, G. J. (2003). Apoptosis in the myelodysplastic syndromes. *Curr. Hematol. Rep.*, **2**, 186–92.

36. Raza, S., Dar, S., Andric, T. *et al.* (1999). Biologic characteristics of 164 patients with myelodysplastic syndromes. *Leuk. Lymphoma*, **33**, 281–7.

37. Allampallam, K., Shetty, V., Mundle, S. *et al.* (2002). Biological significance of proliferation, apoptosis, and monocyte/macrophage cells in bone marrow biopsies of 145 patients with myelodysplastic syndrome. *Int. J. Hematol.*, **75**, 289–97.

38. Yoshida, Y. and Mufti, G. J. (1999). Apoptosis and its significance in MDS: controversies revisited. *Leuk. Res.*, **23**, 777–85.

39. Raza, A., Mundle, S., Shetty, V. *et al.* (1996). Novel insights into the biology of myelodysplastic syndromes: excessive apoptosis and the role of cytokines. *Int. J. Hematol.*, **63**, 265–78.

40. Turk, B. E., Jiang, H., and Liu, J. O. (1996). Binding of thalidomide to alpha 1-acid glycoprotein may be involved in its inhibition of tumor necrosis factor alpha production. *Proc. Natl Acad. Sci. U.S.A.*, **93**, 7552–6.

41. Raza, A., Meyer, P., Dutt, D. *et al.* (2001). Thalidomide produces transfusion independence in long-standing refractory anemias of patients with myelodysplastic syndromes. *Blood*, **98**, 958–65.

42. Knudson, A. G. Jr. (1971). Mutation and cancer: statistical study of retinoblastoma. *Proc. Natl Acad. Sci. U.S.A.*, **68**, 820–3.

43. French, J. E., Lacks, G. D., Trempus, C. *et al.* (2001). Loss of heterozygosity frequency at the *Trp53* locus in *p53*-deficient (+/−) mouse tumors is carcinogen and tissue-dependent. *Carcinogenesis*, **22**, 99–106.

44. Fero, M. L., Rivkin, M., Tasch, M. *et al.* (1996). A syndrome of multiorgan hyperplasia with features of gigantism, tumorigenesis, and female sterility in *p27(Kip1)*-deficient mice. *Cell*, **85**, 733–44.

45. Song, W. J., Sullivan, M. G., Legare, R. D. *et al.* (1999). Haploinsufficiency of *CBFA2* causes familial thrombocytopenia with propensity to develop acute myelogenous leukaemia. *Nat. Genet*, **23**, 166–75.

46. Michaud, J., Wu, F., Osato, M. *et al.* (2002). In vitro analyses of known and novel *RUNX1/AML1* mutations in dominant familial platelet disorder with predisposition to acute myelogenous leukemia: implications for mechanisms of pathogenesis. *Blood*, **99**, 1364–72.

47. Pierre, R. V. and Hoagland, H. C. (1972). Age-associated aneuploidy: loss of Y chromosome from human bone marrow cells with aging. *Cancer*, **30**, 889–94.

48. United Kingdom Cancer Cytogenetics Group (UKCCG) (1992). Loss of the Y chromosome from normal and neoplastic bone marrows. *Genes Chromosomes Cancer*, **5**, 83–8.

49. Wiktor, A., Rybicki, B. A., Piao, Z. S. *et al.* (2000). Clinical significance of Y chromosome loss in hematologic disease. *Genes Chromosomes Cancer*, **27**, 11–16.

50. Wattel, E., Lai, J. L., Hebbar, M. *et al.* (1993). De novo myelodysplastic syndrome (MDS) with deletion of the long arm of chromosome 20: a subtype of MDS with distinct hematological and prognostic features? *Leuk. Res.*, **17**, 921–6.

51. Kurtin, P. J., Dewald, G. W., Shields, D. J., and Hanson, C. A. (1996). Hematologic disorders associated with deletions of chromosome 20q: a clinicopathologic study of 107 patients. *Am. J. Clin. Pathol.*, **106**, 680–8.

52. Bench, A. J., Nacheva, E. P., Hood, T. L. *et al.* (2000). Chromosome 20 deletions in myeloid malignancies: reduction of the common deleted region, generation of a PAC/BAC contig and identification of candidate genes. UK Cancer Cytogenetics Group (UKCCG). *Oncogene*, **19**, 3902–13.

53. Wang, P. W., Eisenbart, J. D., Espinosa, III R. *et al.* (2000). Refinement of the smallest commonly deleted segment of chromosome 20 in malignant myeloid diseases and development of a PAC-based physical and transcription map. *Genomics*, **67**, 28–39.

54. Thirman, M. J. and Larson, R. A. (1996). Therapy-related myeloid leukemia. *Hematol. Oncol. Clin. North Am.*, **10**, 293–320.

55. West, R. R., Stafford, D. A., White, A. D., Bowen, D. T., and Padua, R. A. (2000). Cytogenetic abnormalities in the myelodysplastic syndromes and occupational or environmental exposure. *Blood*, **95**, 2093–7.

56. Larson, R. A., Le Beau, M. M., Vardiman, J. W., and Rowley, J. D. (1996). Myeloid leukemia after hematotoxins. *Environ. Health Perspect.*, **104** (suppl. 6), 1303–17.

57. Aul, C., Bowen, D. T., and Yoshida, Y. (1998). Pathogenesis, etiology and epidemiology of myelodysplastic syndromes. *Haematologica*, **83**, 71–86.

58. Pedersen-Bjergaard, J., Andersen, M. K., and Christiansen, D. H. (2000). Therapy-related acute myeloid leukemia and myelodysplasia after high-dose chemotherapy and autologous stem cell transplantation. *Blood*, **95**, 3273–9.

59. McCarthy, C. J., Sheldon, S., Ross, C. W., and McCune, W. J. (1998). Cytogenetic abnormalities and therapy-related myelodysplastic syndromes in rheumatic disease. *Arthritis Rheum.*, **41**, 1493–6.

60. Hayes, R. B., Yin, S. N., Dosemeci, M. *et al.* (1997). Benzene and the dose-related incidence of hematologic neoplasms in China. Chinese Academy of Preventive Medicine–National Cancer Institute Benzene Study Group. *J. Natl Cancer Inst.*, **89**, 1065–71.

61. Fenaux, P., Lucidarme, D., Lai, J. L., and Bauters, F. (1989). Favorable cytogenetic abnormalities in secondary leukemia. *Cancer*, **63**, 2505–8.

62. Rowley, J. D. and Olney, H. J. (2002). International workshop on the relationship of prior therapy to balanced chromosome aberrations in therapy-related myelodysplastic syndromes and acute leukemia: overview report. *Genes Chromosomes Cancer*, **33**, 331–45.

63. Boultwood, J., Lewis, S., and Wainscoat, J. S. (1994). The 5q− syndrome. *Blood*, **84**, 3253–60.

64. Fairman, J., Chumakov, I., Chinault, A. C., Nowell, P. C., and Nagarajan, L. (1995). Physical mapping of the minimal region of loss in 5q− chromosome. *Proc. Natl Acad. Sci. U.S.A.*, **92**, 7406–10.

65. Zhao, N., Stoffel, A., Wang, P. W. *et al.* (1997). Molecular delineation of the smallest commonly deleted region of chromosome 5 in malignant myeloid diseases to 1–1.5 Mb and preparation of a PAC-based physical map. *Proc. Natl Acad. Sci. U.S.A.*, **94**, 6948–53.

66. Jaju, R. J., Boultwood, J., Oliver, F. J. *et al.* (1998). Molecular cytogenetic delineation of the critical deleted region in the 5q− syndrome. *Genes Chromosomes Cancer*, **22**, 251–6.

67. Horrigan, S. K., Arbieva, Z. H., Xie, H. Y. *et al.* (2000). Delineation of a minimal interval and identification of 9 candidates for a tumor suppressor gene in malignant myeloid disorders on 5q31. *Blood*, **95**, 2372–7.

68. Le Beau, M. M., Espinosa, III R., Neuman, W. L. *et al.* (1993). Cytogenetic and molecular delineation of the smallest commonly deleted region of chromosome 5 in malignant myeloid diseases. *Proc. Natl Acad. Sci. U.S.A.*, **90**, 5484–8.

69. Boultwood, J., Fidler, C., Strickson, A. J. *et al.* (2002). Narrowing and genomic annotation of the commonly deleted region of the 5q− syndrome. *Blood*, **99**, 4638–41.

70. Paulsson, K., Sall, T., Fioretos, T., Mitelman, F., and Johansson, B. (2001). The incidence of trisomy 8 as a sole chromosomal aberration in myeloid malignancies varies

in relation to gender, age, prior iatrogenic genotoxic exposure, and morphology. *Cancer Genet. Cytogenet.*, **130**, 160–5.

71. Maserati, E., Aprili, F., Vinante, F. *et al.* (2002). Trisomy 8 in myelodysplasia and acute leukemia is constitutional in 15–20% of cases. *Genes Chromosomes Cancer*, **33**, 93–7.

72. Mastrangelo, R., Tornesello, A., Mastrangelo, S., Zollino, M., and Neri, G. (1995). Constitution trisomy 8 mosaicism evolving to primary myelodysplastic syndrome: a new subset of biologically related patients? *Am. J. Hematol.*, **48**, 67–8.

73. Matsuda, A., Yagasaki, F., Jinnai, I. *et al.* (1998). Trisomy 8 may not be related to the pathogenesis of myelodysplastic syndromes: disappearance of trisomy 8 in a patient with refractory anaemia without haematological improvement. *Eur. J. Hematol.*, **60**, 260–1.

74. Kardos, G., Baumann, I., Passmore, S. J. *et al.* (2003). Refractory anemia in childhood: a retrospective analysis of 67 patients with particular reference to mono-somy 7. *Blood*, **102**, 1997–2003.

75. Luna-Fineman, S., Shannon, K. M., and Lange, B. J. (1995). Childhood monosomy 7: epidemiology, biology, and mechanistic implications. *Blood*, **85**, 1985–99.

76. Emanuel, P. D. (1999). Myelodysplasia and myeloproliferative disorders in childhood: an update. *Br. J. Haematol.*, **105**, 852–63.

77. Martinez-Climent, J. A. and Garcia-Conde, J. (1999). Chromosomal rearrange-ments in childhood acute myeloid leukemia and myelodysplastic syndromes. *J. Pediatr. Hematol. Oncol.*, **21**, 91–102.

78. Bjork, J., Albin, M., Mauritzson, N. *et al.* (2000). Smoking and myelodysplastic syndromes. *Epidemiology*, **11**, 285–91.

79. Kere, J. (1989). Chromosome 7 long arm deletion breakpoints in preleukemia: mapping by pulsed field gel electrophoresis. *Nucleic Acids Res.*, **17**, 1511–20.

80. Johnson, E. J., Scherer, S. W., Osborne, L. *et al.* (1996). Molecular definition of a narrow interval at 7q22.1 associated with myelodysplasia. *Blood*, **87**, 3579–86.

81. Le Beau, M. M., Espinosa, III R., Davis, E. M. *et al.* (1996). Cytogenetic and molecular delineation of a region of chromosome 7 commonly deleted in malignant myeloid diseases. *Blood*, **88**, 1930–5.

82. Fischer, K., Frohling, S., Scherer, S. W. *et al.* (1997). Molecular cytogenetic delin-eation of deletions and translocations involving chromosome band 7q22 in myeloid leukemias. *Blood*, **89**, 2036–41.

83. Liang, H., Fairman, J., Claxton, D. F. *et al.* (1998). Molecular anatomy of chromo-some 7q deletions in myeloid neoplasms: evidence for multiple critical loci. *Proc. Natl Acad. Sci. U.S.A.*, **95**, 3781–5.

84. Tosi, S., Scherer, S. W., Giudici, G. *et al.* (1999). Delineation of multiple deleted regions in 7q in myeloid disorders. *Genes Chromosomes Cancer*, **25**, 384–92.

85. Döhner, K., Brown, J., Hehmann, U. *et al.* (1998). Molecular cytogenetic characterization of a critical region in bands 7q35–q36 commonly deleted in malignant myeloid disorders. *Blood*, **92**, 4031–5.

86. Lewis, S., Abrahamson, G., Boultwood, J. *et al.* (1996). Molecular characterization of the 7q deletion in myeloid disorders. *Br. J. Haematol.*, **93**, 75–80.

87. Kratz, C. P., Emerling, B. M., Donovan, S. *et al.* (2001). Candidate gene isolation and comparative analysis of a commonly deleted segment of 7q22 implicated in myeloid malignancies. *Genomic*, **77**, 171–80.

88. Johansson, B., Mertens, F., and Mitelman, F. (1993). Cytogenetic deletion maps of hematologic neoplasms: circumstantial evidence for tumor suppressor loci. *Genes Chromosomes Cancer*, **8**, 205–18.

89. Wang, P., Spielberger, R. T., Thangavelu, M. *et al.* dic(5;17): a recurring abnormality in malignant myeloid disorders associated with mutations of *TP53*. *Genes Chromosomes Cancer*, **20**, 282–91.

90. Lai, J. L., Preudhomme, C., Zandecki, M. *et al.* (1995). Myelodysplastic syndromes and acute myeloid leukemia with 17p deletion. An entity characterized by specific dysgranulopoiesis and a high incidence of *P53* mutations. *Leukemia*, **9**, 370–81.

91. Merlat, A., Lai, J. L., Sterkers, Y. *et al.* (1999). Therapy-related myelodysplastic syndrome and acute myeloid leukemia with 17p deletion. A report on 25 cases. *Leukemia*, **13**, 250–7.

92. Sankar, M., Tanaka, K., Kumaravel, T. S. *et al.* (1998). Identification of a commonly deleted region at 17p13.3 in leukemia and lymphoma associated with 17p abnormality. *Leukemia*, **12**, 510–16.

93. Rowley, J. D. (2000). Molecular genetics in acute leukemia. *Leukemia*, **14**, 513–17.

94. Bain, B. J., Moorman, A. V., Johansson, B., Mehta, A. B., and Secker-Walker, L. M. (1998). Myelodysplastic syndromes associated with 11q23 abnormalities. European 11q23 workshop participants. *Leukemia*, **12**, 834–9.

95. Secker-Walker, L. M., Moorman, A. V., Bain, B. J., and Mehta, A. B. (1998). Secondary acute leukemia and myelodysplastic syndrome with 11q23 abnormalities. EU Concerted Action 11q23 Workshop. *Leukemia*, **12**, 840–4.

96. Bloomfield, C. D., Archer, K. J., Mrozek, K. *et al.* (2002). 11q23 balanced chromosome aberrations in treatment-related myelodysplastic syndromes and acute leukemia: report from an international workshop. *Genes Chromosomes Cancer*, **33**, 362–78.

97. Rowley, J. D., Reshmi, S., Sobulo, O. *et al.* (1997). All patients with the t(11;16)(q23;p13.3) that involves *MLL* and *CBP* have treatment-related hematologic disorders. *Blood*, **90**, 535–41.

98. Le Beau, M. M., Albain, K. S., Larson, R. A. *et al.* (1986). Clinical and cytogenetic correlations in 63 patients with therapy-related myelodysplastic syndromes and

acute nonlymphocytic leukemia: further evidence for characteristic abnormalities of chromosomes no. 5 and 7. *J. Clin. Oncol.*, **4**, 325–45.

99. Smith, S. M., Le Beau, M. M., Huo, D. *et al.* (2003). Clinical-cytogenetic associations in 306 patients with therapy-related myelodysplasia and myeloid leukemia: the University of Chicago series. *Blood*, **102**, 42–52.

100. Cortes, J., O'Brien, S., Kantarjian, H. *et al.* (1994). Abnormalities in the long arm of chromosome 11 (11q) in patients with de novo and secondary acute myelogenous leukemias and myelodysplastic syndromes. *Leukemia*, **8**, 2174–8.

101. Super, H. J., McCabe, N. R., Thirman, M. J. *et al.* (1993). Rearrangements of the *MLL* gene in therapy-related acute myeloid leukemia in patients previously treated with agents targeting DNA-topoisomerase II. *Blood*, **82**, 3705–11.

102. Look, A. T. (1997). Oncogenic transcription factors in the human acute leukemias. *Science*, **278**, 1059–64.

103. Golub, T. R., Barker, G. F., Lovett, M., and Gilliland, D. G. (1994). Fusion of PDGF receptor beta to a novel *ETS*-like gene, *TEL*, in chronic myelomonocytic leukemia with t(5;12) chromosomal translocation. *Cell*, **77**, 307–16.

104. Ross, T. S., Bernard, O. A., Berger, R., and Gilliland, D. G. (1998). Fusion of huntington interacting protein 1 to platelet-derived growth factor beta receptor (PDGR-beta-R) in chronic myelomonocytic leukemia with t(5;7)(q33;q11.2). *Blood*, **91**, 4419–26.

105. Magnusson, M. K., Meade, K. E., Brown, K. E. *et al.* (2001). Rabaptin-5 is a novel fusion partner to platelet-derived growth factor beta receptor in chronic myelomonocytic leukemia. *Blood*, **98**, 2518–25.

106. Kulkarni, S., Heath, C., Parker, S. *et al.* (2000). Fusion of H4/D10S170 to the platelet-derived growth factor receptor beta in *BCR-ABL* negative myeloproliferative disorders with a t(5;10)(q33;q21). *Cancer Res.*, **60**, 3592–8.

107. Abe, A., Emi, N., Tanimoto, M. *et al.* (1997). Fusion of the platelet-derived growth factor receptor beta to a novel gene *CEV14* in acute myelogenous leukemia after clonal evolution. *Blood*, **90**, 4271–7.

108. Rubin, C. M., Larson, R. A., Bitter, M. A. *et al.* (1987). Association of a chromosomal 3;21 translocation with the blast phase of chronic myelogenous leukemia. *Blood*, **70**, 1338–42.

109. Rubin, C. M., Larson, R. A., Anastasi, J. *et al.* (1990). t(3;21)(q26;q22): A recurring chromosomal abnormality in therapy-related myelodysplastic syndrome and acute myeloid leukemia. *Blood*, **76**, 2594–8.

110. Nucifora, G., Begy, C. R., Kobayashi, H. *et al.* (1994). Consistent intergenic splicing and production of multiple transcripts between *AML1* at 21q22 and unrelated genes at 3q26 in (3;21)(q26;q22) translocations. *Proc. Natl Acad. Sci. U.S.A.*, **91**, 4004–8.

111. Sitailo, S., Sood, R., Barton, K., and Nucifora, G. (1999). Forced expression of the leukemia-associated gene *EVI1* in ES cells: a model for myeloid leukemia with 3q26 rearrangements. *Leukemia*, **13**, 1639–45.

112. Sood, R., Talwar-Trikha, A., Chakrabarti, S. R., and Nucifora, G. (1999). MDS1/EVI1 enhances TGF-beta1 signaling and strengthens its growth-inhibitory effect but the leukemia-associated fusion protein AML1/MDS1/EVI1, product of the t(3;21), abrogates growth-inhibition in response to TGF-beta1. *Leukemia*, **13**, 348–57.

113. Martinelli, G., Ottaviani, E., Buonamici, S. *et al.* (2003). Association of 3q21q26 syndrome with different *RPN1EVI1* fusion transcripts. *Haematologica*, **88**, 1221–8.

114. Pekarsky, Y., Rynditch, A., Wieser, R., Fonasch, C., and Gardiner, K. (1997). Activation of a novel gene in 3q21 and identification of intergenic fusion transcripts with ecotropic viral insertion site I in leukemia. *Cancer Res.*, **57**, 3914–19.

115. Raynaud, S. D., Baens, M., Grosgeorge, J. *et al.* (1996). Fluorescence in situ hybridization analysis of t(3;12)(q26;p13): a recurring chromosomal abnormality involving the *TEL* gene (*ETV6*) in myelodysplastic syndromes. *Blood*, **88**, 682–9.

116. Block, A. M. W., Carroll, A. J., Hagemeijer, A. *et al.* (2002). Rare recurring balanced chromosome abnormalies in therapy-related myelodysplastic syndromes and acute leukemia: report from an international workshop. *Genes Chromosomes Cancer*, **33**, 401–12.

117. Lepelley, P., Soenen, V., Preudhomme, C. *et al.* (1995). *BCL-2* expression in myelodysplastic syndromes and its correlation with hematological features, *p53* mutations and prognosis. *Leukemia*, **9**, 726–30.

118. Ridge, S. A., Worwood, M., Oscier, D., Jacobs, A., and Padua, R. A. (1990). *FMS* mutations in myelodysplastic, leukemic, and normal subjects. *Proc. Natl Acad. Sci. U.S.A.*, **87**, 1377–80.

119. Kiyoi, H., Towatari, M., Yokota, S. *et al.* (1998). Internal tandem duplication of the *FLT3* gene is a novel modality of elongation mutation which causes constitutive activation of the product. *Leukemia*, **12**, 1333–7.

120. Horiike, S., Yokota, S., Nakao, M. *et al.* (1997). Tandem duplications of the *FLT3* receptor gene are associated with leukemic transformation of myelodysplasia. *Leukemia*, **11**, 1442–6.

121. Tidow, N., Kasper, B., and Welte, K. (1998). Clinical implications of G-CSF receptor mutations. *Crit. Rev. Oncol. Hematol.*, **28**, 1–6.

122. Saunthararajah, Y., Nakamura, R., Nam, J. M. *et al.* (2002). HLA-DR15 (DR2) is overrepresented in myelodysplastic syndrome and aplastic anemia and predicts a response to immunosuppression in myelodysplastic syndrome. *Blood*, **100**, 1570–4.

123. Arland, M., Fiedler, W., Samalecos, A., and Hossfeld, D. K. (1994). Absence of point mutations in a functionally important part of the extracellular domain of the

C-KIT proto-oncogene in a series of patients with acute myeloid leukemia (AML). *Leukemia*, **8**, 498–501.

124. Siitonen, T., Savolainen, E. R., and Koistinen, P. (1994). Expression of the c-*KIT* proto-oncogene in myeloproliferative disorders and myelodysplastic syndromes. *Leukemia*, **8**, 631–7.

125. Zochbauer, S., Gsur, A., Gotzl, M. *et al.* (1994). *MDR1* gene expression in myelodysplastic syndrome and in acute myeloid leukemia evolving from myelodysplastic syndrome. *Anticancer Res.*, **14**, 1293–5.

126. Bueso-Ramos, C. E., Manshouri, T., Haidar, M. A. *et al.* (1995). Multiple patterns of *MDM-2* deregulation in human leukemias: implications in leukemogenesis and prognosis. *Leuk. Lymphoma*, **17**, 13–18.

127. Faderl, S., Kantarjian, H. M., Estey, E. *et al.* (2000). The prognostic significance of p16(INK4a)/p14(ARF) locus deletion and MDM-2 protein expression in adult acute myelogenous leukemia. *Cancer*, **89**, 1976–82.

128. Ogata, K. and Tamura, H. (2000). Thrombopoietin and myelodysplastic syndromes. *Int. J. Hematol.*, **72**, 173–7.

129. Bouscary, D., Preudhomme, C., Ribrag, V. *et al.* (1995). Prognostic value of C-MPL expression in myelodysplastic syndromes. *Leukemia*, **9**, 783–8.

130. Shannon, K. M., O'Connell, P., Martin, G. A. *et al.* (1994). Loss of the normal *NF1* allele from the bone marrow of children with type 1 neurofibromatosis and malignant myeloid disorders. *N. Engl. J. Med.*, **330**, 597–601.

131. Gallagher, A., Darley, R. L., and Padua, R. (1997). The molecular basis of myelodysplastic syndromes. *Haematologica*, **82**, 191–204.

132. Padua, R. A. and West, R. R. (2000). Oncogene mutation and prognosis in the myelodysplastic syndromes. *Br. J. Haematol.*, **111**, 873–4.

133. Christiansen, D. H., Andersen, M. K., and Pedersen-Bjergaard, J. (2003). Methylation of *p15INK4B* is common, is associated with deletion of genes on chromosome arm 7q and predicts a poor prognosis in therapy-related myelodysplasia and acute myeloid leukemia. *Leukemia*, **17**, 1813–19.

134. Loh, M. L., Vattikuti, S., Schubbert, S. *et al.* (2003). Somatic mutations in *PTPN11* implicate the protein tyrosine phosphatase SHP-2 in leukemogenesis. *Blood*, **103**, 2325–31.

135. Counter, C. M., Gupta, J., Harley, C. B., Leber, B., and Bacchetti, S. (1995). Telomerase activity in normal leukocytes and in hematologic malignancies. *Blood*, **85**, 2315–20.

136. Norrback, K. F. and Roos, G. (1997). Telomeres and telomerase in normal and malignant haematopoietic cells. *Eur. J. Cancer*, **33**, 774–80.

137. Xu, D., Gruber, A., Peterson, C., and Pisa, P. (1998). Telomerase activity and the expression of telomerase components in acute myelogenous leukaemia. *Br. J. Haematol.*, **102**, 1367–75.

138. Li, B., Yang, J., Andrews, C. *et al.* (2000). Telomerase activity in preleukemia and acute myelogenous leukemia. *Leuk. Lymphoma*, **36**, 579–87.

139. Misawa, S. and Horiike, S. (1996). *TP53* mutations in myelodysplastic syndrome. *Leuk. Lymphoma*, **23**, 417–22.

140. Kita-Sasai, Y., Horiike, S., Misawa, S. *et al.* (2001). International prognostic scoring system and *TP53* mutations are independent prognostic indicators for patients with myelodysplastic syndrome. *Br. J. Haematol.*, **115**, 309–12.

141. Cilloni, D., Gottardi, E., Messa, F. *et al.* (2003). Significant correlation between the degree of *WTI* expression and the international prognostic scoring system score in patients with myelodysplastic syndromes. *J. Clin. Oncol.*, **21**, 1988–95.

5

Molecular mechanisms and gene expression patterns in myelodysplastic syndromes

Wolf-Karsten Hofmann[1] and H. Phillip Koeffler[2]

[1]University Hospital "Benjamin Franklin," Berlin, Germany
[2]Cedars Sinai Research Institute, UCLA School of Medicine, Los Angeles, CA

Introduction

The underlying causes of primary myelodysplastic syndrome (MDS) are still being defined. Analysis of cytogenetic abnormalities, glucose-6-phosphate dehydrogenase isoenzymes, restriction-linked polymorphisms, and X-linked DNA polymorphisms of the androgen receptor has shown that MDS is a clonal abnormality of the hematopoietic stem cell characterized by defective maturation and in advanced stages of uncontrolled proliferation.[1] Lymphocytes are probably not usually involved in the clonal hematopoiesis in MDS,[2] but precursors of red blood cells (RBC), platelets, neutrophils, monocytes, eosinophils, and basophils are members of the abnormal clone. One proposal for the multistep pathogenesis of MDS is shown in Figure 5.1. After initial damage of the progenitor cell by a toxin or a spontaneous mutation, several additional alterations may affect these cells, providing them with a growth advantage. These alterations can influence expression of cell cycle-related genes and transcription factors as well as tumor suppressor genes.

The defects of the hematopoietic stem cells in myelodysplastic syndrome are not well characterized. First, one of the major (technical) problems is that most of the experiments that utilize clinical samples from MDS patients are performed with low-density, non-adherent bone marrow cells. This may be adequate for high-risk MDS and acute myeloid leukemia (AML) evolved from MDS because of the more uniform blast population. In contrast, in low-risk MDS, the bone marrow cells are very heterogeneous. Therefore,

Myelodysplastic Syndromes: Clinical and Biological Advances, ed. Peter L. Greenberg. Published by Cambridge University Press. © Cambridge University Press 2006.

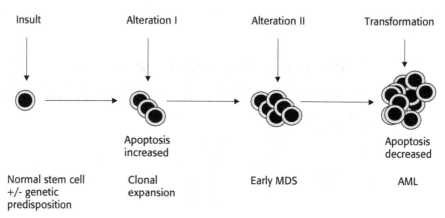

Fig. 5.1   Multistep pathogenesis in myelodysplastic syndromes (MDS). The initial genetic insult on the hematopoietic stem cell can be caused by chemicals, radiation, cytotoxic drugs, or random endogenous mutations. The accumulation of several alterations which may affect cell cycle control, transcription, or tumor suppressors results in the expansion of the MDS clone. These cells undergo increased apoptosis. The progression to leukemia is probably not dependent on the order of occurrence of genetic alterations but is dependent on the genes that are altered. The final step, leukemic transformation, may be enhanced by alteration of additional genes including tumor suppressor genes and/or by hypermethylation of critical targets. The later stage of leukemogenesis is associated with a decreased apoptosis. AML, acute myeloid leukemia.

molecular abnormalities that are characteristic of the malignant cells are much more difficult to find in low-risk MDS compared to high-risk MDS or AML. Second, the lack of suitable experimental models for MDS, e.g., cell lines or animal systems, hampers progress in understanding the biology of this disease. Therefore, new approaches to elucidate the underlying abnormalities are needed.

We and others[3,4] have shown that to characterize the cellular and molecular defects using clinical samples from patients with MDS requires the analysis of freshly isolated and unstimulated (steady-state) CD34+ bone marrow cells. Since expression of CD34 is a marker for hematopoietic stem cells, the experiments to detect abnomalities have focused on the CD34+ cells from patients with MDS.[3,5,6] Even those highly purified cells may demonstrate a broad biological variability, especially in low-risk MDS because the CD34+ cells in this subgroup of MDS may not always be monoclonal.

Table 5.1 Presence of genetic alterations in bone marrow cells from patients with myelodysplastic syndrome (MDS) and their frequency

Gene	Chromosome	MDS subtype	Alteration	Frequency
$AML1^{36}$	21q22.3	All	Mutation	5%
$CHK2^{44}$	22q12.1	RA	Mutation	Rare
$G\text{-}CSF^{31,32}$	17q11.2–q12	MDS/CN	Mutation	10%
$NF1^{28}$	17q11.2	JCMML	Mutation	30%
$p15^{INK4b48,49}$	9p21	RAEB > RA	Methylation	20–40%
$p16^{INK4a47}$	9p21	All	Methylation	Rare
$p53^{40,41}$	17p13.1	RAEB, CMML	Mutations	10%
$PTPN11^{30}$	12q24.1	RAEB	Mutation	20%
RAS^{39}	1p13.2	All, JCMML	Mutation	10–40%

RA, refractory anemia; CN, congenital neutropenia; JCMML, juvenile chronic myelomonocytic leukemia; RAEB, refractory anemia with excess of blasts.

Genetic instability as detected by microsatellite instability in early MDS may also contribute to the clonal expansion of the MDS cells.[7] One study suggested that a disproportionate number of individuals who develop therapy-related MDS/AML have a germline mutation of one of their mismatch repair genes, making them predisposed to MDS/AML after toxic exposure.[8] However, other studies have been unable to substantiate these findings.[9–11] The most frequent genetic alterations in MDS are listed in Table 5.1.

The recently available microarray technology is a powerful new tool to assess the expression of a large number of genes in a single experiment. The initial use of array technology in medical science was to characterize global gene expression profiles during physiological changes or disease progression. The aim of those studies was to accelerate the identification of diagnostic and prognostic markers and to identify novel tumor-specific markers for certain malignant diseases. Furthermore, experience has shown that microarray analyses can provide sufficient data to detect genes or gene patterns that are associated with alterations of specific cellular pathways or signal cascades.[12] The development of strategies for the analysis of differentially expressed genes provides the tools to correlate expression data of unknown genes with expression patterns for genes known to be involved in regulation of the biology of the cell.

Specific syndromes in MDS associated with distinct molecular alterations

Inactivation of tumor suppressor genes is a crucial event in oncogenesis. A proposed mechanism for inactivation of genes either associated with normal differentiation and/or genes involved in regulation of the cell cycle is that one allele of the gene sustains a mutation and then the normal remaining allele is lost through a variety of possible means such as deletion or recombination.[13] MDS is often associated with cytogenetic deletions such as −5/5q−, −7/7q−, suggesting that genes located at these sites behave as tumor suppressor genes and their alteration is a contributing cause of MDS.[14,15] As illustrated below, several specific syndromes are characterized by significant genetic defects resulting in characteristic phenotypical changes. We anticipate that these list will continue to grow rapidly.

5q− syndrome

This clinically distinct entity involves a deletion of the long arm of chromosome 5 and is characterized by a female preponderance, thrombocytosis, macrocytic, fairly severe anemia often requiring RBC transfusions, prominent megaloblastoid erythroid hyperplasia in the bone marrow, and megakaryocytes which are large, often greater than 30 μm in diameter, and which often have a single eccentric round nucleus.[16] Interestingly, the rate of leukemic transformation in individuals with 5q− syndrome is only 25% after an observation period of 15 years.[17] The underlying molecular lesion in 5q− syndrome is still unknown. The critical segment may be at chromosome 5q31.[18,19] The human *GRAF* gene located in this region can fuse to the *MLL* gene, disrupting both alleles,[20] but the significance of this gene in the 5q− syndrome is unclear. Also, the loss of one allele of one or many genes on 5q (haploinsufficiency) could contribute to the 5q− abnormality, similar to what occurs in the familial platelet disorder with predisposition to AML (see below).

In striking contrast to this syndrome is the occurrence of loss of chromosome 5 or 5q− in therapy-related MDS which presages an almost inevitable leukemic transformation. This may be associated with loss of other regions of 5q compared to the region in the 5q− syndrome as well as other cytogenetic abnormalities.

12p syndrome

Individuals with CMML may have rearrangements at 12p.[21] These individuals can have a fusion of the *TEL* gene (translocation, ETS, leukemia – ETS-related oncogene, normally located on 12p13) with a second partner, platelet-derived growth factor receptor-β (*PDGFRβ*, located on 5q31), resulting in a fusion of the transmembrane and tyrosine kinase portion of *PDGFRβ* to the helix–loop–helix (HLH) region of the *TEL* gene.[22] The *TEL* region may cause homodimerization of the chimeric protein with activation of the tyrosine kinase of *PDGFRβ*, resulting in secondary growth signals. In addition, *PDGFRβ* rarely fuses to one of several other genes, including Huntingtoin-interacting protein 1 (HIP-1), possibly causing a myeloproliferative disorder,[23] often associated with eosinophilia. The physician should recognize these abnormalities in patients with MDS because they may respond to treatment with imatinib mesylate (STI571, Glivec).

Juvenile chronic myelomonocytic leukemia

Juvenile chronic myelomonocytic leukemia (JCMML) is another syndrome of MDS, and it is marked by monosomy 7. These individuals are usually males, younger than 5 years of age, who may have splenomegaly, hepatomegaly, leukemic skin infiltration, and leukocytosis with increased numbers of monocytes in the peripheral blood, as well as thrombocytopenia and anemia.[24,25] Their myeloid hematopoietic progenitor cells have spontaneous growth in soft agar culture with increased sensitivity to myeloid growth factors, including granulocyte–macrophage colony-stimulating factor (GM-CSF). These patients have a poor prognosis unless allografting is performed.[26]

Often, individuals with JCMML have one of three mutations that could result in hyperactivity of the RAS pathway. In 10–15% of children, JCMML is associated with neurofibromatosis type 1 (NF-1). The NF-1 tumor suppressor gene encodes neurofibromin, which regulates the growth of immature myeloid cells by accelerating guanosine triphosphate hydrolysis of RAS proteins.[27] The NF-1 gene was found to be inactivated by mutation in 30% of children with JCMML, including those without a clinical diagnosis of NF-1.[28] RAS mutations occur in about 20% of children with JCMML.[29]

Recently[30] it was shown that children with JCMML in association with the Noonan syndrome have mutations in the *PTPN11* gene encoding for a non-receptor protein tyrosine phosphatase (SHP-2). Further analyses revealed the presence of mutations of *PTPN11* in patients with advanced MDS (20% in refractory anemia with excess of blasts, RAEB) but not in early-stage MDS (refractory anemia, RA). At present, the impact of *PTPN11* mutations on hematopoietic disturbances in MDS is not completely clear but it may serve as a prognostic marker for the course of MDS.

MDS associated with either congenital neutropenia or familial platelet disorder with predisposition to AML (FPD/AML)

In severe congenital neutropenia, maturation of myeloid progenitor cells is arrested. About 25% of individuals with congenital neutropenia have a mutation in the granulocyte colony-stimulating factor (G-CSF) receptor gene at a site that interrupts signals required for the maturation of myeloid cells and 50% of these patients develop MDS.[31,32] The MDS clone usually has monosomy 7 (75%) and often has an *N-ras* mutation (40%). The majority of patients with congenital neutropenia have a mutation in the neutrophil elastase gene (*ELA2*).[33] These mutations may increase apoptosis and/or compromise myeloid differentiation, but how they increase the risk for development of MDS/AML is unclear.

Another congenital abnormality associated with development of MDS is FPD/AML. This abnormality results from the mutation of only one allele of the *AML1* gene (also called core-binding factor A2 (*CBFA2*)). Haploinsufficiency of the *AML1* gene causes an autosomal dominant congenital platelet defect and thrombocytopenia.[34,35] These individuals usually have normal peripheral blood red and white cell counts, but analysis of either their bone marrow or peripheral blood cells shows a decrease in megakaryocytic, erythroid, and myeloid progenitor cells. These individuals are predisposed to the acquisition of additional mutations that cause MDS/AML (e.g. +8, 5q−, 11q−, 20q−), but the remaining normal *AML1* allele in the abnormal clone does not become altered. This syndrome prompted investigators to examine the frequency of mutation of this gene in the "general population" of MDS patients. Data suggest that *AML1* mutations occur in 5% (2/37 cases) of cases of MDS[36] and this mutant gene can act as dominant negative inhibitor by competing with wild-type *AML1* for interaction with core-binding factor-β

(CBF-β).[36] Inactivation of transcriptional regulation by *AML1* is a recurring theme in the development of MDS and AML. For example, the AML-*ETO* fusion product found in the t(8;21) AML is associated with silencing of *AML1*. Inversion or deletion of chromosome 16 fuses CBF-β to the myosin heavy chain, which prevents its heterodimerization with *AML1*, resulting in an inactivated *AML1*.[37]

Alteration of signal transduction and cell cycle-related genes in MDS

Known abnormalities of signal transduction genes in MDS include point mutations of *ras* (frequency of 10–15%). *N-ras* is most frequently mutated, with a point mutation occuring at codon 12, 13, or 61.[38,39] Mutations of this gene result in an activated protein which stimulates its downstream targets such as *RAF* and *MAPK*. MDS with mutant *N-ras* may be associated with a worse prognosis.[39] Of interest, activation of the *ras* pathway is most frequently associated with an abnormality that has a monocytoid-like differentiation, including mutated *ras* in chronic myelomonocytic leukemia (CMML) and mutated *NF1* or *PTPN11* in JCMML. Lessons learned from JCMML suggest that *ras*, *NF1*, or *PTPN11* may be mutated, causing an altered *ras* pathway and if one of these genes is mutated, rarely will the other two be altered.

Alterations of the *p53* gene occur in about 10% of MDS.[40,41] Changes are usually missense mutations of one allele, with the second allele being lost. Patients whose abnormal clone has an isochromosome 17q often have a *p53* mutation in their cells. These mutations usually prevent the protein from being able to bind to DNA, thus losing its ability to transactivate target genes such as the cyclin-dependent kinase inhibitor (CDKI) *p21*[WAF2]. Mutations of *p53* are associated with progression of the disease and poor prognosis. Recently, somatic point mutations of several myeloid transcription factors have been demonstrated in patients with AML and MDS, including *AML1* (mentioned above) and *c-ebpα*.[36,42,43]

One other reason for the abnormal proliferation associated with a block of differentiation in MDS may be the disturbance of the mitotic checkpoint *CHK2*.[44] Elimination of checkpoints may result in cell death, infidelity in the distribution of either chromosomes or other organelles between dividing cells, or increased susceptibility to environmental perturbations such as DNA-damaging agents.[45]

Epigenetic changes

One of the mechanisms to regulate gene transcription is DNA methylation. Many genes have repeated sequences of CG nucleotides (CpG islands) within the promotor sequence. Such CpG islands are the target for methylation resulting in either decreased or absent binding of transcription factors to the methylated binding site. As a consequence, the gene will not be transcriptional-activated. DNA methylation is a part of the normal regulation of gene expression, but aberrant DNA methylation may cause gene silencing of a number of important tumor suppressor genes or cell cycle-controlling genes. Given the principle that malignant transformation of cells may be caused by the biallelic disruption of genes which have a control function (such as the cell cycle or regulation of apoptosis), the first hit may be mutation of one allele whereas the second hit may be gene silencing of the other allele by abnormal DNA methylation. This is an alternative means[46] for the inactivation of tumor suppressor genes in addition to point mutations or gene deletions.

Important genes for cell cycle regulation are the CDKIs $p15^{INK4B}$ and $p16^{INK4A}$. These two genes are rarely mutated or deleted,[47] but transcription of the $p15^{INK4B}$ gene is often silenced due to abnormal methylation of its promoter region,[48–50] particularly in MDS with excess of blasts.

Gene expression analysis by microarrays in MDS

Recently, we and others have shown that microarray analyses can provide sufficient data to detect genes or gene patterns which are associated with alterations of specific cellular pathways or signal cascades in tumor cells,[12,51–55] including MDS.[4,56] The technique of gene expression profiling can also be used for subclassification of leukemias[57,58] and lymphomas.[59] The approach to predict prognosis or risk type of MDS using gene expression data is a long way from practice,[60] but the ability to predict who will do well and who will not may have a strong impact on the further classification and risk definition of MDS.

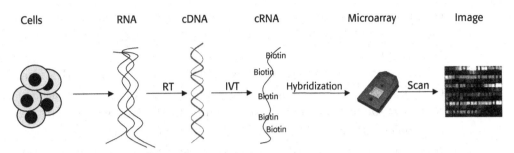

Fig. 5.2   Principle of oligonucleotide microarray hybridization. After extraction of RNA, double-strand cDNA is synthesized and used to produce cRNA by in vitro transcription. The labeled cRNA is hybridized to the oligonucleotide microarray at 45 °C for 16 h. After washing and staining, the image is scanned with an argon-ion confocal laser, with 488 nm emission and detection at 570 nm. RT, reverse transcription; IVT, in vitro transcription.

Technique of global gene expression analysis

CD34+ cell selection and nucleic acid preparation

Fresh bone marrow is processed immediately after aspiration to select the CD34+ cells within 2 h. CD34+ cells can be purified by several techniques, including high-gradient magnetic cell separation (MACS) using superpara-magnetic streptavidin microparticles. The yield and purity of the positively selected CD34+ cells are evaluated by flow cytometry.

The quality of RNA extracted from MDS-CD34+ cells is critical for any microarray experiment. The Bioanalyzer system (Agilent, Waldbronn, Germany) is used to evaluate the quality of the RNA to ensure that the gene expression measured by microarray assay is not affected by degradation of the RNA extracted from the purified CD34+ cells. Figure 5.2 summarizes the principle of the oligonucleotide microarray technique.

Microarrays

Two main methods are available to perform global gene expression analysis. The initial experiments were done using cDNA technology.[61] The principle of this technique is that, for each of the genes to be analyzed (up to 20 000 per chip), a short cDNA fragment is spotted on a glass slide which will be used for hybridization with the target RNA. The newer approach is oligonucleotide microarrays (such as the GeneChip system, Affymetrix Inc., Santa Clara, CA). The advantages of the cDNA technique are high specificity and low cost; the disadvantage is the need of a reference RNA for hybridization of each of the samples, which lessens the impact of this technique for routine application.

The experiments in bone marrow cells from patients with MDS were carried out with both techniques; the more broadly accepted approach (in particular for hybridizing very small amounts of RNA) seems to be the oligonucleotide technique. The detailed protocol for the sample preparation and microarray processing is available from www.affymetrix.com. Because of the limited number of CD34+ cells and the low content of RNA in hematopoietic stem cells, a double in vitro transcription technique (nanogram-scale assay) has been established. To assay 50 ng of total RNA, the standard Affymetrix target amplification protocol has been modified, using the first-round cRNA product to generate a double-stranded cDNA that is then used for a second round of in vitro transcription for synthesis of the biotinylated cRNA.

Selection of differentially expressed genes in CD34+ cells from MDS patients compared to normal individuals

Using several levels of statistical restrictions, as described previously,[51] we directly compared the gene expression in CD34+ cells from normal individuals to those from patients with low-risk as well as high-risk MDS (International Prognostic Scoring System (IPSS)[17]) We found a number of genes to be highly differentially expressed, including those involved in cell growth and signaling, as well as those that are probably involved in the regulation of hematopoiesis.[51] The step-by-step characterization of the differentially expressed genes in CD34+ MDS cells extends our knowledge about altered cellular pathways and generates new hypotheses about the pathogenesis of MDS,[56] including an enhanced susceptibility of hematopoietic stem cells in MDS to external damage, which may be the initial hit followed by an alteration of cell cycle control or hematopoietic differentiation (see below).

We found that the expression of the radiation-inducible immediate-early response gene (*IEX1*) was decreased in low-risk MDS. *IEX1* was initially identified in human squamous carcinoma cells, and its expression was induced by radiation.[62] In addition, several of the downregulated genes in low-risk MDS (*MIG2, STIP1*) code for proteins which protect cells from stresses caused by mutagens or other factors. Our data suggest that CD34+ cells from MDS patients lack certain defensive proteins that may result in their increased susceptibility to cell damage.

One gene that was significantly overexpressed in low-risk MDS compared to normal controls as detected by microarray analysis was delta-like 1 (*DLK1*), a secreted protein that has epidermal growth factor motifs. Overexpression of *DLK1* was previously described in high-risk MDS.[4] The function of this gene in hematopoiesis is not known, but it is genomically imprinted and only expressed from the paternal allele.[63] We found that this gene was markedly upregulated in our series of low-risk MDS cases compared with normal CD34+ marrow cells. For biologic validation of gene expression data of *DLK1*, 13 myeloid cell lines were investigated; it was found that *DLK1* was expressed in human erythroleukemia and megakaryoblastic cell lines. Induction of differentiation of K562 cells toward more mature erythroid precursors resulted in decreased *DLK1* expression.

Prediction of disease risk using CD34+ cells from patients with MDS

The first description of MDS-specific genes which were found overexpressed in CD34+ cells from patients with MDS compared with leukemic cells from patients with AML was published in 2001.[4] Twenty genes (including *DLK1*) were selected by direct comparison of expression data in MDS versus AML. Hierarchical cluster analysis demonstrated that the selected genes could be clearly distinguished in the MDS samples from the AML samples.[4] Furthermore, a recent study showed that gene expression profiles specific for subtypes of MDS according to the French–American–British (FAB) classification can be used to distinguish bone marrow samples from patients with RA from those with RAEB.[64]

We have used two independend data sets created from a total of 19 patients with MDS to predict the risk groups of those patients at the time of initial diagnosis.[51] Using the first data set (11 patients, sample numbers 275–286, Plate 10a), we identified by class membership prediction 11 genes, including genes associated with signal transduction in tumor cells and transcription factors (Table 5.2) whose expression can be used to differentiate with high accuracy between low-risk MDS, high-risk MDS, and normal individuals (numbers 271–274, Plate 10a). To verify the power of the genes selected by class membership prediction, we used the 11 genes for hierarchical

Table 5.2 Genes selected by class membership prediction analysis to be predictive for distinguishing between normal individuals, low-risk, and high-risk myelodysplastic syndromes

Gene	Acc.	Map	Description
TACSTD2	J04152	1p32	Tumor-associated Ca^{2+} signal transducer 2
UQCRC1	L16842	3p21.3	Ubiquinol-cytochrome C reductase core protein 1
TNNC1	M37984	3p21.3	Troponin C, slow
KDELR	M88458	7p	Endoplasmic reticulum protein retention receptor
CLC	L01664	19q13.1	Charcot–Leyden crystal
ATF3	L19871	1	Activating transcription factor 3
H-PLK	M55422	7	Krueppel-related zinc finger protein
RGS19	X91809		Regulator of G-protein signaling 19
GNG7	AW051450		Guanine nucleotide-binding protein gamma 7
FARP1	AI701049		Ferm, arhgef, and pleckstrin domain-containing protein
TPD52L2	U44429	6q22–q23	Tumor protein D52-like 2

Acc., Gene bank accession number; Map, chromosomal position.

clustering with Spearman's confidence correlation (Plate 10a). We generated three clusters. All of the controls (normal CD34+ cells) were in one cluster (with a maximum of two subclusters). Furthermore, all the high-risk and low-risk MDS were separated into different clusters with a maximum of three subclusters.

In a second experiment, we used the 11 predictive genes in a clustering analysis in an independent data set obtained from CD34+ cells from patients with low-risk and high-risk MDS (sample numbers 3000–13591, Plate 10b). The aim of this additional experiment was to evaluate the predictive power of the 11 selected genes in a new series of patient samples. As shown in Plate 10b, we found two clusters corresponding to the IPSS high-risk and low-risk classifications, demonstrating the power of the selected genes for risk-group prediction.

The search for genes specific for different stages of MDS is underway. Different studies revealed different lists of genes which are associated with either low-risk or high-risk MDS.[4,51,64] One reason for this may be that the "real MDS target cell" is not yet defined. At least one gene – *DLK1* – was detected to be overexpressed in low-risk MDS in all studies. At this time, we propose that *DLK1* may contribute to the block of differentiation of hematopoietic progenitor cells in MDS and may give the abnormal clone a growth advantage (unpublished data).

Summary and future directions

The discovery of underlying mechanisms causing primary MDS requires further work. Different molecular alterations which have been described suggest that it is a multistep alteration to the hematopoietic stem cells that include genes involved in cell cycle control and mitotic checkpoints as well as growth factor receptors. Secondary signal proteins and transcription factors which give the cell a growth advantage over its normal counterpart may also be affected. The accumulation of such defects may finally cause the leukemic transformation of MDS.

As a hope for the future, microarray analysis can detect gene expression profiles which are strongly associated with different risk-groups in MDS. Therefore, we believe that the prognosis of this disease may be predicted using gene expression analysis. We and others have shown that microarray analysis can be used with small amounts of RNA, which can be obtained from cells during a routine diagnostic bone marrow aspirate. This method may facilitate making therapeutic decisions in cases where the diagnosis and/or risk evaluation is not possible based on morphologic and classical cytogenetic data. The results from a number of studies using CD34+ cells as well as other cell types (e.g., granulocytes) from patients with MDS are pending. Furthermore, such analysis of global gene expression provides new insights into alterations of cellular pathways in early hematopoietic stem cells in MDS. This should result in the design or discovery of target-specific drugs for the treatment of MDS.

REFERENCES

1. Parker, J. and Mufti, G. J. (1996). Ras and myelodysplasia: lessons from the last decade. *Semin. Hematol.*, **33**, 206–24.
2. Saitoh, K., Miura, I., Takahashi, N., and Miura, A. B. (1998). Fluorescence in situ hybridization of progenitor cells obtained by fluorescence-activated cell sorting for

the detection of cells affected by chromosome abnormality trisomy 8 in patients with myelodysplastic syndromes. *Blood*, **92**, 2886–92.

3. Hofmann, W. K., Kalina, U., Wagner, S. *et al.* (1999). Characterization of defective megakaryocytic development in patients with myelodysplastic syndromes. *Exp. Hematol.*, **27**, 395–400.

4. Miyazato, A., Ueno, S., Ohmine, K. *et al.* (2001). Identification of myelodysplastic syndrome-specific genes by DNA microarray analysis with purified hematopoietic stem cell fraction. *Blood*, **98**, 422–7.

5. Kalina, U., Hofmann, W. K., Koschmieder, S. *et al.* (2000). Alteration of c-mpl-mediated signal transduction in CD34(+) cells from patients with myelodysplastic syndromes. *Exp. Hematol.*, **28**, 1158–63.

6. Preisler, H. D., Li, B., Chen, H. *et al.* (2001). P15INK4B gene methylation and expression in normal, myelodysplastic, and acute myelogenous leukemia cells and in the marrow cells of cured lymphoma patients. *Leukemia*, **15**, 1589–95.

7. Kaneko, H., Horiike, S., Taniwaki, M., and Misawa, S. (1996). Microsatellite instability is an early genetic event in myelodysplastic syndrome but is infrequent and not associated with TGF-beta receptor type II gene mutation. *Leukemia*, **10**, 1696–9.

8. Ben-Yehuda, D., Krichevsky, S., Caspi, O. *et al.* (1996). Microsatellite instability and *p53* mutations in therapy-related leukemia suggest mutator phenotype. *Blood*, **88**, 4296–303.

9. Tasaka, T., Lee, S., Spira, S. *et al.* (1996). Infrequent microsatellite instability during the evolution of myelodysplastic syndrome to acute myelocytic leukemia. *Leuk. Res.*, **20**, 113–17.

10. Willman, C. L. (1998). Molecular genetic features of myelodysplastic syndromes (MDS). *Leukemia*, **12** (suppl. 1), S2–6.

11. Rimsza, L. M., Kopecky, K. J., Ruschulte, J. *et al.* (2000). Microsatellite instability is not a defining genetic feature of acute myeloid leukemogenesis in adults: results of a retrospective study of 132 patients and review of the literature. *Leukemia*, **14**, 1044–51.

12. Hofmann, W. K., de Vos, S., Tsukasaki, K. *et al.* (2001). Altered apoptosis pathways in mantle cell lymphoma detected by oligonucleotide microarray. *Blood*, **98**, 787–94.

13. Krug, U., Ganser, A., and Koeffler, H. P. (2002). Tumor suppressor genes in normal and malignant hematopoiesis. *Oncogene*, **21**, 3475–95.

14. Chen, Z. and Sandberg, A. A. (2002). Molecular cytogenetic aspects of hematological malignancies: clinical implications. *Am. J. Med. Genet.*, **115**, 130–41.

15. Hirai, H. (2002). Molecular pathogenesis of MDS. *Int. J. Hematol.*, **76** (suppl. 2), 213–21.

16. Thiede, T., Engquist, L., and Billstrom, R. (1998). Application of megakaryocytic morphology in diagnosing 5q– syndrome. *Eur. J. Haematol.*, **41**, 434–7.

17. Greenberg, P., Cox, C., Le Beau, M. M. *et al.* (1997). International scoring system for evaluating prognosis in myelodysplastic syndromes. *Blood*, **89**, 2079–88.

18. Carter, G., Ridge, S., and Padua, R. A. (1992). Genetic lesions in preleukemia. *Crit. Rev. Oncog.*, **3**, 339–64.

19. Willman, C. L., Sever, C. E., Pallavicini, M. G. *et al.* (1993). Deletion of IRF-1, mapping to chromosome 5q31.1, in human leukemia and preleukemic myelodysplasia. *Science*, 1993; **259**, 968–71.

20. Borkhardt, A., Bojesen, S., Haas, O. A. *et al.* (2000). The human *GRAF* gene is fused to MLL in a unique t(5;11)(q31;q23) and both alleles are disrupted in three cases of myelodysplastic syndrome/acute myeloid leukemia with a deletion 5q. *Proc. Natl Acad. Sci. U.S.A.*, **97**, 9168–73.

21. Heim, S. (1992). Cytogenetic findings in primary and secondary MDS. *Leuk. Res.*, **16**, 43–6.

22. Golub, T. R., Barker, G. F., Lovett, M., and Gilliland, D. G. (1994). Fusion of PDGF receptor beta to a novel *ets*-like gene, *tel*, in chronic myelomonocytic leukemia with t(5;12) chromosomal translocation. *Cell*, **77**, 307–16.

23. Apperley, J. F., Gardembas, M., Melo, J. V. *et al.* (2002). Response to imatinib mesylate in patients with chronic myeloproliferative diseases with rearrangements of the platelet-derived growth factor receptor beta. *N. Engl. J. Med.*, **347**, 481–7.

24. Passmore, S. J., Chessells, J. M., Kempski, H. *et al.* (2003). Paediatric myelodysplastic syndromes and juvenile myelomonocytic leukaemia in the UK: a population-based study of incidence and survival. *Br. J. Haematol.*, **121**, 758–67.

25. Emanuel, P. D. (2004). Juvenile myelomonocytic leukemia. *Curr. Hematol. Rep.*, **3**, 203–9.

26. Locatelli, F., Niemeyer, C., Angelucci, E. *et al.* (1997). Allogeneic bone marrow transplantation for chronic myelomonocytic leukemia in childhood: a report from the European working group on myelodysplastic syndrome in childhood. *J. Clin. Oncol.*, **15**, 566–73.

27. Shannon, K. M., O'Connell, P., Martin, G. A. *et al.* (1994). Loss of the normal NF1 allele from the bone marrow of children with type 1 neurofibromatosis and malignant myeloid disorders. *N. Engl. J. Med.*, **330**, 597–601.

28. Side, L. E., Emanuel, P. D., Taylor, B. *et al.* (1998). Mutations of the NF1 gene in children with juvenile myelomonocytic leukemia without clinical evidence of neurofibromatosis, type 1. *Blood*, **92**, 267–72.

29. Flotho, C., Valcamonica, S., Mach-Pascual, S. *et al.* (1999). *RAS* mutations and clonality analysis in children with juvenile myelomonocytic leukemia (JMML). *Leukemia*, **13**, 32–7.

30. Tartaglia, M., Niemeyer, C. M., Fragale, A. *et al.* (2003). Somatic mutations in *PTPN11* in juvenile myelomonocytic leukemia, myelodysplastic syndromes and acute myeloid leukemia. *Nat. Genet.*, **34**, 148–50.

31. Dong, F., Brynes, R. K., Tidow, N. *et al.* (1995). Mutations in the gene for the granulocyte colony-stimulating-factor receptor in patients with acute myeloid leukemia preceded by severe congenital neutropenia. *N. Engl. J. Med.*, **333**, 487–93.

32. Freedman, M. H., Bonilla, M. A., Fier, C. *et al.* (2000). Myelodysplasia syndrome and acute myeloid leukemia in patients with congenital neutropenia receiving G-CSF therapy. *Blood*, **96**, 429–36.

33. Dale, D. C., Person, R. E., Bolyard, A. A. *et al.* (2000). Mutations in the gene encoding neutrophil elastase in congenital and cyclic neutropenia. *Blood*, **96**, 2317–22.

34. Song, W. J., Sullivan, M. G., Legare, R. D. *et al.* (1999). Haploinsufficiency of *CBFA2* causes familial thrombocytopenia with propensity to develop acute myelogenous leukaemia. *Nat. Genet.*, **23**, 166–75.

35. Ho, C. Y., Otterud, B., Legare, R. D. *et al.* (1996). Linkage of a familial platelet disorder with a propensity to develop myeloid malignancies to human chromosome 21q22.1–22.2. *Blood*, **87**, 5218–24.

36. Imai, Y., Kurokawa, M., Izutsu, K. *et al.* (2000). Mutations of the *AML1* gene in myelodysplastic syndrome and their functional implications in leukemogenesis. *Blood*, **96**, 3154–60.

37. Horwitz, M., Benson, K. F., Li, F. Q. *et al.* (1997). Genetic heterogeneity in familial acute myelogenous leukemia: evidence for a second locus at chromosome 16q21–23.2. *Am. J. Hum. Genet.*, **61**, 873–81.

38. Fenaux, P. (2001). Chromosome and molecular abnormalities in myelodysplastic syndromes. *Int. J. Hematol.*, **73**, 429–37.

39. Paquette, R. L., Landaw, E. M., Pierre, R. V. *et al.* (1993). *N-ras* mutations are associated with poor prognosis and increased risk of leukemia in myelodysplastic syndrome. *Blood*, **82**, 590–9.

40. Lai, J. L., Preudhomme, C., Zandecki, M. *et al.* (1995). Myelodysplastic syndromes and acute myeloid leukemia with 17p deletion. An entity characterized by specific dysgranulopoiesis and a high incidence of *p53* mutations. *Leukemia*, **9**, 370–81.

41. Jonveaux, P., Fenaux, P., Quiquandon, I. *et al.* (1991). Mutations in the *p53* gene in myelodysplastic syndromes. *Oncogene*, **6**, 2243–7.

42. Pabst, T., Mueller, B. U., Zhang, P. *et al.* (2001). Dominant-negative mutations of *CEBPA*, encoding CCAAT/enhancer binding protein-alpha (C/EB Palpha), in acute myeloid leukemia. *Nat. Genet.*, **27**, 263–70.

43. Gombart, A. F., Hofmann, W. K., Kawano, S. *et al.* (2002). Mutations in the gene encoding the transcription factor CCAAT/enhancer binding protein alpha in myelodysplastic syndromes and acute myeloid leukemias. *Blood*, **99**, 1332–40.

44. Hofmann, W. K., Miller, C. W., Tsukasaki, K. *et al.* (2001). Mutation analysis of the DNA-damage checkpoint gene *CHK2* in myelodysplastic syndromes and acute myeloid leukemias. *Leuk. Res.*, **25**, 333–8.

45. Dasika, G. K., Lin, S. C., Zhao, S. *et al.* (1999). DNA damage-induced cell cycle checkpoints and DNA strand break repair in development and tumorigenesis. *Oncogene*, **18**, 7883–99.

46. Herman, J. G. and Baylin, S. B. (2003). Gene silencing in cancer in association with promoter hypermethylation. *N. Engl. J. Med.*, **349**, 2042–54.

47. Nakamaki, T., Bartram, C., Seriu, T. *et al.* (1997). Molecular analysis of the cyclin-dependent kinase inhibitor genes, *p15, p16, p18* and *p19* in the myelodysplastic syndromes. *Leuk. Res.*, **21**, 235–40.

48. Uchida, T., Kinoshita, T., Nagai, H. *et al.* (1997). Hypermethylation of the *p15INK4B* gene in myelodysplastic syndromes. *Blood*, **90**, 1403–9.

49. Quesnel, B., Guillerm, G., Vereecque, R. *et al.* (1998). Methylation of the *p15(INK4b)* gene in myelodysplastic syndromes is frequent and acquired during disease progression. *Blood*, **91**, 2985–90.

50. Herman, J. G., Civin, C. I., Issa, J. P. *et al.* (1997). Distinct patterns of inactivation of *p15INK4B* and *p16INK4A* characterize the major types of hematological malignancies. *Cancer Res.*, **57**, 837–41.

51. Hofmann, W. K., de Vos, S., Komor, M. *et al.* (2002). Characterization of gene expression of CD34+ cells from normal and myelodysplastic bone marrow. *Blood*, **100**, 3553–60.

52. DeRisi, J., van den Hazel, B., Marc, P. *et al.* (2000). Genome microarray analysis of transcriptional activation in multidrug resistance yeast mutants. *FEBS Lett.*, **470**, 156–60.

53. Kaminski, N., Allard, J. D., Pittet, J. F. *et al.* (2002). Global analysis of gene expression in pulmonary fibrosis reveals distinct programs regulating lung inflammation and fibrosis. *Proc. Natl Acad. Sci. U.S.A.*, **97**, 1778–83.

54. De Vos, J., Couderc, G., Tarte, K. *et al.* (2001). Identifying intercellular signaling genes expressed in malignant plasma cells by using complementary DNA arrays. *Blood*, **98**, 771–80.

55. Neiman, P. E., Ruddell, A., Jasoni, C. *et al.* (2001). Analysis of gene expression during myc oncogene-induced lymphomagenesis in the bursa of Fabricius. *Proc. Natl Acad. Sci. U.S.A.*, **98**, 6378–83.

56. Lee, Y. T., Miller, L. D., Gubin, A. N. *et al.* (2001). Transcription patterning of uncoupled proliferation and differentiation in myelodysplastic bone marrow with erythroid-focused arrays. *Blood*, **98**, 1914–21.

57. Golub, T. R., Slonim, D. K., Tamayo, P. *et al.* (1999). Molecular classification of cancer: class discovery and class prediction by gene expression monitoring. *Science*, **286**, 531–7.

58. Schoch, C., Kohlmann, A., Schnittger, S. *et al.* (2002). Acute myeloid leukemias with reciprocal rearrangements can be distinguished by specific gene expression profiles. *Proc. Natl Acad. Sci. U.S.A.*, **99**, 10008–13.

59. Alizadeh, A. A., Eisen, M. B., Davis, R. E. *et al.* (2000). Distinct types of diffuse large B-cell lymphoma identified by gene expression profiling. *Nature*, **403**, 503–11.

60. Rosenwald, A., Wright, G., Chan, W. C. *et al.* (2002). The use of molecular profiling to predict survival after chemotherapy for diffuse large-B-cell lymphoma. *N. Engl. J. Med.*, **346**, 1937–47.

61. Schena, M., Shalon, D., Davis, R. W., and Brown, P. O. (1995). Quantitative monitoring of gene expression patterns with a complementary DNA microarray. *Science*, **270**, 467–70.

62. Kondratyev, A. D., Chung, K. N., and Jung, M. O. (1996). Identification and characterization of a radiation-inducible glycosylated human early-response gene. *Cancer Res.*, **56**, 1498–502.

63. Schmidt, J. V., Matteson, P. G., Jones, B. K., Guan, X. J., and Tilghman, S. M. (2002). The *Dlk1* and *Gtl2* genes are linked and reciprocally imprinted. *Genes Dev.*, **14**, 1997–2002.

64. Ueda, M., Ota, J., Yamashita, Y. *et al.* (2003). DNA microarray analysis of stage progression mechanism in myelodysplastic syndrome. *Br. J. Haematol.*, **123**, 288–96.

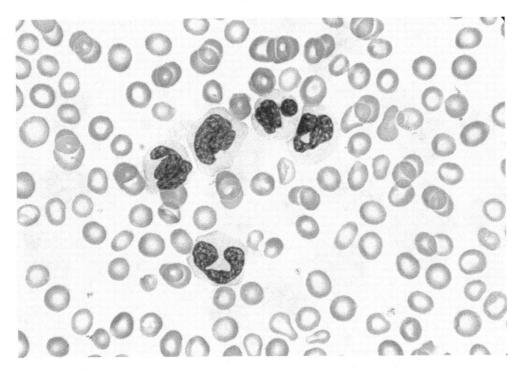

Plate 1 Blood smear from a patient with sideroblastic anemia. The red blood cells demonstrate aniso-cytosis with occasional macrocytes and anisochromasia, a predominant population of normochromic cells, and occasional hypochromic cells.

Plates 1-10 are available for download in colour from www.cambridge.org/9780521182287

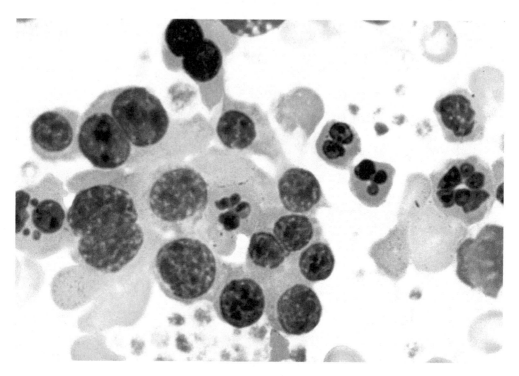

Plate 2 Marrow aspirate showing marked dyserythropoiesis and dysplastic hypogranular neutrophils.

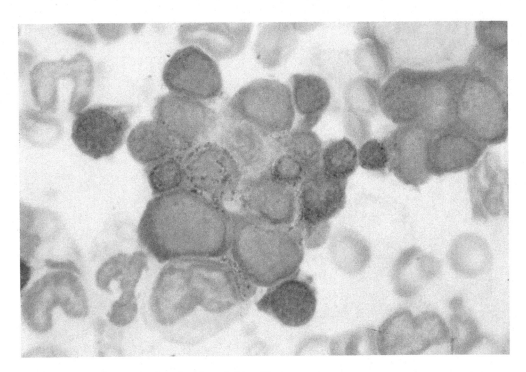

Plate 3 Marrow iron stain showing ringed sideroblasts.

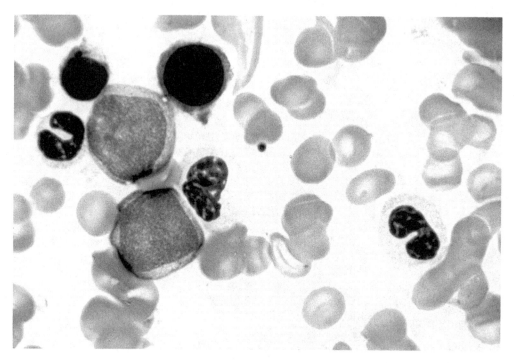

Plate 4 Marrow specimen from a patient with refractory anemia with excess blasts-1 (RAEB-1). Two blasts and three neutrophils with hyposegmented nuclei and hypogranular cytoplasm are shown.

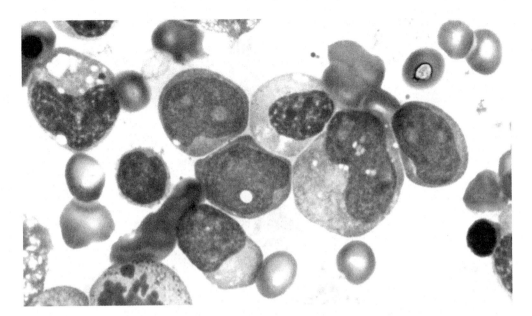

Plate 5 Marrow aspirate specimen showing dysplastic promyelocytes and myelocytes with nuclear–cytoplasmic asynchrony. Cells with nuclear features of a promyelocyte and specific (secondary granules) characteristics of myelocytes, promyelocytes with reduced azurophilic (primary) granules, and myelocytes with clumped nuclear chromatin are present.

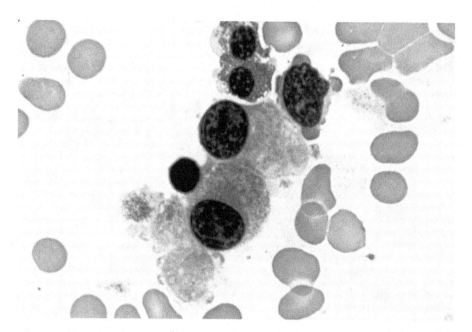

Plate 6 Bone marrow aspirate smear showing a megakaryocyte with a non-lobulated nucleus, from a woman with 5q− syndrome.

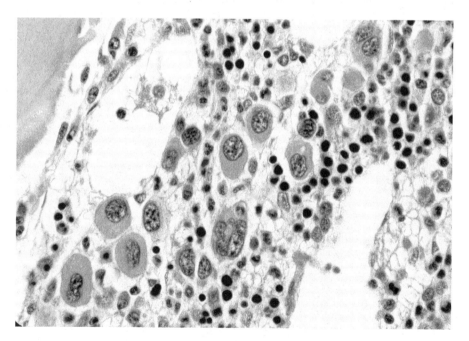

Plate 7 Bone marrow biopsy with numerous megakaryocytes, the majority of which have hypolobulated nuclei, from a woman with 5q− syndrome.

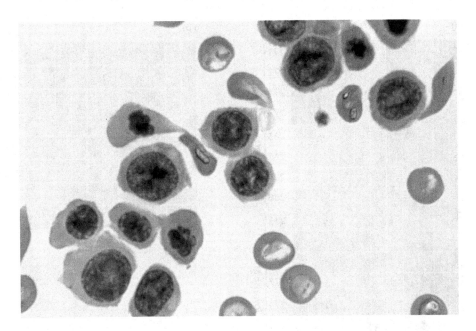

Plate 8 Bone marrow aspirate showing marked dyserythropoiesis in a patient with arsenic intoxication.

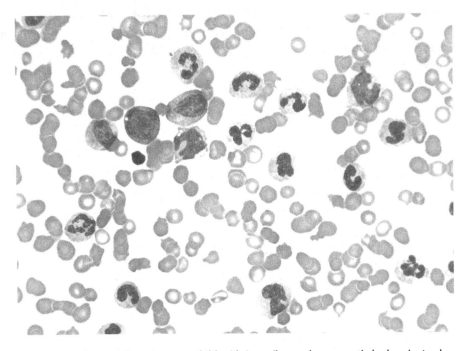

Plate 9 Blood smear from a young child with juvenile myelomonocytic leukemia. Leukocytosis with increased monocytes, neutrophils, and occasional blasts is present.

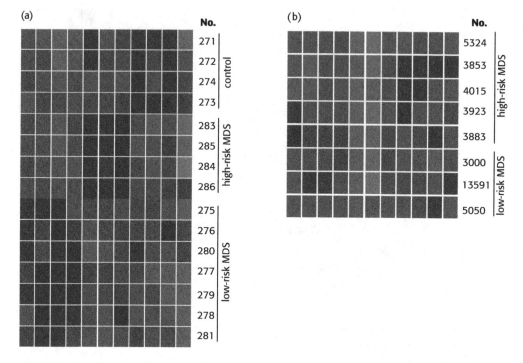

Plate 10 Identification of genes expressed in CD34+ marrow cells, distinguishing between low-risk myelodysplastic syndromes (MDS), high-risk MDS, and healthy individuals. Adapted from Hofmann, W. K., de Vos, S., Komor, M. *et al*. Characterization of gene expression of CD34+ cells from normal and myelodysplastic bone marrow. *Blood*, 2002; **100**, 3553–60. © American Society of Hematology, used with permission.

6

Immunologic mechanisms and treatment of myelodysplastic syndromes

A. John Barrett, Elaine Sloand, and Neal S. Young

National Heart, Lung and Blood Institute, National Institutes of Health, Bethesda, MD, USA

Background

The concept that an immune-mediated response directed against hematopoietic cells can cause failure of the bone marrow leading to pancytopenia arose from early experiences with the use of bone marrow transplants to treat severe aplastic anemia (SAA). In 1976 Mathé et al. in Paris[1] reported a curious case in which a patient transplanted for SAA from a human leukocyte antigen (HLA)-identical sibling donor subsequently achieved full hematologic recovery without any vestige of donor marrow engraftment. Subsequently Jeannet et al.[2] reported sustained autologous hematological recovery in 3 SAA patients receiving antithymocyte globulin (ATG) and a one-haplotype mismatched marrow transplant. At the time the stimulus to autologous hematological recovery was thought to be conferred by the transiently engrafting donor marrow itself, and experiments by Speck & Kissling[3] using mismatched grafts and ATG in aplastic rabbits seemed to support this view. However, Ascensão et al. in 1976[4] made the critical observation that in vitro exposure of aplastic anemia patients' bone marrow to ATG caused a dramatic recovery in granulocyte colony formation, while marrow cells from the patients cocultured with normal marrow suppressed colony formation. Such observations pointed to an immune-mediated mechanism in SAA and stimulated Gluckman et al.[5] to treat SAA patients with ATG alone: of 17 patients, 8 had a prompt and sustained hematological recovery. Subsequent extensive laboratory studies and widespread clinical experience have clearly established that the majority of patients with SAA have immune-mediated T-cell-mediated marrow suppression which can be reversed in a high proportion of cases by immunosuppressive treatment with ATG (reviewed by Young *et al.*)[6].

Encouraged by the hematological responses to immunosuppression seen in SAA patients, several investigators in the 1980s also used ATG to treat the bone marrow failure accompanying hypoplastic myelodysplastic syndromes (MDS). Some of these patients had sustained recovery of their blood counts.[7,8] While treatment to improve outcome in MDS has focused on ways to prevent or treat disease progression to acute leukemia, cytopenia in the absence of any progression to leukemia is the more frequent cause of death in MDS. To test the hypothesis that an immune-mediated process contributed to the marrow failure encountered in both cellular and hypocellular forms of MDS, we treated a series of transfusion-dependent cytopenic MDS patients with immunosuppression.[9] We tested the hypothesis that ATG, administered in a schedule used for treating SAA, could improve cytopenia and reverse red cell transfusion-dependence in patients with MDS. The trial, started in 1994, and a long-term follow-up were reported in 2002.[10] Of 61 patients, 21 (34%) showed hematological responses and became red blood cell transfusion-independent. In 1998 Jonašova *et al.*[11] reported significant and sustained responses to cyclosporin (CSA) in a group of 17 MDS patients with varying degrees of cytopenia. These results indicated that immunosuppressive treatment could improve bone marrow function in some patients with MDS and stimulated trials of immunosuppressive therapy for MDS in other centers.[12,13] The current consensus is that immunosuppressive treatments can produce sustained and significant improvements in bone marrow function in some patients with MDS. These clinical findings have stimulated research into the nature of the immune-mediated pathophysiology in MDS, defining the patient categories most likely to benefit from immunosuppression, and devising optimum immunosuppressive treatment regimens. In this chapter we review the evidence for an immunological process in MDS, summarize clinical results of immunosuppressive treatment, and identify prognostic features that predict response to treatment.

Evidence for an immune-mediated process in MDS

Clinical observations and a growing body of experimental evidence link bone marrow failure in MDS with a T-cell-dominated immune-mediated process.

Response to ATG treatment

The hematological responses to ATG treatment outlined above underlie the assumption that bone marrow failure in MDS is at least in part immune-mediated. The tendency for abnormalities in the T-cell repertoire to normalize following ATG treatment (see below) provides additional circumstantial evidence that hematological recovery in MDS is a result of a modification in immune function. However, in the absence of a clear understanding of the mechanism of ATG treatment, we must be cautious in concluding that the response to these polyclonal and quite complex immunoglobulin preparations is simply due to the reversal of an immune-mediated process through their immunosuppressive action. Other agents such as CSA and corticosteroids appear to have more modest ability to improve marrow function in MDS, suggesting that ATG may have unique modes of action.[14] Recently, for example, Killick et al.[12] showed that ATG favored the persistence of normal CD34 cells in long-term cultures of MDS marrow by a direct (non-T-cell-mediated) effect on MDS progenitors. The nature of this protective mechanism was not identified but it is possible that ATG reduced death from apoptosis by blocking the *fas* receptor on progenitor cells, preventing T-cell engagement via *fas*-ligand.

Association with immune-mediated diseases

There appears to be more than chance association of MDS with immune-mediated tissue disorders, including rheumatoid arthritis, temporal arteritis, polymyalgia rheumatica[15] and immune-mediated vasculitis[16] (reviewed by Hamblin[17]). However, the most compelling evidence for immune-mediated mechanism of marrow failure in MDS comes from the close relationship of the disease with the marrow failure disorder SAA – a condition with an established immune-mediated pathogenesis for bone marrow failure – and with large granular lymphocytic (LGL) lymphoproliferative disease.

Relationship between SAA and MDS

There is considerable overlap between SAA and MDS: patients with SAA can progress to MDS and patients with MDS can have marrow aplasia just as profound as is seen in SAA. Indeed, in some cases this overlap can cause diagnostic confusion and uncertainty as to whether the disease represents SAA or MDS. We proposed that the two disorders SAA and MDS include

Table 6.1 Similarity between severe aplastic anemia (SAA) and myelodysplastic syndrome (MDS)

Feature	SAA	MDS	References
PNH defect	> 50%	18–25%	19
HLA-DR2(15) expression	~30% of patients	~28% of patients	20
Marrow cellularity	< 20% by definition	< 20–100%	21
Marrow CFU-GM content	Low	Low	22,23
Trisomy-8 in marrow	Low	5–10%	24–26
Erythroid dysplasia	Sometimes	Usual	29
Response to I/S	Up to 80%	Up to 30%[a]	9,28
Progression to leukemia	Rare	Common	24

[a] Depending on selection of patients.
PNH, paroxysmal nocturnal hemoglobinuria; HLA, human leukocyte antigen; CFU-GM, colony-forming unit–granulocyte, macrophage; I/S, immunosuppressive therapy.

a subset of individuals with a common immune-mediated etiology for the marrow failure (Table 6.1).[9,18–29]

In this model, MDS may resemble SAA at presentation with near-zero marrow cellularity; the underlying MDS is only revealed when dysplastic features and karyotypic change become evident after hematological recovery. Conversely, individuals with less severe marrow failure present clinically as MDS with a cellular marrow in which dysplastic features can be identified. The immune-mediated process in SAA could itself drive clonal change and development of MDS by selective pressure.[30] Clonal expansions of phosphatidylinositol glycan-class A (PIG-A) mutant stem cells leading to mixed syndromes of SAA/paroxysmal hemoglobinuia (PNH) are believed to be one such marker of immune selection pressure.[31] PNH mutations (revealed by decreased or absence of glycosylphosphoinositol (GPI)-anchored proteins CD55 and CD59 on neutrophils and red cells) have been described in MDS and SAA. PNH abnormalities can be found in up to 25% of patients with MDS and the PNH abnormality is a favorable factor for response to ATG.[32] Current understanding of the PNH defect is that PIG-A gene mutations are present in normal marrow. In a healthy marrow environment these minor clones have no growth advantage and are eclipsed by the majority of normal stem cells. In conditions of bone marrow failure caused by an immune-mediated process such as MDS and SAA, PIG-A mutations result in a failure of the PNH cell to anchor critical cell surface molecules. As a consequence, PNH cells do not express costimulatory molecules essential for provoking a T-lymphocyte cytolytic attack. In a marrow environment, dominated by strong immune-mediated T-cell damage to myeloid precursors, the possession of a PIG-A mutation would provide a selective growth advantage to the PNH clone which expands to become a significant and persisting subclone. More recent data from our laboratory demonstrating that GPI-anchored protein (AP) positive CD34+ cells were more likely to express apoptotic markers than GPI-anchor-deficient is consistent with this hypothesis.[33] In this and other studies,[34] GPI-AP CD34 cells proliferated normally while GPI-AP-deficient cells showed decreased growth in culture. The overrepresentation of HLA DR15 (the major molecular defined subset of the serologically defined HLA DR2 molecule)[19] suggests an etiological link between some patients with SAA and MDS but provides no further clues to etiology at present. Finally, the natural histories of SAA and MDS overlap – about 5% of patients with SAA successfully responding to immunosuppressive (I/S) treatment develop MDS, which can progress to acute leukemia.[35] Some patients, diagnosed as SAA because they have no dysplastic features, possess minor clones of abnormal karyotype (often trisomy 8) in their marrow. These patients best typify the overlap syndrome of profound marrow failure in the presence of an MDS clonal abnormality.

MDS and large granular lymphocyte proliferative diseases

T-cell LGL leukemia is a clonal disorder of CD8+ T cells associated with bone marrow failure. As in SAA and MDS, many patients respond to CSA treatment, suggesting an immune suppression of the marrow by the T-cell clone.[11,36]. In vitro, the suppression of colony-forming unit–granulocyte, macrophage (CFU-GM) and colony-forming unit–erythroid (CFU-E) by the LGL clone further supports an immune-mediated mechanism for the cytopenia. LGL disease is strongly associated with immune-mediated disorders[37,38] – notably rheumatoid arthritis – and may be the mechanism for neutropenia observed in Felty's syndrome. LGL disease is characterized by a circulating T-cell repertoire dominated by a single CD8+ T-cell clone representing a mixed population of effector-memory and end-effector T cells.

Although often described as leukemia, the condition is indolent, typically with a low burden of LGL cells. The condition is therefore more characteristic of a persisting immune response than of a malignancy, although eventually the LGL T-cell clone can proliferate autonomously. LGL T cells are also found circulating in increased numbers in some patients with MDS and SAA.[39] The occurrence of morphologically similar activated T cells in MDS, SAA, and LGL does not in itself link the diseases etiologically; the finding of clonal or oligoclonal CD8+ T-cell expansions in all of these conditions, together with cases of MDS with diagnostic criteria overlapping with LGL disease suggests that the conditions are somehow linked.[40] We recently described a series of 9 patients with MDS with massive CD8+CD56+ T-cell clonal expansions typical of LGL disease; only 2 responded to ATG and CSA, suggesting that the LGL clonal disorder, presumed responsible for the marrow failure, was difficult to suppress. LGL disease has distinct features which separate it from SAA and MDS: HLA DR4 but not DR15[41] is overrepresented in LGL, marrow failure is rarely profound, and the platelet count is usually normal. Possibly committed progenitors rather than pluripotent stem cells are targets of immune attack in LGL disease.

In vitro progenitor cell inhibition

Several investigators have found that lymphocytes from patients with MDS suppress both erythroid (CFU-E) and granulocytic (CFU-GM) progenitor cell growth.[42] These observations were further refined by Molldrem et al.[43], who showed that the suppressive effect was mediated by CD8+ cells through major histocompatibility complex (MHC) class I molecules on the target. The myelosuppressive effect of autologous T cells on CFU-GM was reduced or completely eliminated following treatment with ATG. Whether the immune response affects both normal and MDS cells was recently addressed by Baumann et al.,[42] who studied hematopoietic colony-forming unit generation by MDS and normal marrow in the presence or absence of autologous lymphocytes. Patients with MDS (but not normal individuals) showed an increased ability to sustain progenitor function in long-term culture. These surviving cells appeared to be derived from residual normal progenitors, suggesting that, while the immune response is induced by the abnormal clone, its effect is on the entire marrow.

Tumor necrosis factor-α (TNF-α) is a key cytokine believed to be responsible for these bystander effects. TNF induces apoptosis through TNF-related

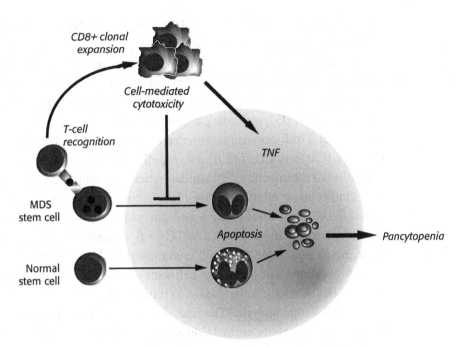

Fig. 6.1   Immune mechanism of pancytopenia in myelodysplastic syndrome (MDS): overexpression of certain myeloid-restricted proteins by MDS progenitor cells leads to their recognition by cytotoxic CD8+ T cells, which undergo clonal expansion. MDS-specific T-cell clones cause direct cytotoxicity to MDS cells as well as apoptosis in normal cells TNF, tumor necrosis factor.

apoptosis-inducing ligand (TRAIL).[44,45] TNF-α production is increased in the marrow of MDS patients and produced, together with interferon-γ (IFN-γ), by the clonally expanded CD8+ T cells in MDS.[46,47] In some series there appears to be a correlation between the French–American–British diagnostic category and TNF expression.[48] These results strongly support the possibility that the bone marrow failure of MDS is mediated by T lymphocytes and provide an immunological explanation for the response of MDS patients to immunosuppression. Figure 6.1 shows a current model of myelosuppressive mechanisms in MDS.

T-cell abnormalities

Better understanding of the significance of T-cell activation markers and the development of techniques to study the T-cell repertoire have advanced our understanding of immune-mediated aspects of MDS. A normal "quiescent" circulating lymphocyte population contains a diverse distribution of thousands of individual clones within 23 currently defined T-cell receptor (TCR) Vβ families. They include balanced CD4+ and CD8+ populations of naive and memory T cells, only a few percent of which express the activation marker CD57, indicating effector T-cell function. During viral infection, clonal T-cell expansions of effector (CD57+, CD27−) and effector-memory (CD57+, CD27+) T cells rapidly emerge and then subside with resolution of the infection.[49,50] Similar patterns of lymphocyte activation are seen in immune-mediated diseases, but, in contrast, the activated expanded clonal T-cell populations can persist for years. Clonal expansions of the T-cell repertoire can be detected by TCR Vβ analysis, which reveals massive enlargement of a single Vβ family containing the clone. Within the Vβ population, the clone can be further defined by complementarity-determining region 3 (CDR3) length analysis – a technique referred to as "spectratyping" or "immunoscope analysis." The analysis is presented as a histogram of CDR3 lengths. Skewing of the normal Gaussian distribution of CDR3 lengths identifies the clonal T-cell population, the clonotype, dominating and expanding a single CDR3 length. Finally, the clone itself can be identified by TCR sequencing.

In MDS, clonal T-cell expansions are commonly found by these techniques.[51–53] The most frequent pattern is one of oligoclonal expansion in CD8+ T cells overexpressing CD57. CD4+ T cells may express activation markers but show no skewing and no consistent Vβ expansion.[41,52] In contrast to LGL disease, where over 90% of circulating CD8+ T cells represent a singe clone, the size of the expanded clone is more usually in the order of 1–10%.[54] While these studies confirm that oligoclonal CD8+ T-cell expansion is common in MDS and likely are causally linked with a myelosuppressive immune-mediated process, to establish that clonal T-cell expansions directly induce myelosuppression requires functional tests such as colony inhibition assays. In our recent work, we focused on immunosuppressive mechanisms in MDS with the cytogenetic abnormality, trisomy-8.[55] Trisomy-8 disease is characterized by large CD8+ clonal T-cell expansions. Myelosuppressive behavior is restricted to the clonally expanded CD8+T cells, which induce apoptotic changes in trisomy-8 cells and inhibit trisomy-8 CFU-GM formation, while leaving the karyotypically normal bone marrow cells relatively unaffected. Furthermore, analysis of surviving colonies in the inhibition assay by fluorescence in situ hybridization (FISH) to identify normal and trisomy-8 colonies showed that the cytotoxic T-cell clones primarily targeted the trisomy-8 progenitors and spared normal CFU-GM (Fig. 6.2).

Trisomy-8 patients usually respond to ATG treatment with significant improvements in blood counts and a reduced transfusion requirement but many require continued treatment with CSA to maintain counts. FISH analysis of marrow from hematological responders showed increased proportions of trisomy-8 cells following treatment and decreased numbers when immunosuppression was discontinued. This indicates that, at least in this MDS subtype, there appear to be trisomy-8-specific T cells that target the cytogenetically abnormal progenitors. Normal marrow may also be targeted and suppressed, either through epitope spreading or as innocent bystanders by cytokines produced by activated T cells. However, it appears that ATG treatment removes an immune block to both MDS and normal marrow cell proliferation.

What are the antigens inducing T-cell responses in MDS?

The antigens produced by MDS cells that induce a T-cell response are unknown. Recent attention has focused on the cancer-embryonic antigen Wilms tumor 1 (*WT1*), which is typically overexpressed in MDS and becomes increasingly expressed as the disease advances. T cells recognizing *WT1* are increased in frequency in MDS.[56–61] Recently dramatic hematological responses were reported in patients with advanced MDS receiving a *WT1* peptide vaccine, suggesting that the antigen is an important target of autoreactive T cells. The primary azurophil granule proteins of granulocyte precursors, elastase, proteinase 3, and cathepsin G, are also aberrantly expressed in MDS.[62] Both elastase and proteinase 3 contain the peptide sequence PR1 found to elicit high-affinity cytotoxic lymphocytes with specificity for myeloid leukemia cells.[63] In trisomy-8 MDS, the presence of three copies of chromosome 8 invites speculation that proteins normally expressed on chromosome 8 are overexpressed because of their increased representation.[64] Both *c-myc* located on chromosome 8 and the gene for cyclin D1 on chromosome 11 are overexpressed in trisomy-8 and are potential candidates for overexpressed autoantigens.

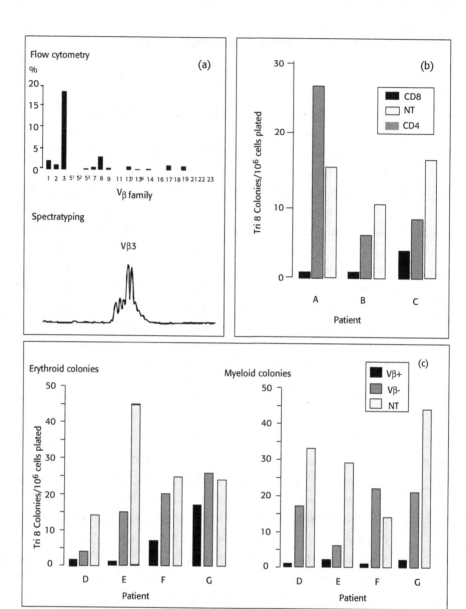

Fig. 6.2   Clonally expanded CD8+ T cells specifically inhibit trisomy-8 hematopoiesis (a) T-cell
receptor analysis in a patient with trisomy 8 myelodysplastic syndrome (MDS) showing
massive expansion of Vβ3 shown by spectratyping to consist of two dominant clono-
types. (b) Specific inhibition of trisomy-8 (Tri 8) granulocyte progenitors (colony-forming
unit–granulocyte, macrophage) (identified by fluorescent in situ hybridization) by CD8+
fractionated T cells, but not by CD4 cells, or non-MDS, unrelated T cells (NT); (3 patients
studied). (c) Specific inhibition of trisomy-8 erythroid and myeloid colony formation by
the selected expanded Vβ family in 4 patients with trisomy-8. Controls are the non-
expanded Vβ families and non-trisomy-8 allogeneic T cells (NT).

Current research focuses on the identification of T cells with specificity for these proteins in MDS. However, there is no evidence directly linking any of these defined proteins with the immune-mediated process in MDS. Finding the antigens recognized by expanded T-cell clones in MDS is challenging but could be achieved by screening these T cells against a universal combinatorial peptide library, representing every possible variation of amino acid sequences in a nine-mer peptide. By identifying target peptides, their parent protein could be identified by sequence matching.

The immune-mediated response to MDS – immune surveillance against a malignant cell?

The occurrence in MDS of an immune response powerful enough to suppress bone marrow function raises the possibility that the clonal stem cell disorder is constrained by a vigilant cell-mediated immune response. Such a T-cell response could control the expansion of dysplastic clones and delay or even prevent progression to leukemia. The expression of a number of tumor-associated antigens by MDS cells supports this hypothesis. This possibility, in turn, raises the concern that immunosuppression could interrupt a protective immune-mediated process that prevents progression of MDS to acute leukemia. It is now clear, for reasons not understood, that leukemic progression is uncommon in ATG responders[18]; in fact, response to ATG is a favorable factor for survival in two studies. It seems unlikely that ATG is itself protective against leukemic progression; more probably, response to ATG occurs in a subgroup of individuals with MDS in whom the disease process is dominated by marrow failure, with little tendency to evolve to leukemia. It still remains to be determined whether immunosuppression favorably influences survival in all MDS subtypes, but currently there is no evidence that ATG has a deleterious effect on survival.

Immune selection could favor the emergence of resistant clones. Trisomy-8 cells are relatively resistant to T-cell-mediated cytotoxicity, raising the possibility that the karyotypic abnormality is selected by immune pressure. We have experimental evidence showing that, although trisomy-8 progenitors express apoptotic markers, they continue to survive and proliferate. Somewhat paradoxically, trisomy-8 patients usually respond favorably to ATG immunosuppression (in a recent analysis, 10 of 17 trisomy-8 patients were responders). After ATG treatment, trisomy-8 cells persist, but hematopoeisis is restored, presumably because suppression of the immune response removed inhibition to residual normal and trisomy-8 cells alike.[65] In the absence of immune suppression, the clonally abnormal trisomy-8 cells can sustain normal hematopoiesis. In this sense, trisomy 8 mimics the chronic phase of chronic myeloid leukemia – a condition where myelopoiesis is normal enough to maintain marrow function, despite the tendency to further clonal progression as the disease advances. Some of the typical morphological changes seen in MDS (hypogranular neutrophils, abnormal megakaryocytes, and dyserythropoiesis) may be, at least in part, the result of T-cell-mediated damage and not intrinsic to the abnormal genome of the MDS cell.

Clinical trials of immunosuppression in MDS

Although in the 1980s a number of case reports indicated that patients with MDS could respond to immunosuppressive treatments, general interest in the use of immunosuppressive therapy in MDS followed the first prospective trials with ATG in 1997[9,10] and with CSA in 1998.[11] There are now published data on over 250 patients treated with immunosuppression in clinical protocols from over 10 centers worldwide.[12–14,16,66–70] Most experience is with ATG-based treatment but some investigators, mainly in Japan, have continued to study CSA.

ATG-based treatments

In 2002, we reported a long-term follow-up of 61 patients with MDS treated with horse ATG.[10] ATG, 40 mg/kg of body weight, was given daily for 4 days. In this non-randomized, single-treatment study, 21 of 61 patients (34%) no longer required red blood cell transfusions within 8 months of treatment. Independence from transfusion was maintained in 17 responders (81%) for a median of 36 months (range, 3–72 months). Ten of 21 patients (47.5%) with severe thrombocytopenia had sustained platelet count increases, and 6 of 11 patients (55%) with severe neutropenia had sustained neutrophil counts of greater than 1×10^9 cells/l. Characteristics favorable for response were younger patient age ($P = 0.005$) and lower platelet counts ($P = 0.038$). Only one of the 21 responders (5%) but 22 of the 40 non-responders (55%) died before the end of the study ($P = 0.008$). One of the 21 responders (5%) and 13 of the 40 non-responders (33%) had disease progression

($P = 0.086$). Thus, ATG response was associated with significantly longer survival and an almost significant decreased time to disease progression. Treatment with ATG also appeared to be beneficial because median survivals of non-responders were similar to those reported from a large multicenter study, while survival of responders was superior. Subsequently, Killick *et al.*[12] treated "low-risk" patients with MDS with ATG. Of 30 patients entering the study, 20 patients (13 with refractory anemia (RA), 4 with RA with excess blasts (RAEB), and 3 with RA with ringed sideroblasts (RARS); mean age 55 years) survived and were evaluable at 6 months. The bone marrow was hypocellular in 8 cases and cytogenetics were abnormal in 4. Patients received horse ATG for 5 days. Ten patients (50%) responded to treatment and became transfusion-independent; 8 of 13 (62%) had RA. The median duration of response was 15.5 months (2–42+ months) at the time of analysis. This study emphasized the favorable response and progression-free survival of patients with less advanced MDS, but there was high mortality and progression to leukemia of patients in the first few months after treatment.

In a trial at the MD Anderson Hospital, Yazji *et al.*[13] described the use of horse ATG 40 mg/kg per day plus methylprednisone 1 mg/kg for 4 days, followed by oral CSA daily for 6 months to treat 31 patients, 18 with RA or RARS, and 13 with more advanced MDS, including 1 with chronic myelomonocytic leukemia (CMML) (median age 59, range 28–79 years). Four (2 RA, 2 RARS) had a complete and 1 (RAEB) a partial remission (16% of total); 3 of these responses were durable remissions (12–60+ months). These rather disappointing findings do not support a potential benefit of combining ATG with other immunosuppressive treatments.

Aivado *et al.*[69] from Dusseldorf treated 10 female patients with low-risk MDS with antilymphocyte globulin (ALG) or ATG; four responded and all had a "non-clonal" marrow identified by X chromosome inactivation patterns (XCIP), evidence of a considerable residual population of normal hematopoiesis. They suggested that such patients responded because immunosuppression improved normal haemopoiesis by relieving immunological pressure on innocent bystanders. In contrast, Steensma *et al.*[70] from the Mayo Clinic found no responses, and considerable toxicity in 8 MDS patients (2 RA and 5 RAEB) treated with ATG, 40 mg/kg per day for

Table 6.2 Clinical trials of antithymocyte globulin (ATG) to treat cytopenias in myelodysplastic syndrome

Center	n	Median age	RA, n (%)	Response n (%)	Response RA %	Median duration response (months)	Comment
National Institutes of Health[10]	61	60	37 (61)	21 (33)	67	> 60	RA, RARS, RAEB-T
London[12]	30	54.5	13 (65)	10 (50)	62	15.5	Only 20 patients evaluable for response
MD Anderson[13]	31	59	18[a] (58)	4 (16)	11	12–60	ATG + CSA + MP
Düsseldorf[69]	10	59	7	4 (40)	28	–	Only non-clonal patients responded
Mayo Clinic[70]	8	71	2	0	0	–	ATG too toxic for general use
Total	140			39 (28%)			

RA, refractory anemia; RARS, RA with ringed sideroblasts; RAEB-T, RA with excess blasts in transformation; ATG, antithymocyte globulin; CSA, ciclosporin; MP, methylprednisolone.
[a]RA + RARS combined.

4 days; they concluded that the side-effects from ATG outweighed any therapeutic advantage in an unselected MDS population and urged that ATG should only be recommended when better prognostic indicators become available. Ganser *et al.* recently reported that treatment of 35 patients with MDS with either rabbit or horse ATG yielded responses only in patients with RA. Geary *et al.* from Manchester UK[71] reported the use of ATG with CSA or oxymetholone in 13 patients presenting with SAA with an abnormal cytogenetic clone, but without morphological features of MDS. All patients ultimately responded to immunosuppression (with or without androgens); 3 patients relapsed into aplasia. No patient transformed to MDS after a median follow-up of 4.1 years and in 4 patients, the cytogenetic clone disappeared after treatment. This study in patients in an overlap category of SAA/MDS supports the hypothesis that the best results occur in the most hypoplastic patients (Table 6.2). In summary, of 140 patients reported,

Table 6.3 Clinical trials of ciclosporin to treat cytopenias in myelodysplastic syndromes

Investigators	n	Response n (%)	Comment
Jonasova et al.[11]	17	14 (82)	Transfusion-independence
Shimamoto et al.[68]	50	30 (60)	Multicenter study
Yamada et al.[72]	18	6 (33)	Cyclosporin + methylprednisone
Miyata et al.[73]	8	4 (50)	
Catalano et al.[66]	11	8 (72)	Prolonged partial responses
Atoyebi et al.[67]	6	0	Unacceptable toxicity
Total	110	62 (56%)	

hematological responses, usually including transfusion-independence, were observed in 39 (28%) cases.

Cyclosporin-based treatments

Jonasova et al.[11] treated 17 cytopenic patients with RA with variable bone marrow cellularity. "Substantial" and sustained haematological response was observed in 14 (82%); anemia improved and all transfusion-dependent patients achieved transfusion-independence. Complete trilineage recovery occurred in 4 patients (23%). CSA was well tolerated in 14 patients but serious side-effects required termination of the therapy in 3, with subsequent loss of the hematological response. In later trials lower response rates to CSA were reported. In a large multicenter study from Japan[68] of 50 patients with variable marrow cellularity (47 RA, 41 of intermediate 1: International Prognostic Scoring System score), hematological improvement occurred in 30 patients (60% all RA). Yamada et al.[72] reported responses to combinations of pulsed methylprednisolone and CSA in 6 of 18 patients (33%), including 3 of 10 patients with RA. Miyata et al.[73] reported improvement in cytopenia in 4 of 8 patients (50%). Prolonged but partial hematologic improvement was seen in 8 of 11 hypoplastic MDS patients treated by Catalano et al.[66] In contrast, Atoyebi et al.[67] found no responses and unacceptable toxicity in 6 patients treated with CSA. Together these findings indicate a potential role for CSA in the treatment of MDS (Table 6.3). Of 110 patients reported, 62 (56%) showed some hematologic response to CSA, but response criteria differ significantly among the studies.

Table 6.4 Predictive factors for a response to immunosuppression with antithymocyte globulin ± other agents[9,10,18,20,74]

Factor	Favorable characteristic	Unfavorable
Age	Younger age, age < 60 years	> 60 years
Transfusion duration	Short interval	Prolonged
HLA-DR	HLA-DR15	Other
MDS subtype	RA, IPSS intermediate-1	RARS, RAEB-T, CMML
Karyotype	Trisomy-8, normal	Other karyotypes
Other	Pancytopenia, PNH hypocellular marrow	Single-lineage cytopenia hypercellular marrow

HLA, human leukocyte antigen; MDS, myelodysplastic syndrome; RA, refractory anemia; IPSS, International Prognostic Scoring System; RARS, RA with ringed sideroblasts; RAEB-T, RA with excess blasts in transformation; CMML, chronic myelomonocytic leukemia; PNH, paroxysmal nocturnal hemoglobinuria clone.

Cytokine antagonists

Several reports of trials using antagonists to TNF-α indicate that the TNF-α receptor blockers, thalidomide and its derivatives are efficacious in a low proportion of patients with MDS. The use of TNF antagonists to treat MDS is dealt with fully in Chapter 7.

Predicting response to immunosuppressive therapy

Analysis of factors predicting outcome has been possible in several large immunosuppressive treatment trials (Table 6.4). In general, severe cytopenia, marrow hypocellularity, younger age, a diagnosis of RA, and absence of karyotypic abnormality are favorable factors for hematological response. Two studies found that patients with PNH clone expansions had a high probability of responding to immunosuppression.[19,32] The presence of PNH clones may be a consequence of immune selection of cells insensitive to T-cell suppression, and thus a reliable marker of immune-mediated cytopenia and therefore hematological response to ATG (see above). In the National Institutes of Health series of 61 patients, the quality of response was better in patients with the lowest platelet and neutrophil counts (Fig. 6.2). Factors predictive for response appear to be the same for treatment with either ATG

Table 6.5 A simplified score for predicting response to antithymocyte globulin-based immunosuppression[74]

Score		Predicted probability of response	
HLA-DR15-negative	HLA-DR15-positive	Category	Response
Patient's age in years + duration of red cell transfusion dependence (months)			
58	> 72	Low	0–40%
50–58	64–72	Intermediate	41–70%
< 50	< 64	High	71–100%

HLA, human leukocyte antigen.

or CSA. There is an impression that ATG achieves responses more frequently than does CSA. However whether ATG is superior to ATG + CSA or CSA alone has not been determined prospectively.

Recently the ability to predict response to immune suppression has been improved by two observations. First, HLA-DR15 either as a single or double allele is an independent factor predicting response.[20] We found that HLA-DR15 was significantly increased in the MDS population when compared with controls or patients with SAA and that a disproportionate number of individuals with HLA-DR15 responded to immunosuppression with ATG or ATG + CSA. A simple algorithm combining patient age and duration of transfusion-dependence in months prior to immunosuppressive treatment, coupled with HLA-DR15 status, can be used to predict response with 90% accuracy (Table 6.5).[74] Previously described prognostic factors, such as a diagnosis of RA, degree of cytopenia, or karyotype, are not incorrect or irrelevant; more likely they are dependent variables incorporated by the predictive formula. Patients with trisomy 8 were generally in the high probability of response group while those with monosomy 7 were in the low probability of response group.[65] The general applicability of the algorithm requires further prospective testing. In a recent analysis[75] we applied the formula to discriminate between different forms of immunosuppression. Seventy-seven patients receiving ATG alone were compared with 32 patients receiving CSA + ATG or 15 receiving CSA alone. The CSA-alone favorable prognostic group had a significantly lower probability of being responders

($P < 0.01$) than did cohorts in which ATG was used, but there was no difference in response rate between those receiving ATG alone and those receiving CSA + ATG. These findings suggest that ATG is a more effective agent than CSA and that further intensification of immunosuppression will not recruit more responders.[65]

Current issues and problems

Response definition

Because different investigators have developed their own definitions for hematological response, detailed comparisons are not possible between reported trials. Several difficulties are encountered in evaluating published data. First is the notorious diversity of age, subtypes, marrow cellularity, and degree of progression contained within the diagnosis MDS which create different case-mixes. Second is the variability within the type and degree of cytopenia encountered in MDS: some patients may have red cell transfusion-dependence without cytopenia in other lineages, while others have pancytopenia. Additionally the degree of cytopenia may be clinically insignificant (e.g., neutrophil counts over 500/mm^3 and platelet counts over 20 000/mm^3) or life-threatening. Finally some investigators describe improvements in blood counts that are not of clinical significance – either because the cytopenias were not severe prior to treatment or because the increase in very low counts observed was insufficient for clinical improvement. Sustained red cell transfusion-dependence remains the most reliable comparator. It would be important to derive broadly accepted criteria for hematological and clinical response to immunosuppression. For example, only clinically significant cytopenias would be included in response definitions (red cell transfusion-dependence, platelets $< 20\,000$/mm^3 with or without transfusion-dependence, neutrophils < 500/mm^3 with or without neutropenic infections). A response in each lineage would then include any of the following, sustained for at least 8 weeks: red cell transfusion-independence, platelet count sustained $> 20\,000$/mm^3, neutrophil response sustained > 500/mm^3. An international working group to standardize criteria in MDS has brought much-needed order to this issue and their guidelines currently provide the best system for reporting response data in MDS.[27,76]

Patient selection, treatment monitoring, and optimization
of immunosuppressive treatment

If generally applicable, the response prediction score should allow us to
focus immunosuppressive treatment on the patient group most likely to
benefit. Other biological markers of immune dysfunction such as clonal
skewing of the CD8+ T-cell repertoire might also help to define patients
in whom cytopenia is immune-mediated and who would therefore respond
to immunosuppressive drugs. Monitoring the T-cell repertoire after treatment may determine the mechanism of treatment response or failure. In
some cases, even after an immune-mediated process is suppressed, marrow
function may remain compromised because of extinction of residual normal hematopoietic progenitors or the inability of dysplastic hematopoiesis
to maintain hematopoietic function. Alternatively, cytopenia could persist
because the immune-mediated response was inadequately or only transiently
suppressed by the treatment. Currently, ATG, ALG, CSA, and TNF inhibitors
all show activity in MDS. New clinical trials are needed to determine whether
combinations of these agents would be more effective.

Summary and future directions

A substantial proportion of patients with MDS have an immune-mediated
process suppression of bone marrow function. Improved hematopoiesis after
immunosuppressive treatment can significantly improve their quality of life.
New algorithms allow the very precise selection of patients likely to benefit from this therapy. However, much remains to be understood about the
nature of the immune-mediated process, in particular the way in which
the immune system interacts with the preleukemia T-cell hematopoietic
progenitor cell clones. These studies should not only allow us to optimize immunosuppressive treatment for the marrow failure of MDS but
may also lead to a better understanding of how the immune system regulates myeloid malignancies. It may thus be possible ultimately to learn from
the natural immune responses to myeloid cells in MDS which key antigens could be targeted by T cells to prevent or treat myeloid leukemias in
future immunotherapy approaches using vaccines or adoptively transferred T
cells.

REFERENCES

1. Mathe, G. and Schwarzenberg, L. (1976). Treatment of bone marrow aplasia by bone marrow graft after conditioning with antilymphocyte globulin. Long term results. *Exp. Hematol.*, **4**, 256–64.

2. Jeannet, M., Speck, B., Rubinstein, A. *et al.* (1976). Autologous marrow reconstitutions in severe aplastic anaemia after ALG pretreatment and HL-A semi-incompatible bone marrow cell transfusion. *Acta Haematol.*, **55**, 129–39.

3. Speck, B. and Kissling, M. (1973). Studies on bone marrow transplantation in experimental ^{32}P-induced aplastic anemia after conditioning with antilymphocyte serum. *Acta Haematol.*, **50**, 193–9.

4. Ascensao, J., Pahwa, R., Kagan, W. *et al.* (1976). Aplastic anaemia: evidence for an immunological mechanism. *Lancet.*, **1**, 669–71.

5. Gluckman, E., Devergie, A., Faille, A. *et al.* (1979). Antilymphocyte globulin treatment in severe aplastic anemia – comparison with bone marrow transplantation. Report of 60 cases. *Haematol. Blood Transfus.*, **24**, 171–9.

6. Young, N., Griffith, P., Brittain, E. *et al.* (1988). A multicenter trial of antithymocyte globulin in aplastic anemia and related diseases. *Blood*, **72**, 1861–9.

7. Biesma, D. H., van den Tweel, J. G., and Verdonck, L. F. (1997). Immunosuppressive therapy for hypoplastic myelodysplastic syndrome. *Cancer*, **79**, 1548–51.

8. Tichelli, A., Gratwohl, A., Wuersch, A., Nissen, C., and Speck, B. (1988). Antilymphocyte globulin for myelodysplastic syndrome. *Br. J. Haematol.*, **68**, 139–40.

9. Molldrem, J. J., Caples, M., Mavroudis, D. *et al.* (1997). Antithymocyte globulin for patients with myelodysplastic syndrome. *Br. J. Haematol.*, **99**, 699–705.

10. Molldrem, J. J., Leifer, E., Bahceci, E. *et al.* (2002). Antithymocyte globulin for treatment of the bone marrow failure associated with myelodysplastic syndromes. *Ann. Intern. Med.*, **137**, 156–63.

11. Jonasova, A., Neuwirtova, R., Cermak, J. *et al.* (1998). Cyclosporin A therapy in hypoplastic MDS patients and certain refractory anaemias without hypoplastic bone marrow. *Br. J. Haematol.*, **100**, 304–9.

12. Killick, S. B., Mufti, G., Cavenagh, J. D. *et al.* (2003). A pilot study of antithymocyte globulin (ATG) in the treatment of patients with 'low-risk' myelodysplasia. *Br. J. Haematol.*, **120**, 679–84.

13. Yazji, S., Giles, F. J., Tsimberidou, A. M. *et al.* (2003). Antithymocyte globulin (ATG)-based therapy in patients with myelodysplastic syndromes. *Leukemia*, **17**, 2101–6.

14. Grigg, A. P. and O'Flaherty, E. (2001). Cyclosporin A for the treatment of pure red cell aplasia associated with myelodysplasia. *Leuk. Lymphoma*, **42**, 1339–42.

15. Billstrom, R., Johansson, H., Johansson, B., and Mitelman, F. (1995). Immune-mediated complications in patients with myelodysplastic syndromes – clinical and cytogenetic features. *Eur. J. Haematol.*, **55**, 42–8.

16. Shimamoto, T. and Ohyashiki, K. (2003). Immunosuppressive treatments for myelodysplastic syndromes. *Leuk. Lymphoma*, **44**, 593–604.

17. Hamblin, T. J. (1987). Myelodysplasia. *Br. J. Hosp. Med.*, **38**, 558–61.

18. Barrett, J., Saunthararajah, Y., and Molldrem, J. (2000). Myelodysplastic syndrome and aplastic anemia: distinct entities or diseases linked by a common pathophysiology? *Semin. Hematol.*, **37**, 15–29.

19. Maciejewski, J. P., Rivera, C., Kook, H., Dunn, D., and Young, N. S. (2001). Relationship between bone marrow failure syndromes and the presence of glycophosphatidyl inositol-anchored protein-deficient clones. *Br. J. Haematol.*, **115**, 1015–22.

20. Saunthararajah, Y., Nakamura, R., Nam, J. M. *et al.* (2002). HLA-DR15 (DR2) is overrepresented in myelodysplastic syndrome and aplastic anemia and predicts a response to immunosuppression in myelodysplastic syndrome. *Blood*, **100**, 1570–4.

21. Tuzuner, N., Cox, C., Rowe, J. M., and Bennett, J. M. (1994). Bone marrow cellularity in myeloid stem cell disorders: impact of age correction. *Leuk. Res.*, **18**, 559–64.

22. Dan, K., An, E., Futaki, M. *et al.* (1993). Megakaryocyte, erythroid and granulocyte-macrophage colony formation in myelodysplastic syndromes. *Acta Haematol.*, **89**, 113–18.

23. Maciejewski, J. P., Kim, S., Sloand, E., Selleri, C., and Young, N. S. (2000). Sustained long-term hematologic recovery despite a marked quantitative defect in the stem cell compartment of patients with aplastic anemia after immunosuppressive therapy. *Am. J. Hematol.*, **65**, 123–31.

24. Maciejewski, J. P., Risitano, A., Sloand, E. M., Nunez, O., and Young, N. S. (2002). Distinct clinical outcomes for cytogenetic abnormalities evolving from aplastic anemia. *Blood*, **99**, 3129–35.

25. Cherry, A. M., Brockman, S. R., Paternoster, S. F. *et al.* (2003). Comparison of interphase FISH and metaphase cytogenetics to study myelodysplastic syndrome: an Eastern Cooperative Oncology Group (ECOG) study. *Leuk. Res.*, **27**, 1085–90.

26. Fenaux, P. (2001). Chromosome and molecular abnormalities in myelodysplastic syndromes. *Int. J. Hematol.*, **73**, 429–37.

27. Cheson, B. D., Bennett, J. M., Kantarjian, H. *et al.* (2001). Myelodysplastic syndromes standardized response criteria: further definition. *Blood*, **98**, 1985.

28. Rosenfeld, S., Follmann, D., Nunez, O., and Young, N. S. (2003). Antithymocyte globulin and cyclosporine for severe aplastic anemia: association between hematologic response and long-term outcome. *J.A.M.A.*, **289**, 1130–5.

29. Shimamoto, T., Iguchi, T., Ando, K. *et al.* (2001). Successful treatment with cyclosporin A for myelodysplastic syndrome with erythroid hypoplasia associated with T-cell receptor gene rearrangements. *Br. J. Haematol.*, **114**, 358–61.

30. Young, N. S. (1992). The problem of clonality in aplastic anemia: Dr Dameshek's riddle, restated. *Blood*, **79**, 1385–92.

31. Young, N. S. and Maciejewski, J. P. (2000). Genetic and environmental effects in paroxysmal nocturnal hemoglobinuria: this little PIG-A goes "why? why? why?" *J. Clin. Invest.*, **106**, 637–41.

32. Dunn, D. E., Tanawattanacharoen, P., Boccuni, P. *et al.* (1999). Paroxysmal nocturnal hemoglobinuria cells in patients with bone marrow failure syndromes. *Ann. Intern. Med.*, **131**, 401–8.

33. Chen, G., Kirby, M., Zeng, W., Young, N. S., and Maciejewski, J. P. (2002). Superior growth of glycophosphatidy linositol-anchored protein-deficient progenitor cells in vitro is due to the higher apoptotic rate of progenitors with normal phenotype in vivo (abstract). *Exp. Hematol.*, **30**, 774–82.

34. Chen, R., Nagarajan, S., Prince, G. M. *et al.* (2000). Impaired growth and elevated *FAS* receptor expression in PIGA(+) stem cells in primary paroxysmal nocturnal hemoglobinuria. *J. Clin. Invest.*, **106**, 689–96.

35. Rosenfeld, S., Follmann, D., Nunez, O., and Young, N. S. (2003). Antithymocyte globulin and cyclosporine for severe aplastic anemia: association between hematologic response and long-term outcome. *J.A.M.A.*, **289**, 1130–5.

36. Gabor, E. P., Mishalani, S., and Lee, S. (1996). Rapid response to cyclosporine therapy and sustained remission in large granular lymphocyte leukemia. *Blood*, **87**, 1199–200.

37. Wallis, W. J., Loughran, T. P., Jr., Kadin, M. E., Clark, E. A., and Starkebaum, G. A. (1985). Polyarthritis and neutropenia associated with circulating large granular lymphocytes. *Ann. Intern. Med.*, **103**, 357–62.

38. Bassan, R., Pronesti, M., Buzzetti, M. *et al.* (1989). Autoimmunity and B-cell dysfunction in chronic proliferative disorders of large granular lymphocytes/natural killer cells. *Cancer*, **63**, 90–5.

39. Akashi, K., Shibuya, T., Taniguchi, S. *et al.* (1999). Multiple autoimmune haemopoietic disorders and insidious clonal proliferation of large granular lymphocytes. *Br. J. Haematol.*, **107**, 670–3.

40. Saunthararajah, Y., Molldrem, J. L., Rivera, M. *et al.* (2001). Coincident myelodysplastic syndrome and T-cell large granular lymphocytic disease: clinical and pathophysiological features. *Br. J. Haematol.*, **112**, 195–200.

41. Battiwalla, M., Melenhorst, J., Saunthararajah, Y. *et al.* (2003). HLA-DR4 predicts haematological response to cyclosporine in T-large granular lymphocyte lymphoproliferative disorders. *Br. J. Haematol.*, **123**, 449–53.

42. Baumann, I., Scheid, C., Koref, M. S. *et al.* (2002). Autologous lymphocytes inhibit hemopoiesis in long-term culture in patients with myelodysplastic syndrome. *Exp. Hematol.*, **30**, 1405–11.

43. Molldrem, J. J., Jiang, Y. Z., Stetler-Stevenson, M. *et al.* (1998). Haematological response of patients with myelodysplastic syndrome to antithymocyte globulin is associated with a loss of lymphocyte-mediated inhibition of CFU-GM and alterations in T-cell receptor Vbeta profiles. *Br. J. Haematol.*, **102**, 1314–22.

44. Greil, R., Anether, G., Johrer, K., and Tinhofer, I. (2003). Tuning the rheostat of the myelopoietic system via *Fas* and TRAIL. *Crit. Rev. Immunol.*, **23**, 301–22.

45. Plasilova, M., Zivny, J., Jelinek, J. *et al.* (2002). TRAIL (Apo2L) suppresses growth of primary human leukemia and myelodysplasia progenitors. *Leukemia*, **16**, 67–73.

46. Koike, M., Ishiyama, T., Tomoyasu, S., and Tsuruoka, N. (1995). Spontaneous cytokine overproduction by peripheral blood mononuclear cells from patients with myelodysplastic syndromes and aplastic anemia. *Leuk. Res.*, **19**, 639–44.

47. Kitagawa, M., Saito, I., Kuwata, T. *et al.* (1997). Overexpression of tumor necrosis factor (TNF)-alpha and interferon (IFN)-gamma by bone marrow cells from patients with myelodysplastic syndromes. *Leukemia*, **11**, 2049–54.

48. Gersuk, G. M., Beckham, C., Loken, M. R. *et al.* (1998). A role for tumour necrosis factor-alpha, *Fas* and *Fas*-ligand in marrow failure associated with myelodysplastic syndrome. *Br. J. Haematol.*, **103**, 176–88.

49. Seaman, M. S., Peyerl, F. W., Jackson, S. S. *et al.* (2004). Subsets of memory cytotoxic T lymphocytes elicited by vaccination influence the efficiency of secondary expansion in vivo. *J. Virol.*, **78**, 206–15.

50. Lima, M., Teixeira, M. A., Queiros, M. L. *et al.* (2003). Immunophenotype and TCR-Vbeta repertoire of peripheral blood T-cells in acute infectious mononucleosis. *Blood Cells Mol. Dis.*, **30**, 1–12.

51. Epperson, D. E., Nakamura, R., Saunthararajah, Y. *et al.* (2001). Oligoclonal T cell expansion in myelodysplastic syndrome: evidence for an autoimmune process. *Leuk. Res.*, **25**, 1075–83.

52. Melenhorst, J. J., Eniafe, R., Follmann, D. *et al.* (2002). Molecular and flow cytometric characterization of the CD4 and CD8 T-cell repertoire in patients with myelodysplastic syndrome. *Br. J. Haematol.*, **119**, 97–105.

53. Plasilova, M., Risitano, A., and Maciejewski, J. P. (2003). Application of the molecular analysis of the T-cell receptor repertoire in the study of immune-mediated hematologic diseases. *Hematology*, **8**, 173–81.

54. Melenhorst, J. J., Eniafe, R., Follmann, D. *et al.* (2003). T-cell large granular lymphocyte leukemia is characterized by massive TCRBV-restricted clonal CD8 expansion and a generalized overexpression of the effector cell marker CD57. *Hematol. J.*, **4**, 18–25.

55. Sloand, E. M., Kim, S., Fuhrer, M. *et al.* (2002). Fas-mediated apoptosis is important in regulating cell replication and death in trisomy 8 hematopoietic cells but not in cells with other cytogenetic abnormalities. *Blood*, **100**, 4427–32.

56. Oka, Y., Tsuboi, A., Murakami, M. *et al.* (2003). Wilms tumor gene peptide-based immunotherapy for patients with overt leukemia from myelodysplastic syndrome (MDS) or MDS with myelofibrosis. *Int. J. Hematol.*, **78**, 56–61.

57. Cilloni, D., Gottardi, E., Messa, F. *et al.* (2003). Significant correlation between the degree of *WT1* expression and the International Prognostic Scoring System Score in patients with myelodysplastic syndromes. *J. Clin. Oncol.*, **21**, 1988–95.

58. Elisseeva, O. A., Oka, Y., Tsuboi, A. *et al.* (2002). Humoral immune responses against Wilms tumor gene *WT1* product in patients with hematopoietic malignancies. *Blood*, **99**, 3272–9.

59. Hosoya, N., Miyagawa, K., Mitani, K., Yazaki, Y., and Hirai, H. (1998). Mutation analysis of the *WT1* gene in myelodysplastic syndromes. *Jpn J. Cancer Res.*, **89**, 821–4.

60. Rosenfeld, C., Cheever, M. A., and Gaiger, A. (2003). WT1 in acute leukemia, chronic myelogenous leukemia and myelodysplastic syndrome: therapeutic potential of *WT1* targeted therapies. *Leukemia*, **17**, 1301–12.

61. Tamaki, H., Ogawa, H., Ohyashiki, K. *et al.* (1999). The Wilms' tumor gene *WT1* is a good marker for diagnosis of disease progression of myelodysplastic syndromes. *Leukemia*, **13**, 393–9.

62. Klasa, R. J., List, A. F., and Cheson, B. D. (2001). Rational approaches to design of therapeutics targeting molecular markers. *Hematology (Am. Soc. Hematol. Educ. Program)*, 443–62.

63. Kochenderfer, J. N. and Molldrem, J. J. (2001). Leukemia vaccines. *Curr. Oncol. Rep.*, **3**, 193–200.

64. Virtaneva, K., Wright, F. A., Tanner, S. M. *et al.* (2001). Expression profiling reveals fundamental biological differences in acute myeloid leukemia with isolated trisomy 8 and normal cytogenetics. *Proc. Natl Acad. Sci. U.S.A.*, **98**, 1124–9.

65. Sloand, E. M., Mainwaring, L., Fuhrer, M. *et al.* (2005). Preferential suppression of trisomy 8 versus normal hematopoietic cell growth by autologous lymphocytes in patients with trisomy 8 versus normal hematopoietic cell growth by autholo-gous lymphocytes in patients with trisomy 8 myelodysplastic syndrome. *Blood*, **106**, 841–51.

66. Catalano, L., Selleri, C., Califano, C. *et al.* (2000). Prolonged response to cyclosporin-A in hypoplastic refractory anemia and correlation with in vitro studies. *Haematologica*, **85**, 133–8.

67. Atoyebi, W., Bywater, L., Rawlings, L., Brunskill, S., and Littlewood, T. J. (2002). Treatment of myelodysplasia with oral cyclosporin. *Clin. Lab. Haematol.*, **24**, 211–14.

68. Shimamoto, T., Tohyama, K., Okamoto, T. *et al.* (2003). Cyclosporin A therapy for patients with myelodysplastic syndrome: multicenter pilot studies in Japan. *Leuk. Res.*, **27**, 783–8.

69. Aivado, M., Rong, A., Stadler, M. *et al.* (2002). Favourable response to antithymocyte or antilymphocyte globulin in low-risk myelodysplastic syndrome patients with a 'non-clonal' pattern of X-chromosome inactivation in bone marrow cells. *Eur. J. Haematol.*, **68**, 210–16.

70. Steensma, D. P., Dispenzieri, A., Moore, S. B., Schroeder, G., and Tefferi, A. (2003). Antithymocyte globulin has limited efficacy and substantial toxicity in unselected anemic patients with myelodysplastic syndrome. *Blood*, **101**, 2156–8.

71. Geary, C. G., Harrison, C. J., Philpott, N. J. *et al.* (1999). Abnormal cytogenetic clones in patients with aplastic anaemia: response to immunosuppressive therapy. *Br. J. Haematol.*, **104**, 271–4.

72. Yamada, T., Tsurumi, H., Kasahara, S. *et al.* (2003). Immunosuppressive therapy for myelodysplastic syndrome: efficacy of methylprednisolone pulse therapy with or without cyclosporin A. *J. Cancer Res. Clin. Oncol.*, **129**, 485–91.

73. Miyata, A., Yasuda, Y., Fujii, S., and Kikuchi, T. [Outcome of immunosuppressive therapy for myelodysplastic syndromes: results of 12 cases from a single institution.] *Rinsho Ketsueki*, **43**, 911–17.

74. Saunthararajah, Y., Nakamura, R., Wesley, R., Wang, Q. J., and Barrett, A. J. (2003). A simple method to predict response to immunosuppressive therapy in patients with myelodysplastic syndrome. *Blood*, **102**, 3025–7.

75. Stadler, M., Germing, U., Kliche, K. O. *et al.* (2004). A prospective, randomised, phase II study of horse antithymocyte globulin vs rabbit antithymocyte globulin as immune-modulating therapy in patients with low-risk myelodysplastic syndromes. *Leukemia*, **18**, 460–5.

76. Cheson, B. D., Bennett, J. M., Kantarjian, H. *et al.* (2000). Report of an international working group to standardize response criteria for myelodysplastic syndromes. *Blood*, **96**, 3671–4.

7

Biologically targeted therapies for myelodysplastic syndromes

Andrew J. Buresh[1] and Alan F. List[2]

[1] University of Arizona Medical Center, Tucson, AZ, USA
[2] University of South Florida, Tampa, FL, USA

Introduction

The management of patients with myelodysplastic syndrome (MDS) remains a challenge distinct from that of most other hematologic malignancies. Therapeutic goals vary among individuals and are influenced by hematological features, prognosis, and age. No single treatment is uniformly effective or addresses the clinical needs for all patients. The standard of care ranges from amelioration of hematological deficits with blood product transfusions and administration of recombinant growth factors, to aggressive chemotherapy and stem cell transplantation for younger individuals with more aggressive disease. Enthusiasm for participation in clinical trials and expectations for benefit have never been greater for patients with MDS. Advancements in the development of novel therapeutics have been accelerated by the elucidation of molecular targets integral to propagation of the malignant clone, disease progression, or disease-specific survival signals. Availability of treatments to the practicing clinician which offer the prospect to alter quality of life meaningfully or the natural history of disease is severely lacking. Preliminary experience with the most promising new therapeutics suggests that some may indeed for the first time offer sustained benefit and raise hopes that the relentless progression of disease and its complication may be curtailed.

Treatment of myelodysplasia and the therapeutic dilemma

Management decisions for patients with MDS must take into account the threat posed by the disease itself, as gauged by prognostic risk factors and the

Myelodysplastic Syndromes: Clinical and Biological Advances, ed. Peter L. Greenberg. Published by Cambridge University Press. © Cambridge University Press 2006.

Table 7.1 Non-cytokine hematopoietic promoting agents for patients with low/intermediate 1 risk myelodysplastic syndrome categorized by mechanism of action and pharmacologic class

Action and pharmacologic class	Agent
Hematopoietic-inhibitory T cells	
Immunosuppressants	Antilymphocyte serotherapy (antithymocyte globulin, ATG), cyclosporin A
Cytoprotection and oxidative injury	
Organic thiol	Amifostine (Ethyol)
TNF-α antagonists	Etanercept (Enbrel), infliximab (Remicade)
Angiogenic molecules and microenvironment	
Antiangiogenics	Thalidomide (Thalomid), CC-5013 (lenalidomide, RevliMid), bevacizumab (Avastin), arsenic trioxide (Trisenox)
Matrix metalloprotease inhibitor	AG3340 (Prinomastat)

TNF-α, tumor necrosis factor-α.

International Prognostic Scoring System (IPSS) (see Chapter 1),[1] patient age, MDS subtype, comorbidities, and performance status. The choice of therapy reflects the specific goals for patients at different risk levels, as well as patient preference.[2] The MDSs differ from most other hematologic malignancies by their varied natural history, and by the morbidity and mortality caused by the associated cytopenias, which influence outcome even in the absence of AML progression. As such, alleviation of disease-related complications and improvement in quality of life are important goals of therapy for lower-risk patients who can expect prolonged survival, whereas extending survival is the principal objective for those with higher-risk disease.[2] Most patients, regardless of prognostic category, eventually succumb to progressive disease or infectious complications.

Lower-risk MDS and low and intermediate 1 IPSS risk categories

Innovative approaches to restore effective blood cell production in lower-risk disease (i.e., low and intermediate 1 IPSS risk categories) have targeted biological effectors of ineffective hematopoiesis (Table 7.1). In nearly all circumstances, ineffective erythropoiesis represents the most pervasive and responsive hematopoietic deficit. Such targeted therapeutics include immunosuppressive therapy with antithymocyte globulin (ATG) and/or ciclosporin A, the phosphoaminothiol amifostine, angiogenesis inhibitors such as thalidomide or one of its structural analogues, small molecule inhibition of vascular endothelial growth factor (VEGF), inhibitors of tyrosine kinase activity, tumor necrosis factor (TNF) inhibitors, arsenic trioxide, and inhibition of matrix metalloprotease activity. Growth factor therapy, with erythropoietin and/or granulocyte colony-stimulating factor (G-CSF), is discussed in Chapter 8.

Hematopoietic inhibitory T cell: a role for immunosuppressive therapy

Accelerated loss of hematopoietic precursors may in selected patients occur through cellular immune-mediated cytotoxicity, a pathobiology shared with aplastic anemia. Oligoclonal hematopoietic-inhibitory T lymphocytes with class I major histocompatibility complex (MHC) antigen restriction act as cellular effectors of ineffective hematopoiesis.[3] In approximately 11% of patients, clonal expansion of a natural killer (NK)-like cell population with a phenotype (CD8+, CD57+, CD56+) analogous to large granular lymphocytes (LGL) is demonstrable, suggesting pathogenic overlap with LGL leukemia.[4] Recognition that immunologic suppression of progenitor growth may contribute to hematopoietic impairment in hypocellular variants led to recent trials testing immunosuppressive therapy. Earlier studies using corticosteroids were complicated by an unacceptable risk of infection.[5] Nevertheless, clinical response correlated with the capacity of corticosteroids to enhance in vitro growth of myeloid colonies.

Many patients responsive to immunosuppressive therapy harbor hematopoietic-inhibitory T lymphocytes (HIT cells), identifiable prospectively through clinical and biological features.[3,6] Treatment with either ciclosporin A or ATG often yields high response rates in appropriately selected candidates with lower-risk disease.[7-11] Twenty-five transfusion-dependent patients with MDS and less than 20% blasts were successfully treated with a single course of ATG at a dose of 40 mg/kg for 4 days.[9] Barrett et al.[12] updated this experience with 60 MDS patients, showing that one-third of patients with less than 15% blasts became independent of red blood cell transfusions, and 87% of responders were free of progression at 2.5 years.[13]

In a non-randomized, single-treatment study,[11] 34% of patients treated with ATG became transfusion-independent. Response was associated with a statistically significant longer survival and an almost significantly decreased time to disease progression. Controlled studies that compare transfusion and survival outcomes in patients treated with ATG versus patients given usual care or other therapies are needed.[11] In unselected patients, the response rate is low, with significant treatment-associated morbidity.[14] A univariate analysis performed by the National Institutes of Health (NIH) investigators and others identified a number of features as overrepresented in immuno-suppression responders, including hypocellularity, age < 60 years, refractory anemia morphologic category, normal karyotype, paroxysmal nocturnal hemoglobinuria (PNH) antigenic phenotype, duration of red blood cell transfusion-dependence and a human leukocyte antigen (HLA) class II DR15 phenotype.[12,15,16] Multivariate analysis identified only HLA class II phenotype, younger age, and shorter red cell transfusion-dependence as independent variables which may be applied in a predictive model for response estimation.[16] Indeed, this model is supported by results of a randomized phase II trial comparing equine and rabbit ATG showing that patients with refractory anemia and short remission duration have the highest probability of clinical benefit.[17] Given the infection risks and potential mortality of immunosuppressive therapy, proper selection of candidates is paramount.

Protection from oxidative injury

The role of TNF-α as a proapoptotic cytokine raised interest in the investigation of treatment modalities that either neutralize the cytokine or protect hematopoietic precursors from its actions. TNF induces programmed cell death by disrupting mitochondrial membrane potential and respiration to generate excess oxygen free radicals which oxidize DNA and intracellular proteins and activate the intrinsic apoptotic pathway.[18] Indeed, in vitro neutralization of TNF enhances the outgrowth of hematopoietic progenitors in MDS.[19] Elevations in plasma TNF correlate with the extent of oxidative DNA injury and depletion of cellular glutathione in the CD34+ compartment, as well as caspase-3 activity.[18,20] Moreover, laboratory studies indicate a direct correlation between TNF and caspase activity apoptotic hematopoietic cells in MDS,[20] whereas caspase inhibitors suppress TNF-induced apoptosis.

Organic thiols, such as glutathione, the most abundant cellular thiol, represent the primary cellular defense against oxygen free radicals.[21] Evidence for increased oxidative stress in MDS derives from serum elevations of the lipid peroxidation product malondialdehyde and the presence of oxidized bases in the progenitor cell compartment.[22] Potential causes of oxidative stress extend beyond TNF and include mitochondrial dysfunction from iron overload or mitochondrial gene mutation, systemic inflammation, and bone marrow stromal defects. Evidence of biological activity of the antioxidant amifostine in vivo suggests that these pathways may be relevant targets for further therapeutic development in MDS.

Amifostine is a phosphorylated aminothiol that was initially developed by the US Department of Defense as a radioprotective agent.[23] Amifostine is a prodrug that is dephosphorylated to yield the free reduced thiol, WR-1065. This latter form of the compound enters cells by facilitated diffusion, where it acts as an efficient scavenger of reactive oxygen species. Differences in alkaline phosphatase activity between normal and neoplastic cells and structural resemblance to polyamines result in preferential conversion in normal tissues, exerting a selective protective effect.[23] In preclinical models and in vitro studies, amifostine protects primitive hematopoietic progenitors from chemotherapy-induced toxicity and stimulates hematopoiesis by promoting the formation of hematopoietic progenitors.[21,24]

In a proof-of-principle study,[25] patients with MDS received treatment with escalating doses of intravenous amifostine either three times per week or once weekly. Evidence of biological activity was observed using the more frequent dosing schedule, with 78% of neutropenic patients experiencing a > 50% increase in neutrophil count, whereas 43% of patients with thrombocytopenia experienced a similar increment in platelet count, and 33% experienced a 50% or greater decline in red cell transfusions.[25] Hematologic changes were not sustained during treatment hiatus and the quality of response did not approach recent standardized thresholds of the International Working Group.[2]

Using the more frequent dosing schedule, amifostine was investigated in phase II trials using more stringent response criteria, yielding disappointing response rates that ranged from 19% to 25%.[26] A 50% or greater reduction in bone marrow blast percentage or ringed sideroblasts was observed in 39% and 47% of evaluable patients, respectively, which correlated with hematologic response. Common adverse effects include nausea, vomiting, and fatigue following cumulative drug administration. Although these studies indicate that amifostine has biological activity that is not erythroid-restricted, monotherapy activity is low and, given its need for chronic intravenous administration, it is not well suited for MDS.[27–31] Pretreament selection of those patients with reasonable potential for benefit would optimize candidate selection in order to preserve quality of life and medical expense. In one study, in vitro capacity to augment bone progenitor growth was predictive of subsequent clinical response to amifostine.[31]

Combination trials involving amifostine with both cytoprotection and hematopoietic promoters have shown some promise. In one study in which amifostine was administered in a regimen including oral pentoxifylline, ciprofloxacin, and dexamethasone, multilineage improvement in cytopenias was observed in over 60% of patients.[32] Whereas ciprofloxacin is a competitive inhibitor of pentoxifylline metabolism, pentoxifylline is a xanthine derivative that interferes with caspase 3-mediated signaling induced by TNF-α, and dexamethasone downregulates mRNA translation of TNF-α.[32] Improvement in cytopenias was observed in the majority of patients, but the duration of response remains unclear. Thus administration of cytoprotectants in combination with other antiapoptotic agents may ameliorate ineffective hematopoiesis; however, the importance and contribution of each of the components of the treatment regimen remain unknown. Trials combining amifostine with erythropoietin have yielded conflicting results,[33–35] indicating that further investigations will be necessary before amifostine can gain a position in the treatment armamentarium for MDS.[32]

The introduction of novel approaches to selectively inactivate TNF-α facilitated clinical investigations to discern the contribution of the cytokine to MDS disease biology. Two classes of agents emerged as potent strategies to neutralize the cytokine, i.e., use of a recombinant soluble TNF-α receptor and a humanized monoclonal antibody. Etanercept (Enbrel) is a soluble recombinant TNF-receptor fusion protein that binds to TNF-α with high affinity to neutralize cytokine activity in vivo. Although etanercept has potent remitting activity in rheumatoid arthritis,[36] its activity in MDS has been disappointing. With the exception of isolated minor erythropoietic improvement, responses are few and without relation to pretreatment TNF-α concentration.[37–39]

Infliximab is an IgG_1k chimeric humanized anti-TNFα monoclonal antibody containing both a human constant and murine variable region that was initially approved for the treatment of refractory collagen vascular disorders.[40,41] Reports of hematologic benefit in selected patients with high endogenous TNF-α plasma concentrations provided the first evidence of clinical benefit in MDS. Two patients with low- and intermediate 1 risk MDS experienced major and minor erythroid responses, respectively, after infliximab treatment, which was associated with a significant decrease in the percentage of apoptotic marrow precursors.[42]

Antiangiogenic agents

Accumulating evidence indicates that clonal expansion and apoptotic response in MDS arise from an interaction between the malignant clone and its microenvironment. Vascular endothelial growth factor-A (VEGF-A) in particular has emerged as an important diffusible effector involved in this interaction, promoting expansion of the leukemic clone while fostering the generation of proapoptotic cytokines. VEGF-A is expressed and elaborated in concordance with its high affinity, type III receptor tyrosine kinases (VEGFR-1 and/or VEGFR-2) by myeloblasts and monocytes in MDS (Fig. 7.1).[43] The magnitude of medullary neovascularity as measured by microvessel density (MVD) increases proportionately with blast percentage, implicating the myeloblast per se as the principal source of angiogenic molecules.[44–47] Among French–American–British (FAB) subtypes, MVD is highest in refractory anemia with excess blasts in transformation (RAEB-T), chronic myelomonocytic leukemia (CMML), and fibrotic MDS subsets compared to refractory anemia (RA), RARS, and RAEB subsets,[46] indicating quantitatively and qualitatively that medullary angiogenesis parallels progression of MDS.[44] Indeed, central medullary clusters of myeloblasts, i.e., abnormal localized immature precursors (ALIP) express both VEGF and VEGFR-1, providing a biological rationale for the pathogenesis of this adverse morphologic feature. Paracrine induction of inflammatory cytokines from receptor-competent endothelial cells, macrophages, and stromal cells appears to augment ineffective hematopoiesis. In vitro neutralization of VEGF suppresses the generation of TNF from MDS bone marrow stroma while promoting recovery of multipotent and erythroid progenitors.[43] Delineation of the biological implications of VEGF and perhaps other angiogenic

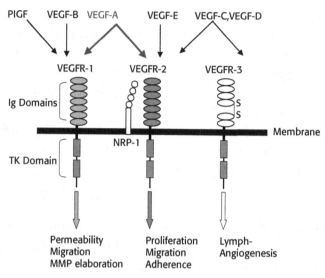

Fig. 7.1   Interaction of vascular endothelial growth factor (VEGF) family members with their cognate receptors on endothelial cells. The VEGF receptors harbor seven extracellular immunoglobulin (Ig)-homology domains. The fifth Ig domain of VEGFR-3 is cleaved after biosynthesis to yield a stable disulfide bond linking the Ig subunits. VEGFR-1 and VEGFR-2 initiate signals essential to the angiogenic response, whereas VEGFR-3 regulates lymph-angiogenesis. NRP-1 binds to the carboxy-terminal sequence of $VEGF_{165}$ to enhance binding of the angiogenic molecule to the VEFGR-2 receptor. TK denotes tyrosine kinase; MMP, matrix metalloproteases; NRP-1, neuropilin-1; PlGF, placental growth factor.

molecules in MDS fostered clinical investigations of antiangiogenic agents that have emerged as a promising class of therapeutics.

Thalidomide (Thalomid, Celgene Inc., Warren, NJ), which displays both antiangiogenic and TNF-inhibitory properties, represents the first agent investigated in this class of therapeutics.[48–50] In a phase II trial of thalidomide performed at the Rush Presbyterian Cancer Institute,[51] 16 of 51 (31%) evaluable patients experienced either red blood cell transfusion-independence or a > 50% decrease in transfusion burden. Sixteen of 83 (19%) of patients responded by intent-to-treat analysis. Improvement in non-erythroid lineages was uncommon. Dose escalation beyond 200 mg/day was limited by cumulative neurological toxicity, and is likely unnecessary. Indeed, the North Central Cancer Treatment Group study N998B that evaluated the tolerance and activity of an alternate schedule of 200 mg/day with escalation to a

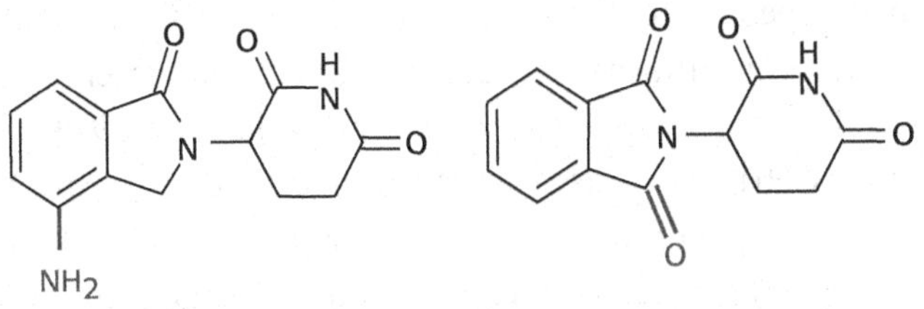

CC5013   thalidomide

Fig. 7.2   Chemical structure of CC5013 and thalidomide. CC5013 differs from its parent compound by the removal of a ketone and addition of an amino group to the glutamate aromatic ring.

maximum daily dose of 1000 mg was compromised by excessive early attrition due to toxicity at a median interval $\leq$ 2.5 months.[52] Median interval to erythroid response was 16 weeks in the Rush trial (range, 12–20 weeks), indicating that prolonged treatment when tolerated appears necessary to maximize hematological benefit. Subsequent institutional studies have confirmed the erythropoietic activity of thalidomide, which, given its necessity for prolonged administration, appears best suited for treatment of patients with lower-risk disease.[53,54] A Celgene-sponsored randomized, placebo-controlled phase trial completed in 2003 should clarify the clinical benefit of low-dose thalidomide in MDS.

More potent analogs of thalidomide that are devoid of neurological toxicity are currently completing phase II investigation.[55,56] These thalidomide analogues have demonstrated 10–1000-fold greater activity than the parent compound in TNF-α inhibition assays and a more potent antiangiogenic effect.[55,56] CC5013 (lenalidomide or Revlimid, Celgene Inc.) is an immunomodulatory derivative (IMiD) of thalidomide (Fig. 7.2) that lacks the neurological toxicities of the parent compound.[57,58] CC5013 inhibits trophic response to VEGF in myeloblasts and endothelial cells, while augmenting heterotypic adhesion of hematopoietic progenitors to bone marrow stroma to promote sustained growth arrest and preferential extinction of myelodysplastic clones.[59] Among 36 MDS patients with symptomatic or transfusion-dependent anemia who completed 8 or more weeks of CC5013 treatment, 24 (67%) experienced an erythroid response according to International Working Group criteria, with 20 patients experiencing sustained transfusion-independence or a 2 g/dl or greater rise in hemoglobin.[60] Hematopoietic-promoting activity appears greatest in patients with low- or intermediate 1 risk disease (72%) or the 5q– deletion (91%). Erythroid responses to CC5013 were associated with complete or partial (> 50%) reduction in the proportion of abnormal metaphases in 11 of 17 informative patients, as well as improved primitive progenitor outgrowth, a reduction in the grade of cytological dysplasia, medullary MVD, and proliferative index. Myeloid and platelet toxicity was dose-limiting, but occurred at all dose levels depending upon cumulative drug exposure, necessitating either dose reduction or treatment interruption. CC5013 is a promising oral therapeutic that may secure a new position in the management of ineffective erythropoiesis in patients with MDS. CC1088, a member of a second functional class of analogues termed selective cytokine-inhibitory drugs or SelCIDs, appears significantly less active in preliminary clinical studies in MDS.

Small molecule inhibitors of the VEGF receptor tyrosine kinases (RTK) which function as target-selective adenosine triphosphate (ATP) mimetics to impair ligand-induced autophosphorylation have had limited investigation in MDS (Table 7.2). SU5416 (Sugen Inc, S. San Francisco, CA) represents the only agent of its class to complete phase II investigation. Like most RTK antagonists, specificity is relative, with activity extending from VEGFR-1 and VEGFR-2 to other type III receptors such as those for the *PDGF, flt3*, and *c-kit* ligands.[61,62] A multicenter trial involving patients with higher-risk MDS or acute myeloid leukemia (AML) yielded minimal reduction in leukemia burden and a corresponding degree of hematological benefit despite increased apoptotic index in the myeloblast population.[63,64] Its insolubility and requirement for twice-weekly intravenous administration limited its clinical development. Investigation of the orally bioavailable congener SU11248 in patients with AML ended prematurely owing to limiting non-hematological organ toxicities.[65] Despite the disappointing early results of this class of agents in myeloid malignancies, clinical investigation of potent and orally active receptor antagonists continues. The Cancer and Leukemia Group B is investigating PTK787 (Novartis, East Hanover, NJ) in patients with lower-risk MDS using a once-daily administration schedule, whereas a more potent RTK inhibitor developed by Agouron Pharmaceuticals (La Jolla, CA), AG13736, is entering phase I and II investigation in patients with advanced MDS or AML.

Table 7.2 Myelodysplastic syndrome (MDS) therapeutics for patients with intermediate-2/high-risk MDS acting through clonal suppression or molecular remodeling

Target and pharmacologic class	Agent
Survival signals	
Receptor tyrosine kinase inhibitors	PTK787
	SU11248
	AG13736, imatinib mesylate (Glivec or Gleevec)
Protein kinase C inhibitor	PKC412
Farnesyl transferase inhibitors	R115777 (tipifarnib, Zarnestra)
	SCH66336 (lonafarnib, Sarasar)
Epigenetic control of gene expression	
DNA methyltransferase inhibitor	5-azacytidine (Vidaza)
	Decitabine (Dacogen)
Histone deacetylase inhibitor	Phenylbutyrate
	Depsipeptide (FR901128)
	MS-275
	Superoxylanilide hydroxaminic acid (SAHA)
	LAQ824, LBH589
	Valproic acid (valproate)
Progenitor maturation	
Pharmacologic differentiators	Cholecalciferol
	Paricalcitrol
	TLK199 (Telintra)

The overproduction of proapoptotic cytokines such as TNF-α, macrophage inflammatory protein-1 (MIP-1), transforming growth factor-beta (TGF-β), interleukin-1 (IL-1), and interferon-gamma (IFN-γ) is demonstrable in both the bone marrow (BM) microenvironment and plasma of patients with MDS.[18,66–70] Monocytes, macrophages, and stromal elements have been identified as the cellular origin of medullary aptogenic cytokine production.[6,70,71] Moreover, abnormal stromal function may contribute to apoptotic loss of hematopoietic precursors by direct cellular contact, rather than the release of soluble factors.[71] The matrix metalloproteases (MMPs) represent a family of zinc-dependent endopeptidases that act as effectors of the angiogenic response, cytokine liberation, and regulators of heterotypic cell adhesion within the microenvironment.[72] MMPs are zymogens, which upon catalytic activation degrade structural components of the extracellular matrix, to disrupt integrin/stromal adhesion signals and promote local liberation of molecules such as VEGF, TNF, and soluble *fas*-ligand by proteolytic cleavage of proteoglycan- or membrane-bound forms.[73–75] AG3340 (Prinomastat; Agouron Pharmaceuticals) is a potent, orally bioavailable, selective inhibitor of MMPs 2 and 9 (gelatinases A and B), and MMP13 (collagenase-3), with weak inhibition of MMP1.[76] In a double-blind, randomized phase II study performed in MDS,[77] arthralgias and joint stiffness were dose-limiting at 15 mg compared to the 5 mg daily dosing schedule (63% versus 33%). Nevertheless, hematological benefit was equivalent: 6 of 26 patients with low- or intermediate-I risk disease experienced red blood cell transfusion-independence that was sustained in some patients beyond 1 year of terminating study treatment (median, 29+ weeks, maximum, 100+ weeks). Although this agent will not continue clinical development, these data, like those of CC5013, provide added proof that angiogenic effectors contribute to ineffective erythropoiesis via their impact on progenitor interaction with the extracellular matrix. Other selective angiogenesis antagonists remain under investigation in MDS. Bevacizumab (Avastin, Genentech, S. San Francisco, CA), a recombinant humanized monoclonal antibody which neutralizes VEGF-A in vivo, is completing phase II investigation and has shown preliminary erythropoietic activity.[78]

Arsenicals have a long history of application in human leukemia, but only recently gained renewed recognition by virtue of activity in acute promyelocytic leukemia. Arsenic trioxide (Trisenox, Cell Therapeutics Inc.) impacts a broad range of cellular targets by virtue of its ability to covalently crosslink and deplete sulfhydryl-rich proteins such as glutathione. Arsenic in its trivalent form inhibits glutathione peroxidase to potentiate peroxide generation, disrupt mitochondrial respiration, repress antiapoptotic proteins, and initiate caspase-mediated apoptotic response.[79–83] Higher arsenic trioxide concentrations are necessary to induce apoptosis and suppress leukemia colony-forming capacity in non-acute promyelocytic leukemia (APL) subtypes of acute myelogenous leukemia (AML) cells.[84,85] In MDS and AML, the antiproliferative effects of ATO also derive from its ability to suppress myeloblast VEGF-A elaboration and cytotoxicity to neovascular endothelium.[86] Not surprisingly, bone marrow specimens from patients with MDS, which, compared to normal progenitors, natively harbor lower glutathione levels,[18] display correspondingly greater susceptibility to ATO-induced apoptosis.[87]

Preliminary results of three clinical trials indicate that ATO has activity in both lower- and higher-risk MDS.[88–90] The doses and schedules applied in these studies varied, ranging from monthly cycles of two sequential weekly treatments of 0.25 mg/kg per day for 5 days followed by a 2-week treatment hiatus, to a dose-intense induction with 0.30 mg/kg per day for 5 days followed by 0.25 mg/kg per day twice-weekly maintenance for 15 weeks. Approximately a quarter of patients have experienced hematological improvement, with few complete or partial remissions. Overall these initial experiences have been encouraging, demonstrating the potential for trilineage hematological improvement with monotherapy that may be sustained for prolonged periods after treatment cessation. Given the manageable toxicity of ATO, combination trials are warranted.

High-risk MDS (IPSS intermediate-2 or high)

Treatment of high-risk MDS remains a major therapeutic challenge. Non-investigational therapies available to the practicing clinician offer little prospect to ameliorate multilineage deficits or prolong survival. Age and performance status generally limit application of intensive chemotherapy as well as consideration of allogeneic stem cell transplant, the only accepted curative therapy for this disease. Clearly, novel targeted therapeutics allowing outpatient administration represent a profound need for most patients with high-risk MDS. Selected agents that have shown promise in clinical investigations are summarized in Table 7.2.

Targeting PDF-receptor and FGF-receptor fusion genes

The World Health Organization's (WHO) recent recommendations to segregate CMML from MDS as a syndrome with overlap myeloproliferative features has gained convincing support from cytogenetic and molecular investigations. Although most cases of chronic myeloproliferative disorders have a normal or aneuploid karyotype, a minority of patients harbor a reciprocal translocation involving chromosomes 5q33 or 8p11 which create novel fusion genes involving the PDGF-β and FGFR1 RTK, respectively.[91–96] These translocations result in the production of constitutively active tyrosine kinase fusion proteins that deregulate hematopoiesis in a manner analogous to the non-receptor oncoprotein kinase, *BCR-ABL*.

Perhaps the most important therapeutic discovery in the management of CMML in recent years is the activity of imatinib in patients harboring reciprocal chromosome translocations involving chromosome 5q33. Although a number of chromosomes and genes may partner in the gene rearrangement, the clinical phenotype is distinct, recognized by the WHO classification as CMML with eosinophilia, but arising from the generation of novel fusion genes involving the PDGF-β receptor with constitutive RTK signaling.[92–97] Transgenic mouse models have shown that these novel RTK fusion genes are singularly responsible for the generation of these myeloproliferative disorders, and are selectively responsive to PDGF kinase inhibitors.[92–98] Imatinib binds to the ATP binding pocket of the PDGF-β receptor analogous to its interaction with *BCR/ABL* to act as a potent inhibitor of receptor kinase activity.[98] Among 5 patients reported to date, each achieved rapid hematological control and sustained complete cytogenetic remission with imatinib monotherapy.[99] In all 5 patients, a normal blood profile was achieved within 4 weeks after treatment began. All responses were durable at 9–12 months of follow-up.

Chemotherapy

The limited life expectancy of patients with higher-risk disease has justifiably placed treatment with cytotoxics in the forefront of management strategies for patients with advanced MDS, albeit with less optimistic expectations for sustained disease control. Chemotherapeutics employed to date range from single-agent topoisomerase I inhibitors to traditional AML chemotherapy combinations employing DNA-targeted agents that are anchored by cytarabine and either topoisomerase I or II interactive agents.[100–102]

A recently completed phase III trial and a retrospective analysis of the MD Anderson Cancer Center (Houston, TX) experience indicate that the topotecan and cytarabine combination popularized in recent years offers no significant advantage over standard anthracycline-containing regimens, and in fact may have inferior remission durability.[101,102] Despite a comparatively high remission rate and reduced induction mortality in the older population compared to historical experiences, fewer than 10% of patients can be expected to remain in remission beyond 2 years.

Selective targeting of leukemic myeloid progenitors using the CD33-selective, calichemicin-conjugated humanized monoclonal antibody gemtuzumab ozogamicin (Mylotarg; Wyeth), was hoped to lessen systemic toxicities of conventional cytotoxics while preserving remitting activity. In a multicenter trial evaluating single versus day-1 and -14 dosing in advanced MDS, gemtuzumab ozogamicin demonstrated limited benefit as a single agent with associated prolonged myelosuppression and associated infectious risk.[103] A second single-institution study yielded similar disappointing results.[104]

Low-dose cytarabine or melphalan monotherapy offers an outpatient alternative to intensive remission induction therapy with reduced treatment-related morbidity, but may result in prolonged myelosuppression while inducing hematologic and pathologic remissions in fewer than 30% of patients.[105–108] Low-dose cytarabine has received the most scrutiny, yielding response rates ranging from 10 to 25% in phase II trials but offering no benefit compared to supportive care in a National Cancer Institute-sponsored intergroup study that involved all FAB types.[105]

Melphalan has been suggested to exert some differentiation effects on leukemic cells in addition to its cytotoxic effects. Twenty-one elderly patients with high-risk MDS or secondary AML were treated with 2 mg melphalan orally once a day. There were 7 (30%) complete responses and 2 (10%) partial responses, occurring within 4–16 weeks and lasting for 12–55 weeks. Retreatment was successful in most at relapse. Treatment was generally well tolerated with minimal complications except for mild and transient initial worsening of cytopenias observed in most patients.[107] In another study, 21 patients with high-risk MDS (6 RAEB, 15 RAEB-T) were given low-dose daily oral melphalan. Seven patients achieved complete remission, 1 partial, and 4 had minor responses. Complete remission patients included those with a normal karyotype and hypocellular marrow.[108] Despite these encouraging results, for most patients with high-risk MDS, therapy with low-dose cytarabine, melphalan, or oral etoposide is suboptimal.

Strategies targeting biological features that confer native chemotherapy resistance have emerged as a promising approach to improve the results of standard induction chemotherapy. P-glycoprotein (Pgp) is a highly conserved plasma membrane glycoprotein encoded by the *MDR1* gene that functions as an ATP-dependent multidrug exporter with broad specificity for natural product-derived antineoplastics, and an inhibitor of caspase-dependent programmed cell death.[109–113] Pgp is natively overexpressed by myeloblasts in RAEB-T and secondary AML, and is associated with a higher probability of induction failure and inferior disease-free survival.[114–116]

A randomized phase III trial performed by the Southwest Oncology Group showed that concurrent treatment with the Pgp inhibitor ciclosporin A and infusional daunorubicin following cytarabine significantly reduces induction resistance in high-risk patients and significantly prolongs duration of remission and increased overall survival.[117] Patients with RAEB-T or secondary AML experienced the greatest benefit, with overall survival (ciclosporin A, 28% versus control, 0%) and disease-free survival (ciclosporin A, 60% versus control, 0%) at 2 years that has been unmatched by any other chemotherapeutic regimen. Similar trends were reported in a French cooperative group study that employed quinine as a Pgp modulator,[118] indicating that this targeted induction strategy may significantly extend survival for selected individuals who are candidates for more intensive therapy. Additional clinical studies using ciclosporin A and newer generations of Pgp antagonists are in progress,[119] raising hopes that this early lead may give rise to a significant advance in the treatment of MDS and associated leukemias.

Epigenetic gene regulation

Less aggressive approaches that target potentially reversible molecular signals implicated in progression of disease have shown considerable promise. While genetic changes such as mutation and deletions are otherwise irreversible features of the neoplastic profile, heritable epigenetic modifications of DNA or chromatin represent neoplastic regulatory processes that disrupt gene expression and are potentially reversible. Methylation of cytosine residues within gene promoters by DNA methyltransferases (DMT) represents a universal feature of the neoplastic phenotype that promotes recruitment of transcriptional corepressors and histone deacetylases and consequent condensation of chromatin that disrupts transcription factor access and DNA binding. In MDS in particular, hypermethylation of cytosine clusters occurs within the *p15* proto-oncogene, i.e., cytosine-guanine islands, and silences expression of the gene coincident with increasing leukemia burden.[120,121] In vitro, inhibitors of DMTs produce global genomic hypomethylation with corresponding derepression of previously silenced genes and terminal differentiation in leukemia cell lines.[122] Two such agents, the DMT inhibitors 5-azacytidine (5-AzaC; Vidaza, Pharmion) and 5-aza-2'-deoxycytidine (decitabine; Dacogen, Supergen), have undergone the most extensive clinical investigation with preliminary proof of principle.[123–127] Both 5-AzaC and decitabine are pyrimidine analogues that on incorporation into DNA[121] inhibit DMT activity in dividing cells.[124,125,128] 5-AzaC represents the first of these two agents to complete phase III investigation.[126] In this trial, performed by the Cancer and Leukemia Group B (CALGB), 191 symptomatic MDS patients were randomized to receive treatment with subcutaneous 5-AzaC, 75 mg/m^2 per day for 7 consecutive days every 28 days or best supportive care alone for 16 weeks. Patients in the supportive-care arm whose disease progressed to a more advanced stage were permitted to cross over to 5-AzaC treatment before the completion of the 16-week observation period. Although this trial preceded the development of the International Working Group response criteria, hematologic benefit was reported in 60% of patients on the 5-AzaC arm, which included complete (7%) and partial (16%) responses, and single or multilineage hematologic improvement (37%). Hematologic improvement in the supportive-care arm was observed in only 5% of patients. Median time to leukemic transformation or death was significantly extended with 5-AzaC treatment, from 13 months in the observation arm to 21 months ($P < 0.007$). Landmark analysis was performed due to the cross-over nature of the study, and showed a median survival of 18 months for 5-AzaC compared to 11 months for supportive care only. Quality-of-life assessment measurements showed improvement in physical function, symptoms, and psychological state for those patients who received treatment with 5-AzaC.[129]

5-AzaC displays limited solubility, thereby necessitating immediate administration after reconstitution, and large volume (approximately 4 ml) that can cause discomfort at the injection site. 5-Aza-2-deoxycytidine (decitabine) is more readily soluble, displays greater stability after reconstitution, and is a more potent inhibitor of DMT. A randomized phase III trial of similar design to the CALGB study evaluated intravenous decitabine and completed enrollment in April 2003. Although the results of this trial are not as yet available, data from phase II investigations provided proof of principle that this agent can restore *p15* expression with a corresponding high rate of cytogenetic and hematologic remitting activity,[127] with an acceptable toxicity profile. Both agents have proceeded with expedited US Food and Drug Administration review in 2004 and 5-AzaC has been approved as the first agent to receive an indication for the treatment of patients with MDS.

Histone deacetylase inhibitors

Epigenetic gene silencing after promoter methylation involves the recruitment of histone deacetylases to create a nuclear corepressor histone deacetylase complex. An open chromatin configuration, which is necessary for transcription factor binding, is maintained by reversible modifications to lysine tails of core histones by acetylation, methylation, or phosphorylation. Histone deacetylases catalyze the removal of acetyl groups from histone proteins, thereby altering electrostatic pressures that normally maintain an open chromatin conformation that is necessary for gene transcription. Older agents that inhibit histone deacetylation, such as phenylbutyrate and depsipeptide, have been replaced with newer, more potent alternatives that are currently under investigation.[13]

Four classes of histone deacetylase inhibitors in clinical development include the cyclic peptides (e.g., depsipeptide, FK228), the short-chain fatty acids (e.g., phenylbutyric and valproic acids), the hydroxamic acids (e.g., superoxylanilide hydroxaminic acid and trichostatin A) and the benzamides (e.g., MS-275; Berlex). Histone deacetylase inhibitors have shown potent differentiating capacity in preclinical studies of acute myeloid leukemia. Trichostatin A induces proerythroblast differentiation in 34% of clinical AML cells in vitro.[130,131] Preliminary clinical investigations indicate that depsipeptide has promising remitting activity in T-cell lymphoma.[132] Valproic acid, an orally bioavailable antiepileptic agent, was recently also demonstrated to act as an effective inhibitor of histone deacetylase in neoplastic cells at concentrations achievable in vivo.[134-136] Preclinical investigations in AML indicate that valproate can restore expression of silenced genes in AML cells.[137] Clinical studies investigating phenylbutyrate and valproate either as single agents or in combination with DMT inhibitors are currently ongoing in both MDS and AML.[138]

Differentiation agents

The development of pharmacologic inducers of hematopoietic differentiation has been limited by the challenge of identifying relevant cellular targets whose function can be modified by synthetic small molecules. The activity of *all*-trans retinoic acid (ATRA) in acute promyelocytic leukemia represents the ideal of this therapeutic strategy. However, fusion genes analogous to the role of promyelocytic leukemia/retinoic acid receptor alpha fusion protein (PML/RAR) that are implicated in dysregulation of myeloid maturation in MDS have yet to be identified. The retinoids have not yielded the hematologic potential hoped for in MDS, but may have a role in select patients, such as the pediatric syndrome of juvenile myelomonocytic leukemia (JMML). Isotretinoin attenuates the spontaneous in vitro proliferation of myeloid progenitors characteristic of this disease.[139] In one report, 6 of 10 JMML patients treated with isotretinoin experienced a complete or partial remission characterized by normalization of the white blood cell count and resolution of organomegaly.[140] Although treatment was well tolerated and responses were sustained, all patients had a normal karyotype and otherwise favorable prognostic features. It remains to be seen whether isotretinoin has remitting activity in high-risk patients. Neutrophil responses were observed in 42% of patients with neutropenia, and platelet responses were seen in 67% of patients with thrombocytopenia. Further studies with this combination regimen are indicated.

TLK199 (Telintra, Telik, San Francisco, CA) is a novel liposomal glutathione derivative that promotes granulopoiesis in both in vitro and animal models. TLK199 is the tripeptide diethylester, gamma-glutamyl ethyl ester (S-benzyl) cysteinyl-R(−)-phenylglycyl ethyl ester hydrochloride, and a selective inhibitor of glutathione S-transferase P1–1 (GST P1–1), a member of a family of enzymes that until recently were believed to function exclusively in cellular defense and drug detoxification.[141–145] Recent investigations indicate that GST P1–1 is a negative growth regulator which upon inhibition promotes the proliferation and differentiation of myeloid precursors.[143,145,146] After intracellular de-esterification, the active diacid form, TLK117, is released to inhibit GST P1-1 and activate the mitogen-activated protein kinase pathway, which is believed to be responsible for its hematopoietic-promoting activity.[143] Indeed, in animal models, TLK199 accelerates myeloid recovery from chemotherapy-induced neutropenia as well as treatment with the myeloid growth factor G-CSF.[145] Preliminary results of a phase I/II trial in MDS have shown hematologic improvement in two or more lineages in 3 of 8 evaluable patients.[146] While investigations with this agent continue, oral bioavailable analogs are also being explored.

Farnesyl transferase inhibitors: targeting survival signaling

The *ras* gene superfamily encodes guanosine triphosphate hydrolases (GTPase) that serve as critical regulatory elements in signal transduction, cellular proliferation, and maintenance of the malignant phenotype. The three *ras* proto-oncogenes (H, N, and K) encode four 21-Kda G-proteins, including two alternatively spliced *K-Ras* products that are posttranslationally modified before incorporation into the inner leaflet of the plasma membrane. Farnesylation of carboxy-terminal consensus sequences by farnesyl protein transferase (FPT) represents the first and rate-limiting posttranslational modification of Ras-GTPases that is requisite for membrane association and transforming activity.[147] FPT catalyzes the transfer of a 15-carbon farnesyl group from farnesyl diphosphate to the C-terminal tetrapeptide CAAX (C, cysteine; A, any aliphatic amino acid; X, any amino acid) sequence of the Ras protein. These G-proteins normally cycle between two conformations induced by binding of either guanosine diphosphate (GDP) or guanosine triphosphate (GTP), the rate of which is controlled by GTPase regulatory proteins (Fig. 7.3). GTPase-activating proteins (GAP) accelerate GTP hydrolysis, whereas guanosine exchange factors (GEF) promote GDP dissociation from the G-protein.

The most common Ras allele mutated in adult MDS and AML is *N-ras* and, to a lesser extent, *K-ras*.[148] *N-ras* mutations have been preferentially associated with the monocytic component of MDS and increased risk of progression to AML.[149,150] Point mutations in the *ras* proto-oncogenes occur at critical regulatory sites (e.g., codons 12, 13, and 61) which inactivate the GTPase response normally stimulated by GAP binding, thereby extending the half-life of the Ras-GTP-bound mutant.

Activating point mutations of the *ras* proto-oncogene are detected in fewer than 20% of unselected patients with MDS, but are common in CMML.[91,149–151] *ras* mutations may occur as an early or late event in MDS; however the relation to risk of disease progression remains uncertain.[150,151] Although some reports support a correlation between *N-ras* mutations and cytogenetic patterns characteristic of MDS (5q−, −7, and +8), such mutations are also demonstrable in the absence of karyotypic abnormalities.[150,151] The clear exception is the morphologic subtype, CMML. Constitutive activation of the *ras*/mitogen-activated protein kinase pathway is demonstrable in 40–70% of cases of adult CMML, resulting either from activating point

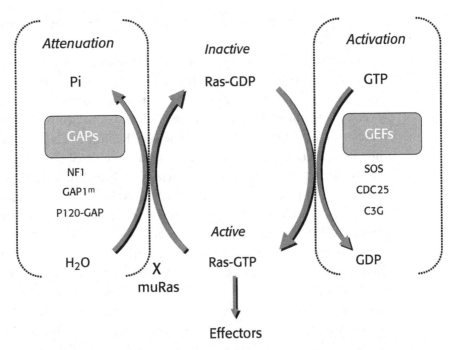

Ras activation cycle. Trophic signals activate guanine exchange factors (GEFs) such as SOS and CDC25 to accelerate the rate of guanosine diphosphate (GDP) dissociation, stabilize the Ras protein in its nucleotide free state, and facilitate guanosine triphosphate (GTP) binding. GTPase-activating proteins (GAPs) accelerate GTP hydrolysis and inorganic phosphate removal (Pi), thereby inactivating Ras. Sustained Ras activation may occur in mutant Ras proteins in which GTPase response to GAP binding is inactivated, or by mutational inactivation of GAPs.

mutations of *ras* alleles or from reciprocal translocations deregulating receptor tyrosine kinases.[96,148,149] While *ras* mutations are detected in fewer than 20% of cases of JMML (90), 30% of patients harbor inactivating mutations of the neurofibromatosis-1 gene (*NF1*), which encodes a GAP that negatively regulates *ras* by accelerating GTP hydrolysis.[152]

The FPT inhibitors (FTI) represent a novel class of potent, orally bioavailable inhibitors of *ras* and other prenylation-dependent molecules. Modulation of multiple cancer-specific pathways has been proposed to explain the wide range of antiproliferative, antiangiogenic, and proapoptotic activity noted with these agents. These diverse actions, coupled with a minimal impact on normal cells and the potential for oral delivery, make FTIs attractive agents for testing in MDS and other hematologic malignancies.[153]

Preliminary results of phase I/II studies in MDS and CMML indicate promising hematopoietic promoting activity that extends to non-erythroid lineages.[154–156] R115777 (tipifarnib, Zarnestra; Janssen Pharmaceuticals, Beerse, Belgium and Spring House, PA) and lonafarnib (SCH66336 or Sarasar; Schering-Plough Research Institute, Kenilworth, NJ) are the leading non-peptide, heterocyclic oral FTIs that have completed phase I and II clinical studies in hematological malignancies.[153–159] In a phase I trial performed exclusively in patients with MDS, 6 of 20 evaluable patients, including 2 of 4 patients with *ras* mutations, experienced hematological improvement or a partial remission using the 3 : 1-week syncopated schedule. Myelosuppression and fatigue were dose-limiting, with the maximum tolerated dose defined as 400 mg/m^2 twice daily.[155] A concurrent phase II trial performed by MD Anderson investigators using a more dose-intensive and protracted schedule (600 mg twice daily for 4 of each 6-week cycle) yielded an unacceptably high frequency of early treatment withdrawal due to drug intolerance (41%). Two complete remissions and one partial remission (19%) were reported in patients lacking mutant *ras* alleles among the 16 patients completing two or more cycles of therapy.[154]

Clinical trials of lonafarnib have employed a continuous-dosing schedule. In a phase I study of lonafarnib administered in patients with advanced chronic myelogenous leukemia, MDS, CMML, or acute leukemia, clinical benefit or hematological improvement according to International Working Group criteria was observed in 5 (29%) of 17 evaluable patients, including red blood cell transfusion-independence, reduction in monocytosis, and major platelet responses in 3 of 5 patients with CMML.[158] Diarrhea and hypokalemia were dose-limiting at 300 mg twice daily. Trough plasma concentrations of lonafarnib exceeded 1000 ng/ml at the 200-mg dose level, and were sufficient to inhibit FPT in vivo. An expanded phase II trial was recently completed which included advanced MDS (RAEB, RAEB-T) or CMML.[159] A total of 15–30 patients were accrued to each cohort using a Simon two-stage design. Disease response was assessed using International Working Group criteria. Forty-two patients were evaluable for response. Overall, 12 of 42 (29%) patients responded by International Working Group criteria

(4/17 MDS, 8/25 CMML). Two patients (5%: 1 MDS, 1 CMML) achieved a complete remission. Hematologic improvement was observed in 10 additional patients (3 MDS, 7 CMML). In these 10 patients, there were 5 major platelet responses, 4 major and 5 minor erythroid responses and 1 major neutrophil response. Of the 23 patients who were red blood cell transfusion-dependent at study entry, 4 (17%: 3 MDS, 1 CMML) achieved red blood cell transfusion-independence, and 4 (17%: 1 MDS, 3 CMML) achieved at least a 50% decrease in red blood cell transfusion requirements. Of the 22 patients who were platelet transfusion-dependent and/or had platelet counts < 30000/mm^3 at baseline, 4 (18%) achieved platelet transfusion-independence. Of the 37 patients who had bone marrow blasts > 5% at baseline, 16 (43%) showed a 50% or greater reduction in bone marrow blasts.[159] A phase III randomized trial is planned to investigate the clinical benefit and frequency of platelet response to lonafarnib in patients with CMML or advanced MDS with severe thrombocytopenia. Although initially intended to interrupt mutant *ras*-induced constitutive signaling, it is clear from the trials completed to date that clinical benefit is independent of mutation status, indicating that inhibition of wild-type *ras* or other farnesylated molecules may be of greater relevance to the activity of the FTIs in MDS and CMML.

Despite the promise of this novel class of therapeutics, a note of caution has been raised by the recent description of leukemia differentiation complicating treatment with lonafarnib. Three patients with proliferative CMML (white blood cell count > 12 000/l) experienced rapid and sustained leukocytosis, which in 2 cases was complicated by pulmonary infiltrates that resolved either after study drug withdrawal or treatment with dexamethasone.[157] The latter findings closely resemble the leukemia differentiation syndrome reported with retinoid therapy for APL, and may be linked to the unique ability of lonafarnib and perhaps other FPT inhibitors to activate beta-1 and beta-2 integrins and promote both heterotypic and homotypic adhesion of CMML cells.[160] Overall, the frequency of leukemoid response to lonafarnib treatment was higher in patients with proliferative (≥ 12 000/l) compared to non-proliferative CMML (54% versus 11%; $P = 0.025$). Close clinical monitoring of patients with proliferative variants receiving FTI treatment may be warranted, with consideration for early introduction of cytoreductive therapy.

Summary and future directions

Over the past two decades, the number of patients diagnosed with MDS has steadily risen owing to the extended survival of our aging population. With current advances in our understanding of the pathobiology of MDS and prognostic models to guide therapy appropriately, patients now have access to an array of promising novel therapeutics with greater expectation for benefit. The identification of relevant biologic targets in MDS has raised expectations for the development of effective disease-specific therapies. Enrollment in clinical trials should be encouraged for patients in whom standard therapy offers the prospect for low probability of success.

REFERENCES

1. Greenberg, P., Cox, C., Le Beau, M. *et al.* (1997). International scoring system for evaluating prognosis in myelodysplastic syndromes. *Blood*, **89**, 2079–88.
2. Cheson, B. D., Bennett, J. M., Kantarjian, H. *et al.* (2000). Report of an international working group to standardize response criteria for myelodysplastic syndromes. *Blood*, **96**, 3671–4.
3. Molldrem, J., Jiang, Y. Z., Stetler-Stevenson, M. *et al.* (2000). Haematological response of patients with myelodysplastic syndrome to antithymocyte globulin is associated with a loss of lymphocyte-mediated inhibition of CFU-GM and alterations in T-cell receptor V-beta profiles. *Br. J. Haematol.*, **28**, 148–55.
4. Saunthararajah, Y., Molldrem, J. L., Rivera, M. *et al.* (2001). Coincidence of myelodysplastic syndrome with large granular lymphocytic leukemia. *Br. J. Haematol.*, **112**, 195–200.
5. Bagby, G. C. Jr, Gabourel, J. D., and Linman, J. W. (1980). Glucocorticoid therapy in the preleukemic syndrome (hemopoietic dysplasia): identification of responsive patients using in-vitro techniques. *Ann. Intern. Med.*, **92**, 55–8.
6. Flores-Figueroa, E., Gutierrez-Espindola, G., Montesinos, J. J. *et al.* (2002). In vitro characterization of hematopoietic microenvironment cells from patients with myelodysplastic syndrome. *Leuk. Res.*, **26**, 677–86.
7. Biesma, D. H., van den Tweel, J. G., Verdonck, L. F. (1997). Immunosuppressive therapy for hypoplastic myelodysplastic syndrome. *Cancer*, **79**, 1548–51.
8. Jonasova, A., Neuwirtova, R., Cermak, J. *et al.* (1998). Cyclosporin A therapy in hypoplastic MDS patients and certain refractory anemias without hypoplastic bone marrow. *Br. J. Hematol.*, **100**, 304–9.
9. Molldrem, J. J., Caples, M., Mavroudis, D. *et al.* (1997). Antithymocyte globulin for patients with myelodysplastic syndrome. *Br. J. Hematol.*, **99**, 699–705.

10. Okada, M., Okamoto, T., Yamada, S. *et al.* (1999). Good response to cyclosporine therapy in patients with myelodysplastic syndromes having the HLA-DRB1–1501 allele. *Blood*, **94**, (suppl. 1), 306a.

11. Molldrem, J. J., Leifer, E., Baheci, E. *et al.* (2002). Antithymocyte globulin for treatment of bone marrow failure associated with myelodysplastic syndrome. *Ann. Intern. Med.*, **137**, 156–63.

12. Barrett, A. J., Molldrem, J. J., Saunthrajarian, Y. *et al.* (1998). Prolonged transfusion independence and disease stability in patients with myelodysplastic syndrome responding to antithymocyte globulin. *Blood*, **92** (suppl. 1), 713a, abstract 2932.

13. Cheson, B. D., Zwiebel, J. A., Dancey, J., and Murgo, A. (2000). Novel therapeutic agents for the treatment of myelodysplastic syndromes. *Semin. Oncol.*, **27**, 560–77.

14. Steensma, D. P., Dispenzieri, A., Moore, S. B. *et al.* (2003). Antithymocyte globulin has limited efficacy and substantial toxicity in un-selected anemic patients with myelodysplastic syndrome. *Blood*, **101**, 2156–8.

15. Saunthararajah, Y., Nakamura, R., Nam, J. M. *et al.* (2002). HLA-DR15 (DR2) is over-represented in myelodysplastic syndrome and aplastic anemia and predicts a response to immunosuppression in myelodysplastic syndrome. *Blood*, **100**, 1570–4.

16. Saunthararajah, Y., Nakamura, R., Wesley, R., Wang, Q., and Barret, A. J. (2003). A simple method to predict response to immunosuppressive therapy in patients with myelodysplastic syndrome. *Blood*, **102**, 3025–7.

17. Stadler, M., Germing, U., Kliche, K.-O. *et al.* (2004). A prospective, randomised, phase II study of horse antithymocyte globulin vs rabbit antithymocyte globulin as immune-modulating therapy in patients with low-risk myelodysplastic syndromes. *Leukemia*, **18**, 449–59.

18. Peddie, C. M., Wolf, C. R., McLellan, L. I. *et al.* (1997). Oxidative DNA damage in CD34+ myelodysplastic cells is associated with intracellular redox changes and elevated plasma tumor necrosis factor-α concentration. *Br. J. Haematol.*, **99**, 625–31.

19. Gersuk, G. M., Lee, J. W., Beckham, C. A. *et al.* (1998). Fax (CD95) receptor and fas ligand expression in bone marrow cells from patients with myelodysplastic syndrome. *Blood*, **88**, 1122–3.

20. Mundle, S. D., Reza, S., Ali, A. *et al.* (1999). Correlation of tumor necrosis factor alpha (TNF alpha) with high caspase 3-like activity in myelodysplastic syndromes. *Cancer Lett.*, **140**, 201–7.

21. Romano, M. F., Lamberti, A., Bisogni, R. *et al.* (1999). Amifostine inhibits hematopoietic progenitor cell apoptosis by activating NF-κB/Rel transcription factors. *Blood*, **94**, 4060–6.

22. Farquhar, M. J. and Bowen, D. T. (2003). Oxidative stress and the myelodysplastic syndromes. *Int. J. Hematol.*, **77**, 342–50.

23. Santini, V. (2001). Amifostine: chemotherapeutic and radiotherapeutic protective effects. *Expert Opini. Pharmacother.*, **2**, 479.

24. List, A. F., Heaton, R., Glinsmann-Gibson, B., and Capizzi, R. L. (1998). Amifostine stimulates formation of multipotent and erythroid bone marrow progenitors. *Leukemia*, **12**, 1596–602.

25. List, A. F., Brasfield, F., Heaton, R. *et al.* (1997). Stimulation of hematopoiesis by amifostine in patients with myelodysplastic syndrome. *Blood*, **90**, 3364–9.

26. List, A. F. (2002). New approaches to the treatment of myelodysplasia. *Oncologist*, **7** (suppl. 1), 39–49.

27. Grossi, A., Fabbri, A., Santini, V. *et al.* (2000). Amifostine in the treatment of low-risk myelodysplastic syndromes. *Haematologica*, **85**, 367–71.

28. Hofmann, W. K., Seipelt, G., Ottmann, O. G. *et al.* (2000). Effect of treatment with amifostine used as a single agent in patients with refractory anemia on clinical outcome and serum tumor necrosis factor alpha levels. *Ann. Hematol.*, **79**, 255–8.

29. Tsiara, S. N., Kapsali, H. D., Panteli, K., Christou, L., and Bourantas, K. L. (2001). Preliminary results of amifostine administration in combination with recominant human erythropoietin in patients with myelodysplastic syndrome. *J. Exp. Clin. Cancer Res.*, **20**, 35–8.

30. Invernizzi, R., Pecci, A., Travaglino, E. *et al.* (2002). Clinical and biological effects of treatment with amifostine in myelodysplastic syndromes. *Br. J. Haematol.*, **118**, 246–50.

31. Viniou, N., Terpos, E., Galanopoulos, A. *et al.* (2002). Treatment of anemia in low-risk myelodysplastic syndromes with amifostine: in vitro testing of response. *Ann. Hematol.*, **81**, 182–6.

32. Raza, A., Qavi, H., Lisak, L. *et al.* (2000). Patients with myelodysplastic syndrome benefit from palliative therapy with amifostine, pentoxyfylline, and ciprofloxacin with or without dexamethasone. *Blood*, **95**, 580–7.

33. Grossi, A., Musto, P., Santini, V. *et al.* (2002). Combined therapy with amifostine plus erythropoietin for the treatment of myelodysplastic syndrome. *Haematologica*, **87**, 322–3.

34. Neumeister, P., Jaeger, G., Eibl, M. *et al.* (2001). Amifostine in combination with erythropoietin and G-CSF promotes multilineage hematopoiesis in patients with myelodysplastic syndrome. *Leuk. Lymphoma*, **40**, 345–9.

35. Tefferi, A., Elliot, M. A., and Hook, C. C. (2001). Amifostine alone and in combination with erythropoietin for the treatment of favorable myelodysplastic syndrome. *Leuk. Res.*, **25**, 183–5.

36. Fleischmann, R. M., Baumgartner, S. W., Tindall, E. A. *et al.* (2003). Response to etanercept (enbrel) in elderly patients with rheumatoid arthritis: a retrospective analysis of clinical trial results. *J. Rheumatol.*, **30**, 691.

37. Deeg, H. J., Gotlib, J., Beckham, C. et al. (2002). Soluble TNF receptor fusion protein (etanercept) for the treatment of myelodysplastic syndrome: a pilot study. *Leukemia*, **16**, 162.

38. Maciejewski, J. P., Risitano, A. M., Sloand, E. M. et al. (2002). A pilot study of the recombinant soluble human tumour necrosis factor receptor (*p75*)-Fc fusion protein in patients with myelodysplastic syndrome. *Br. J. Haematol.*, **117**, 119.

39. Rosenfeld, C. and Bedell, C. (2002). Pilot study of recombinant human soluble tumor necrosis factor receptor (TNFR: Fc) in patients with low risk myelodysplastic syndrome. *Leuk. Res.*, **26**, 721.

40. St Clair, E. W. (2002). Infliximab treatment for rheumatic disease: clinical and radiological efficacy. *Ann. Rheum. Dis.*, **61** (suppl. 2), ii67.

41. Braun, J., Sieper, J., Breban, M. et al. (2002). Anti-tumour necrosis factor alpha therapy for ankylosing spondylitis: international experience. *Ann. Rheum. Dis.*, **61** (suppl. 3), iii51.

42. Stasi, R. and Amadori, S. (2002). Infliximab chimaeric anti-tumour necrosis factor alpha monoclonal antibody treatment for patients with myelodysplastic syndromes. *Br. J. Haematol.*, **116**, 334.

43. Bellamy, W. T., Richter, L., Sirjani, D. et al. (2001). Vascular endothelial cell growth factor is an autocrine promoter of abnormal localized immature myeloid precursors and leukemia progenitor formation in myelodysplastic syndromes. *Blood*, **97**, 1427–34.

44. Korkolopoulou, P., Apostolidou, E., Pavlopoulos, P. M. et al. (2001). Prognostic evaluation of the mircovascular network in myelodysplastic syndromes. *Leukemia*, **15**, 1369–76.

45. Aguayo, A., O'Brien, S., Keating, M. et al. (2000). Clinical relevance of intracellular vascular endothelial growth factor levels in B-cell chronic lymphocytic leukemia. *Blood*, **96**, 768–70.

46. Pruneri, G., Bertolini, F., Soligo, D. et al. (1999). Angiogenesis in myelodysplastic syndromes. *Br. J. Cancer*, **81**, 1398–401.

47. Aguayo, A., Kantarjian, H., Manshouri, T. et al. (2000). Angiogenesis in acute and chronic leukemias and myelodysplastic syndromes. *Blood*, **96**, 2240–5.

48. Sampaio, E. P., Sarno, E. N., Gallily, R., Cohn, Z. A., and Kaplan, G. (1991). Thalidomide selectively inhibits tumor necrosis factor alpha production by stimulated human monocytes. *J. Exp. Med.*, **173**, 699–703.

49. Moreira, A. L., Sampaio, E. P., Zmuidzinas, A. et al. (1993). Thalidomide exerts its inhibitory action on tumor necrosis factor alpha by enhancing mRNA degradation. *J. Exp. Med.*, **177**, 1675.

50. Turk, B. E., Jiang, H., and Liu, J. O. (1996). Binding of thalidomide to alpha$_1$-acid glycoprotein may be involved in its inhibition of tumor necrosis factor alpha production. *Proc. Natl Acad. Sci. U.S.A.*, **93**, 7552.

51. Raza, A., Meyer, P., Dutt, D. *et al.* (2001). Thalidomide produces transfusion independence in long-standing refractory anemias of patients with myelodysplastic syndromes. *Blood*, **98**, 958–65.

52. Moreno-Aspitia, A., Geyer, S., Li, C. *et al.* (2002). N998B: multicenter phase II trial of thalidomide (Thal) in adult patients with myelodysplastic syndromes (MDS). *Blood*, **100**, 96a.

53. Zorat, F., Shetty, V., Dutt, D. *et al.* (2001). The clinical and biological effects of thalidomide in patients with myelodysplastic syndrome. *Br. J. Haematol.*, **115**, 881–94.

54. Steins, M. B., Padro, T., Bieker, R. *et al.* (2002). Efficacy and safety of thalidomide in patients with acute myeloid leukemia. *Blood*, **99**, 834.

55. Corral, L. G., Haslett, P. A., Muller, G. W. *et al.* (1999). Differential cytokine modulation and T cell activation by two distinct classes of thalidomide analogues that are potent inhibitors of TNF alpha. *J. Immunol.*, **163**, 380–6.

56. Davies, F. E., Raje, N., Hideshima, T. *et al.* (2001). Thalidomide and immunomodulatory derivatives augment natural killer cell cytotoxicity in multiple myeloma. *Blood*, **98**, 210–16.

57. Richardson, P. G., Schlossman, R. L., Weller, E. *et al.* (2002). Immunomodulatory drug CC-5013 overcomes drug resistance and is well tolerated in patients with relapsed multiple myeloma. *Blood*, **100**, 3063.

58. List, A. F., Kurtin, S. E., Glinsmann-Gibson, B. J. *et al.* (2002). High erythropoietic remitting activity of the immunomodulatory thalidomide analog, CC5013, in patients with myelodysplastic syndrome (MDS). *Blood*, **100**, 96a.

59. List, A. F., Tate, W., Glinsmann-Gibson, B., and Baker, A. (2002). The immunomodulatory thalidomide analog CC5013 inhibits trophic response to VEGF in AML cells by abolishing cytokine-induced *PI3-Akt* activation. *Blood*, **100**, 139a.

60. List, A. F., Kurtin, S. E., Roe, D. J. *et al.* (2005). Efficacy of lenalidomide in myelodysplastic syndromes. *N. Engl. J. Med.*, **352**, 11–19.

61. Smolich, B. D., Yuen, H. A., West, K. A. *et al.* (2001). The antiangiogenic protein kinase inhibitors SU5416 and SU6668 inhibit the SCF receptor (*c-kit*) in a human myeloid leukemia cell line and in acute myeloid leukemia blasts. *Blood*, **97**, 1413–21.

62. Spiekermann, K., Dirschinger, R. J., Schwab, R. *et al.* (2003). The protein tyrosine kinase inhibitor SU5614 inhibits *FLT3* and induces growth arrest and apoptosis in AML-derived cell lines expressing a constitutively activated *FLT3*. *Blood*, **101**, 1494.

63. Giles, F. J., Stopeck, A. T., Silverman, L. R. *et al.* (2003). SU5416, a small molecule tyrosine kinase receptor inhibitor, has biologic activity in patients with refractory acute myeloid leukemia or myelodysplastic syndromes. *Blood*, **102**, 795–801.

64. Albitar, M., Smolich, B. D., Cherrington, J. M. *et al.* (2001). Effects of SU5416 on angiogenic factors, proliferation and apoptosis in patients with hematological malignancies. *Blood*, **98**, 110a (abstract).

65. Foran, J., Paquette, R., Copper, M. *et al.* (2002). A phase I study of repeated oral dosing with SU11248 for the treatment of patients with acute myeloid leukemia who have failed or are not eligible for conventional chemotherapy. *Blood*, **100**, 558a.

66. Raza, A., Gezer, S., Mundle, S. *et al.* (1995). Apoptosis in bone marrow biopsy samples involving stromal and hematopoietic cells in 50 patients with myelodysplastic syndromes. *Blood*, **86**, 268–76.

67. Dai, C., Price, J. O., Brunner, T. *et al.* (1998). Fas ligand is present in human erythroid colony-forming cells and interacts with *Fas* induced by interferon α to produce erythroid cell apoptosis. *Blood*, **85**, 1243–55.

68. Maciejewski, J., Selleri, C., Anderson, S. *et al.* (1995). *Fas* antigen expression on CD34+ human marrow cells is induced by interferon-α and tumor necrosis factor-α and potentiates cytokine-mediated hematopoietic suppression in vitro. *Blood*, **85**, 3183–90.

69. Raza, A., Mundle, S., Shetty, V. *et al.* (1996). Novel insights into biology of myelodysplastic syndromes: excessive apoptosis and the role of cytokines. *Int. J. Hematol.*, **63**, 265–78.

70. Kitagawa, M., Saito, I., Kuwata, T. *et al.* (1991). Overexpression of tumor necrosis factor ((TNF)-α and interferon (INF)-γ by bone marrow cells from patients with myelodysplastic syndromes. *Leukemia*, **11**, 2049–54.

71. Tauro, S., Hepburn, M. D., Peddie, C. M. *et al.* (2002). Functional disturbance of marrow stromal microenvironment in the myelodysplastic syndromes. *Leukemia*, **16**, 785–90.

72. Liekens, S., DeClercq, E., and Neyts, J. (2001). Angiogenesis: regulators and clinical applications. *Biochem. Pharmacol.*, **61**, 253–70.

73. Gearing, A. J. H., Beckett, P., Christodoulou, M. *et al.* (1994). Processing of tumor necrosis factor-α precursor by metalloproteinases. *Nature*, **370**, 555–7.

74. Black, R. A., Rauch, C. T., Kozlosky, C. J. *et al.* (1997). A metalloproteinase disintegrin that releases tumor necrosis factor-alpha from cells. *Nature*, **385**, 729–33.

75. Kayagaki, N., Kawasaki, A., Ebata, T. *et al.* (1995). Metalloproteinase-mediated release of human *Fas* ligand. *J. Exp. Med.*, **182**, 1777–83.

76. Price, A., Shi, Q., Morris, D. *et al.* (1999). Marked inhibition of tumor growth in a malignant glioma tumor model by a novel synthetic matrix metalloproteinase inhibitor AG3340. *Clin. Cancer Res.*, **5**, 845–54.

77. List, A. F., Kurtin, S., Callander, N. *et al.* (2002). Randomized, double-blind phase II study of the matrix metalloprotease (MMP) inhibitor, AG3340 (Prinomastat) in patients with myelodysplastic syndrome. *Blood*, **100**, 789a.

78. Gotlib, J., Jamieson, C., List, A. *et al.* (2003). Phase II study of bevacizumab (anti-VEGF humanized monoclonal antibody) in patients with myelodysplastic syndrome (MDS). *Blood*, **102** (suppl. 1), 425a.

79. Miller, W. H. Jr, Schipper, H. M., Lee, J. S., Singer, J., and Waxman, S. (2002). Mechanisms of action of arsenic trioxide. *Cancer Res.*, **62**, 3893.

80. Lehmann, S., Bengtzen, S., Paul, A., Christensson, B., and Paul, C. (2001). Effects of arsenic trioxide (As_2O_3) on leukemic cells from patients with non-M_3 acute myelogenous leukemia: studies of cytotoxicity, apoptosis and the pattern of resistance. *Eur. J. Haematol.*, **66**, 357.

81. Li, Y. M. and Broome, J. D. (1999). Arsenic targets tubulins to induce apoptosis in myeloid leukemia cells. *Cancer Res.*, **59**, 776.

82. Kroemer, G. and de The, H. (1999). Arsenic trioxide, a novel mitochondriotoxic anticancer agent? *J. Natl Cancer Inst.*, **91**, 743.

83. Jing, Y., Dai, J., Chalmers-Redman, R. M. E., Tatton, W. G., and Waxman, S. (1999). Arsenic trioxide selectively induces acute promyelocytic leukemia cell apoptosis via a hydrogen peroxide-dependent pathway. *Blood*, **94**, 2102.

84. Rojewski, M. T., Baldus, C., Knauf, W., Thiel, E., and Schrezenmeier, H. (2002). Dual effects of arsenic trioxide (As_2O_3) on non-acute promyelocytic leukaemia myeloid cell lines: induction of apoptosis and inhibition of proliferation. *Br. J. Haematol.*, **116**, 555.

85. Lehmann, S., Bengtzen, S., Paul, A., Christensson, B., and Paul, C. (2001). Effects of arsenic trioxide (As_2O_3) on leukemic cells from patients with non-M_3 acute myelogenous leukemia: studies of cytotoxicity, apoptosis and the pattern of resistance. *Eur. J. Haematol.*, **66**, 357.

86. Roboz, G. J., Dias, S., Lam, G. *et al.* (2000). Arsenic trioxide induces dose- and time-dependent apoptosis of endothelium and may exert an antileukemic effect via inhibition of angiogenesis. *Blood*, **96**, 1525.

87. Donelli, A., Chiodino, C., Panissidi, T., Roncaglia, R., and Torelli, G. (2000). Might arsenic trioxide be useful in the treatment of advanced myelodysplastic syndromes? *Haematologica*, **85**, 1002–3.

88. List, A. F., Schiller, G. J., Mason, J., Douer, D., and Paradise, C. (2002). Trisenox® (arsenic trioxide, ATO) in patients (pts) with myelodysplastic syndromes (MDS): preliminary findings in a phase II clinical study. *Blood*, **100**, 790a.

89. Raza, A., Lisak, L. A., Tahir, S. *et al.* (2002). Trilineage responses to arsenic trioxide (Trisenox®) and thalidomide in patients with myelodysplastic syndromes (MDS), particularly those with inv(3)(q21q26.2). *Blood*, **100**, 795a.

90. Vey, N., Dreyfus, F., Guerci, A. *et al.* (2003). Trisenox (arsenic trioxide) in patients (pts) with myelodysplastic syndromes (MDS): preliminary results of a phase I/II study. *Blood*, **104**, 401a.

91. Flotho, C., Valcamonica, S., Mach-Pascual, S. *et al.* (1999). *RAS* mutations and clonality analysis in children with juvenile myelomonocytic leukemia (JMML). *Leukemia*, **13**, 32.

92. Tomasson, M. H., Sternberg, D. W., Williams, I. R. *et al.* (2000). Fatal myeloproliferation, induced in mice by TEL/PDGFbetaR expression, depends on PDGFbetaR tyrosines 579/581. *J. Clin. Invest.*, **105**, 423–32.

93. Ross, T. S., Bernard, O. A., Berger, R. *et al.* (1998). Fusion of huntingtin interacting protein 1 to platelet-derived growth factor beta receptor (PDGFbetaR) in chronic myelomonocytic leukemia with t(5:7)(q33;q11.2). *Blood*, **91**, 4419–26.

94. Schwaller, J., Anastasiadou, E., Cain, D. *et al.* (2001). *H4(D10S170)*, a gene frequently rearranged in papillary thyroid carcinoma, is fused to the platelet-derived growth factor receptor beta gene in atypical chronic myeloid leukemia with t(5;10)(q33;q22). *Blood*, **97**, 3918.

95. Magnusson, M. K., Meade, K. E., Brown, K. E. *et al.* (2001). Rabaptin-5 is a novel fusion partner to platelet-derived growth factor beta receptor in chronic myelomonocytic leukemia. *Blood*, **98**, 2518–25.

96. Cross, N. C. P. and Reiter, A. (2002). Tyrosine kinase fusion genes in chronic myeloproliferative diseases. *Leukemia*, **16**, 1207–12.

97. Golub, T. R., Barker, G. F., Lovett, M., and Gilliland, D. G. (1994). Fusion of PDGF receptor beta to a novel ets-like gene, *tel*, in chronic myelomonocytic leukemia with t(5; 12) chromosomal translocation. *Cell*, **77**, 307–16.

98. Tomasson, M. H., Williamson, I. R., Hasserjian, R. *et al.* (1999). TEL/PDGFbetaR induces hematologic malignancies in mice that respond to a specific tyrosine kinase inhibitor. *Blood*, **93**, 1707–14.

99. Apperley, J. F., Gardembas, M., Melo, J. V. *et al.* (2002). Response to imatinib mesylate in patients with chronic myeloproliferative diseases with rearrangements of the platelet-derived growth factor receptor beta. *N. Engl. J. Med.*, **347**, 481–7.

100. Wattel, E., De Botton, S., Lai, J. L. *et al.* (1997). Long-term follow-up of de novo myelodysplastic syndromes treated with intensive chemotherapy; incidence of long-term survivors and outcome of partial responders. *Br. J. Haematol.*, **98**, 983–91.

101. Estey, E. H., Thall, P. F., Cortes, J. E. *et al.* (2001). Comparison of idarubicin + ara-C, fludarabine + ara-C, and topotecan + ara-C based regimens in treatment of newly diagnosed acute myeloid leukemia, refractory anemia with excess blasts in transformation, or refractory anemia with excess blasts. *Blood*, **98**, 3575–83.

102. Guilhot, F., Bouabdallah, R., Desablens, B. *et al.* (2002). Topotecan, cytosine arabinoside and G-CSF (TAG) versus idarubicin, cytosine arabinoside and G-CSF (IDAG) in patients with myelodysplastic syndrome (MDS) or MDS in transformation: a randomized phase III study. *Blood*, **100**, 98a.

103. Raza, A., Fenaux, P., Erba, H. *et al.* (2002). Preliminary analysis of a randomized phase 2 study of the safety and efficacy of 1 vs. 2 doses of gemtuzumab ozogamicin (Mylotarg) in patients with high risk myelodysplastic syndrome. *Blood*, **100**, (suppl. 1), 793a.

104. Estey, E. H., Thall, P. F., Giles, F. J. *et al.* (2002). Gemtuzumab ozogamicin with or without interleukin-11 in patients 65 years of age or older with untreated acute myeloid leukemia and high-risk myelodysplastic syndrome: comparison with idarubicin plus continuous-infusion, high-dose cytosine arabinoside. *Blood*, **99**, 4343.

105. Miller, K. B., Kim, K., Morrison, F. S. *et al.* (1992). The evaluation of low-dose cytarabine in the treatment of myelodysplastic syndromes: a phase-III intergroup study. *Ann. Hematol.*, **65**, 162–8 (erratum appears in *Ann. Hematol.* 1993; **66**, 164).

106. Hellstrom-Lindberg, E., Robert, K. H., Gahrton, G. *et al.* (1992). A predictive model for the clinical response to low dose ara-C: a study of 102 patients with myelodysplastic syndrome or acute leukemia. *Br. J. Haematol.*, **81**, 503–11.

107. Denzlinger, C., Bowen, D., Benz, D. *et al.* (2000). Low-dose melphalan induces favourable responses in elderly patients with high-risk myelodysplastic syndromes or secondary acute myeloid leukaemia. *Br. J. Hematol.*, **108**, 93–5.

108. Omoto, E., Deguchi, S., Takaba, S. *et al.* (1996). Low-dose melphalan for treatment of high-risk myelodysplastic syndromes. *Leukemia*, **10**, 609–14.

109. Ueda, K., Cardarelli, C., Gottesman, M. M., and Pastan, I. (1987). Expression of a full-length cDNA for the human "*MDR1*" gene confers resistance to colchicine, doxorubicin, and vinblastine. *Proc. Natl Acad. Sci. U.S.A.*, **84**, 3004–8.

110. Naito, M., Tsuge, H., Kuroko, C. *et al.* (1993). Enhancement of cellular accumulation of cyclosporine by anti-P-glycoprotein monoclonal antibody MRK-16 and synergistic modulation of multidrug resistance. *J. Natl Cancer Inst.*, **85**, 311–16.

111. Pallis, M. and Russell, N. (2000). P-glycoprotein plays a drug-efflux-independent role in augmenting cell survival in acute myeloblastic leukemia and is associated with modulation of a sphingomyelin-ceramide apoptotic pathway. *Blood*, **95**, 2897–904.

112. Johnstone, R. W., Cretney, E., and Smyth, M. J. (1999). P-glycoprotein protects leukemia cells against caspase-dependent, but not caspase-independent, cell death. *Blood*, **93**, 1075–85.

113. Smyth, M. J., Krasovskis, E., Sutton, V. R., and Johnstone, R. W. (1998). The drug efflux protein, P-glycoprotein, additionally protects drug-resistant tumor cells from multiple forms of caspase-dependent apoptosis. *Proc. Natl Acad. Sci. U.S.A.*, **95**, 7024–9.

114. List, A. F., Spier, C. M., Cline, A. *et al.* (1991). Expression of the multidrug resistance gene product (P-glycoprotein) in myelodysplasia is associated with a stem cell phenotype. *Br. J. Haematol.*, **78**, 28–34.

115. Samdani, A., Vijapurkar, U., Grimm, M. A. *et al.* (1996). Cytogenetics and p-glycoprotein (PGP) are independent predictors of treatment outcome in acute myeloid leukemia (AML). *Leuk. Res.*, **202**, 175–80.

116. Leith, C. P., Kopecky, K. J., Godwin, J. *et al.* (1997). Acute myeloid leukemia in the elderly: assessment of multidrug resistance (MDR1) and cytogenetics distinguishes

biologic subgroups with remarkably distinct responses to standard chemotherapy. A Southwest oncology group study. *Blood*, **89**, 3323–9.

117. List, A. F., Kopecky, K. J., Willman, C. L. *et al.* (2001). Benefit of cyclosporine modulation of drug resistance in patients with poor-risk acute myeloid leukemia: a Southwest oncology group study. *Blood*, **98**, 3212–20.

118. Wattel, E., Solary, E., Hecquet, B. *et al.* (1998). Quinine improves the results of intensive chemotherapy in myelodysplastic syndromes expressing p-glycoprotein: results of a randomized study. *Br. J. Haematol.*, **102**, 1015–24.

119. Mahadevan, D. and List, A. F. (2004). Targeting the multidrug resistance-1 transporter: molecular regulation and implications for trials in AML. *Blood*, **104**, 1940–51.

120. Uchida, T., Kinoshita, T., Nagai, H. *et al.* (1997). Hypermethylation of the *P15INK3B* gene in myelodysplastic syndromes. *Blood*, **90**, 1403–9.

121. Quesnel, B., Guillerm, G., Vereecque, R. *et al.* (1998). Methylation of the *p15INK4B* gene in myelodysplastic syndromes is frequent and acquired during disease progression. *Blood*, **91**, 2985–90.

122. Saiki, J. H., McCredie, K. B., Vietti, T. J. *et al.* (1978). 5-Azacytidine in acute leukemia. *Cancer*, **42**, 2111–14.

123. Silverman, L. R., Holland, J. F., Weinberg, R. S. *et al.* (1993). Effects of treatment with 5-azacytidine on the in vivo and in vitro hematopoiesis in patients with myelodysplastic syndromes. *Leukemia*, **7** (suppl. 1), 21–9.

124. Silverman, L. R., Holland, J. F., Nelson, D. *et al.* (1991). Trilineage response of myelodysplastic syndromes to subcutaneous azacytidine. *Proc. Am. Soc. Clin. Oncol.*, **10**, 222a (abstract).

125. Chitambar, C. R., Libnoch, J. A., Matthaeus, W. G. *et al.* (1991). Evaluation of continuous infusion of low-dose 5-azacytidine in the treatment of myelodysplastic syndromes. *Am. J. Hematol.*, **37**, 100–4.

126. Silverman, L. R., Demakos, E., Peterson, B. *et al.* (2002). Randomized controlled trial of azacytidine in patients with the myelodysplastic syndrome: a study of the cancer and leukemia group B. *J. Clin. Oncol*, **20**, 2429–40.

127. Daskalakis, M., Nguyen, T. T., Nguyen, C. *et al.* (2002). Demethylation of a hypermethylated *P15/INK4B* gene in patients with myelodysplastic syndrome by 5-aza-2'-deoxycytidine (decitabine) treatment. *Blood*, **100**, 2957–64.

128. Silverman, L. R., Davis, R. B., Holland, J. F. *et al.* (1989). 5-Azacytidine as a low-dose continuous infusion is an effective therapy for patients with myelodysplastic syndromes. *Proc. Am. Soc. Clin. Oncol.*, **8**, 198 (abstract 768).

129. Kornblith, A. B., Herndon, II J. E., Silverman, L. R. *et al.* (2002). Impact of azacytidine on the quality of life of patients with myelodysplastic syndrome treated in a randomized phase III trial: a cancer and leukemia group B study. *J. Clin. Oncol.*, **20**, 2441–52.

130. Kosugi, H., Towatari, M., Hatano, S. *et al.* (1999). Histone deacetylase inhibitors are the potent inducer/enhancer of differentiation in acute myeloid leukemia: a new approach to anti-leukemia therapy. *Leukemia*, **13**, 1316.

131. Ferrara, F. F., Fazi, F., Bianchini, A. *et al.* (2001). Histone deacetylase-targeted treatment restores retinoic acid signaling and differentiation in acute myeloid leukemia. *Cancer Res.*, **61**, 2.

132. Piekarz, R. L., Robey, R., Sandor, V. *et al.* (2001). Inhibitor of histone deacetylation, depsipeptide (FR901228), in the treatment of peripheral and cutaneous T-cell lymphoma: a case report. *Blood*, **98**, 2865.

133. Cote, S., Rosenauer, A., Bianchini, A. *et al.* (2002). Response to histone deacetylase inhibition of novel PML/RARalpha mutants detected in retinoic acid-resistant APL cells. *Blood*, **100**, 2586.

134. Gottlicher, M., Minucci, S., Zhu, P. *et al.* (2001). Valproic acid defines a novel class of HDAC inhibitors inducing differentiation of transformed cells. *EMBO J.*, **20**, 6969.

135. Phiel, C. J., Zhang, F., Huang, E. Y. *et al.* (2001). Histone deacetylase is a direct target of valproic acid, a potent anticonvulsant, mood stabilizer, and teratogen. *J. Biol. Chem.*, **276**, 36734.

136. Koyama, N., Koschmieder, S., Tyagi, S. *et al.* (2002). Differential effects of histone deacetylase inhibitors on interleukin-18 gene expression in myeloid cells. *Biochem. Biophys. Res. Commun.*, **292**, 937.

137. Jiemjit, A., Trujillo, M., and Gore, S. (2002). Induction of re-expression of silenced genes in acute myeliod leukaemia by valproic acid. *Blood*, **100**, 540a (abstract).

138. Ferrero, D., Campa, E., Campana, S., Dellacasa, C., and Boccadoro, M. (2002). Preliminary experience with valproic acid in association to differentiative agents and low dose chemotherapy in poor prognosis AML. *Blood*, **100**, 267b (abstract).

139. Castleberry, R. P., Emanuel, P. D., Zuckerman, K. S. *et al.* (1994). A pilot study of isotretinoin in the treatment of juvenile chronic myelogenous leukemia. *N. Engl. J. Med.*, **331**, 1680–4.

140. Stasi, R., Brunetti, M., Terzoli, E., and Amadori, S. (2002). Sustained response to recombinant human erythropoietin and intermittent *all*-trans retinoic acid in patients with myelodysplastic syndromes. *Blood*, **99**, 1578.

141. Lyttle, M. H., Hocker, M. D., Hui, H. C. *et al.* (1994). Isozyme-specific glutathione-S-transferase inhibitors: design and synthesis. *J. Med. Chem.*, **37**, 189–94.

142. Ruscoe, J. E., Rosario, L. A., Wang, T. *et al.* (2001). Pharmacologic or genetic manipulation of glutathione S-transferase P1–1 (GSTpi) influences cell proliferation pathways. *J. Pharmacol. Exp. Ther.*, **298**, 339–45.

143. Morgan, A. S., Stanboli, A., and Sanderson, P. E. (1996). TER199 increases bone marrow (BM) CFU-GM and peripheral platelet and neutrophil counts in myelosuppressed rodents. *Blood*, **88**, 134b.

144. Tew, K. D. (1994). Glutathione-associated enzymes in anticancer drug resistance. *Cancer Res.*, **54**, 4313–20.

145. Meng, F., Broxmeyer, H. E., Toavs, D. K. *et al.* (2001). TLK199: a novel, small molecule myelostimulant. *Proc. Annu. Meeting Am. Assoc. Cancer Res.*, **42**, 214 (abstract 1144).

146. Faderl, S., Kantarjian, H., Estey, E. *et al.* (2003). Hematologic improvement following treatment with TLK199 (a novel glutathione analog inhibitor of GST (1–1) in myelodysplastic synrome: interim results of a phase I/IIa study. *Blood*, **102** (suppl. 1), 426a.

147. Reuter, C. W. M., Morgan, M. A., and Bergmann, L. (2000). Targeting the ras signaling pathway: a rational, mechanism-based treatment for hematologic malignancies? *Blood*, **96**, 1655–69.

148. Tobal, K., Pagluca, A., Bhatt, B. *et al.* (1990). Mutation of the human FMS gene (M-CSF receptor) in myelodysplastic syndromes and acute myeloid leukemia. *Leukemia*, **4**, 486–9.

149. Hirsch-Ginsberg, C., LeMaistre, A. C., Kantarjian, H. *et al.* (1990). Ras mutations are rare events in Philadelphia chromosome-negative *bcr* gene rearrangement-negative chronic myelogenous leukemia, but are prevalent in chronic myelomonocytic leukemia. *Blood*, **76**, 1214–19.

150. Melani, C., Haliassos, A., Chomel, J. C. *et al.* (1990). *Ras* activation in myelodysplastic syndromes: clinical and molecular study of the chronic phase of the disease. *Br. J. Haematol.*, **74**, 408.

151. Padua, R. A., Guinn, B. A., Al-Sabah, A. I. *et al.* (1998). *RAS, FMS* and *p53* mutations and poor clinical outcome in myelodysplasias: a 10-year follow-up. *Leukemia*, **12**, 887.

152. Side, L. E., Emanuel, P. D., Taylor, B. *et al.* (1998). Mutations of the *NF1* gene in children with juvenile myelomonocytic leukemia without clinical evidence of neurofibromatosis, type 1. *Blood*, **92**, 267–72.

153. Karp, J. E., Lancet, J. E., Kaufmann, S. H. *et al.* (2001). Clinical and biologic activity of the farnesyl transferase inhibitor R115777 in adults with refractory and relapsed acute leukemias: a phase I clinical-laboratory correlative trial. *Blood*, **97**, 3361–9.

154. Kurzrock, R., Albitar, M., Cortes, J. E. *et al.* (2004). Phase II study of R115777, a farnesyl transferase inhibitor, in myelodysplastic syndrome. *J. Clin. Oncol.*, **22**, 1287–92.

155. Kurzrock, R., Kantarjian, H. M., Cortes, J. E. *et al.* (2003). Farnesyltransferase inhibitor R115777 in myelodysplastic syndrome: clinical and biologic activities in the phase 1 setting. *Blood*, **102**, 4527–34.

156. Liu, M., Bryant, M. S., Chen, J. *et al.* (1998). Antitumor activity of SCH 66336, an orally bioavailable tricyclic inhibitor of farnesyl protein transferase, in human tumor xenograft models and Wap-*ras* transgenic mice. *Cancer Res.*, **58**, 4947–56.

157. Buresh, A., Perentesis, J., Rimsza, L. *et al.* (2004). Hyperleukoytosis complicating treatment with lonafarnib in patients with chronic myelomonocytic leukemia. *Leukemia*, **19**, 308–10.

158. Cortes, J., Holyoake, T., Silver, R. *et al.* (2002). Continuous oral lonafarnib (Sarasar^{TM}) for the treatment of patients with advanced hematologic malignancies: a phase II study. *Blood*, **100**, 793a.

159. Feldman, E., Cortes, J., Holyoake, T. *et al.* (2003). Continuous oral lonafarnib (Sarasar ^{TM}) for the treatment of patients with myelodysplastic syndrome. *Blood*, **102**, abstract 1531.

160. List, A. F., Tache-Tallmadge, C., Tate, W. *et al.* (2003). Lonafarnib (Sarasar^{TM}) modulates integrin affinity to promote homotypic and heterotypic adhesion of chronic myelomonocytic leukemia (CMML) cells. *Proc. Am. Assoc. Cancer Res.*, **44**, 39a.

8

Supportive care in myelodysplastic syndromes: hemopoietic cytokine and iron chelation therapy

Jason Gotlib[1] and Peter L. Greenberg[1,2]

[1] Stanford University Cancer Center, Stanford, CA, USA
[2] VA Palo Alto Health Care System, Palo Alto, CA, USA

Myelodysplastic syndromes (MDS) comprise a heterogeneous spectrum of clonal myeloid hemopathies characterized by bone marrow failure, morphologic dysplasia, and a variable tendency to evolve into acute myeloid leukemia (AML). In low-risk MDS, excessive intramedullary apoptosis of hematopoietic progenitors and ineffective hematopoiesis contribute to the paradoxical finding of hypercellular marrows in the setting of chronic refractory cytopenias. Evolution to AML occurs in approximately 30% of MDS cases, and is frequently associated with reversion of marrow myeloid precursors to a leukemic phenotype. The in vitro and in vivo study of the proliferative and differentiation abnormalities involved in MDS hematopoiesis has been facilitated by the development of recombinant hemopoietic growth factors (HGFs). Refractory cytopenias are major causes of morbidity in MDS. Thus, supportive care to manage these consequences of the marrow failure in MDS is the mainstay of treatment for these individuals.

Symptomatic anemia is a critical clinical problem in MDS. Cytokine therapy with recombinant erythropoietin (rEPO) has resulted in erythroid responses in a proportion of individuals with MDS, which can be substantially increased in selected patients with addition of recombinant granulocyte colony-stimulating factor (rG-CSF). Identification of the clinical and histopathologic features which predict response to these HGFs permits tailoring of these treatments to appropriate subsets of MDS patients. Due to the combination of ineffective erythropoiesis and the relatively large amount of red blood cell (RBC) transfusions MDS patients receive to treat their

Myelodysplastic Syndromes: Clinical and Biological Advances, ed. Peter L. Greenberg. Published by Cambridge University Press. © Cambridge University Press 2006.

hypoproductive anemia, a substantial proportion of these individuals have iron overload. Until now, limited investigation has been been dedicated to the pathological mechanisms, clinical consequences, and treatment of transfusional hemosiderosis and hemochromatosis in MDS. Desferroxiamine (Desferal), a predominantly subcutaneously administered iron chelator, has been used, although inconsistently, to treat iron overload in MDS. With the recent development of oral iron chelators, which hold promise as effective and convenient alternatives to desferroxiamine, and the emergence of non-invasive methods for measuring liver iron content, iron overload has emerged as a fertile area of study in MDS and other transfusion-dependent chronic anemias.

MDS and in vitro hematopoiesis

In vitro culture systems have proven valuable for analyzing the proliferative and differentiative effects of various HGFs on hemopoietic stem cells and committed progenitors. These in vitro assays are relevant to the study of MDS in which defective differentiation leads to ineffective hematopoiesis.[1] The colony-forming capacities of pluripotent hemopoietic stem cells (colony-forming unit–granulocyte, erythroid, macrophage, megakaryocyte (CFU-GEMM)), and their progeny, committed progenitor cells (granulocyte-macrophage (CFU-GM), burst-forming unit–erythroid (BFU-E), CFU–erythroid (CFU-E), and CFU–megakaryocyte (CFU-Mk)), are low or absent in most MDS (and AML) patients.[1–5]

Diminished production and responsiveness to HGFs constitute the two principal hemopoietic regulatory derangements found in MDS.[1] Marrow cells and peripheral blood T cells from MDS patients produce decreased amounts of several cytokines, including granulocyte–macrophage colony-stimulating factor (GM-CSF), interleukin-3 (IL-3), macrophage colony-stimulating factor (M-CSF), and IL-6.[6] Levels of monocyte-derived granulocyte colony-stimulating factor (G-CSF) are decreased in MDS patients, but also in elderly control subjects.[7] In clonogenic cultures, CFU-GM stimulated with G-CSF and GM-CSF are subnormal in a majority of MDS patients.[8] In MDS, GM-CSF and IL-3 generally exhibit greater myeloid proliferative effects in vitro than G-CSF, whereas G-CSF has more potent differentiative effects. These findings are particularly evident in higher-risk MDS patients (e.g., refractory anemia with excess blasts (RAEB)/RAEB in transformation (RAEB-T)) and those with normal karyotypes.[8]

MDS erythroid progenitors show suboptimal responses to erythropoietin (EPO) in vitro.[9,10] Analysis of the relationship between EPO levels and erythroid precursors from MDS patients indicates that the anemia of MDS was not attributable to EPO's inability to induce generation of CFU-E, but was related to the size of the BFU-E population, whose severe deficiency resulted in an insufficient influx of EPO-responsive cells.[10] Despite the relatively low serum EPO levels in MDS, these findings suggested that EPO therapy in MDS patients would have limited clinical benefit because the initial growth requirements and generation of BFU-E from more primitive cells were not regulated solely by this hormone. These in vitro predictions have been borne out in clinical trials where EPO has shown modest efficacy in improving the anemia of MDS patients.

G-CSF synergistically augments the in vitro EPO responsiveness of BFU-E in normal and MDS marrow,[10] and in clinical trials of the hormone combination improved hemoglobin responses were observed, particularly in patients with refractory anemia with ringed sideroblasts (RARS). Investigations using serum-free media and purified CD34+ cells with recombinant HGFs have shown decreased responsiveness of MDS hematopoietic progenitors to G-CSF and EPO.[11] The mechanism(s) underlying the altered responsiveness of MDS precursors to cytokines is unclear. G-CSF and IL-3 binding in MDS have not exhibited significantly different receptor numbers or affinity for the receptors.[12] Postreceptor signaling pathway abnormalities after EPO-binding have been demonstrated in precursors from some MDS patients.[13] These in vitro observations have served as a platform for clinical trial testing of several HGFs in MDS, including EPO, G-CSF/GM-CSF, interleukins, and recombinant thrombopoietic substances.

National Comprehensive Cancer Network (NCCN) guidelines for MDS: supportive care, HGFs, and iron chelation

The majority of MDS patients have symptomatic anemia and associated fatigue. In this primarily elderly population, anemia may aggravate co-morbidities such as cardiac and pulmonary disease. In the evaluation of anemia, other contributing causes should be excluded, including iron, vitamin B_{12} or folate deficiency, hemolysis, blood loss, toxic chemicals (e.g., arsenic, lead) and renal disease.

The community standard for the treatment of MDS remains supportive care, which includes clinical and psychosocial/quality-of-life assessments, and transfusions. Under the NCCN guidelines, leukocyte-reduced RBC transfusions are recommended for MDS patients with symptomatic fatigue.[14] Similarly, platelet transfusions are suggested for severe thrombocytopenia or thrombocytopenia-related bleeding. Antifibrinolytic agents such as aminocaproic acid may be considered for bleeding which is not alleviated by platelet transfusions. For patients who are serologically cytomegalovirus (CMV)-negative and are potential candidates for hemopoietic cell transplantation, use of CMV-negative and irradiated blood products is recommended.

Support with hemopoietic cytokines can be clinically useful for a proportion of patients with symptomatic, refractory cytopenias. Based on data cited below, in anemic MDS patients with EPO levels < 500 U/l and marrows lacking ringed sideroblasts, the NCCN treatment guidelines recommend high doses of subcutaneous (sc) rEPO in the range of 150–300 U/kg per day.[14] If an erythroid response is not observed at the lower doses of this range after 6–8 weeks of treatment, escalation to the higher doses should be considered for an additional 6–8-week period (or may be considered initially). Based on the potential synergistic activity of rEPO + rG-CSF in vitro, a 6–8-week trial of the combination has been recommended for MDS patients whose anemia fails to respond to rEPO alone. Relatively low doses of sc rG-CSF (0.3–3 µg/kg per day) are sufficient to elicit erythroid responses; the rG-CSF dose is titrated to normalize the absolute neutrophil count (ANC) in neutropenic patients, or double the ANC in those with a normal neutrophil count. The combination appears to be particularly effective in patients with EPO levels < 500 U/l, and in individuals with the RARS subtype of MDS who typically demonstrate poor erythroid responses to rEPO alone. The frequent dosing of sc rEPO ± rG-CSF is based on a preponderance of published reports which utilize daily dosing; however, thrice-weekly dosing of sc rEPO ± rG-CSF has recently been shown to be effective (see below). Data have been also been published regarding the clinical utility of once-weekly dosing (see below), although its efficacy compared to more frequent dosing has not been evaluated in a randomized trial. For neutropenic MDS patients with active infections, or a history of recurrent bacterial infections, the NCCN guidelines recommend use of single-agent sc rG-CSF or rGM-CSF.[14] Few data are available regarding the effects of iron overload in MDS patients, and the appropriate time to commence chelation therapy in this population. The current recommendation by the NCCN is to initiate iron chelation with sc nightly desferroxiamine for patients who have received over 20–30 RBC transfusions, monitoring organs particularly susceptible to the toxic effects of iron (e.g., heart, liver, pancreas).[14]

Mechanisms of action of EPO and G-CSF

In response to EPO, DNA synthesis, GATA-1 binding activity and signal transducer and activation of transcription (STAT)-5 activation were found to be absent or severely decreased in MDS compared to normal marrow cells.[13] Another study determined that ineffective erythropoiesis was more strongly correlated with stimulation of *fas*-mediated proapoptotic pathways rather than defective antiapoptotic signaling via the *Jak2*-STAT5 pathway.[15] In some cases, both mechanisms appear to be operative. Investigators have also demonstrated that apoptosis was associated with increased *fas*-ligand production during the stage of erythroid differentiation, a process that could be inhibited by a chimeric Fas-Fc protein.[16] Using marrow cell morphology and fluorescence in situ hybridization (FISH) in cytogenetically categorized MDS patients, rEPO treatment in responding patients resulted in a significantly lower proportion of FISH-abnormal erythroid precursors compared to before EPO treatment.[17] In addition, patients responding to rEPO had a significantly lower percentage of FISH-abnormal erythroid precursors compared to unresponsive individuals. Although not consistently found by all investigators, these results are consistent with rEPO-induced proliferation of residual karyotypically normal erythroid precursors in a proportion of MDS patients.

Studies of apoptosis within MDS marrow progenitor cells have begun to unravel the mechanism whereby rG-CSF synergistically works with rEPO to improve the hemoglobin in MDS patients. In the RARS subgroup, rG-CSF inhibited the increased *fas*-induced apoptosis of MDS bone marrow cells.[18] rG-CSF mediated reductions in caspase-8 and caspase-3-like activity, with concomitant reductions in the amount of late cellular apoptotic changes.

Erythroid progenitor cells from MDS patients also demonstrate spontaneous release of cytochrome c from mitochondria with subsequent activation of caspase-9, an additional apoptotic pathway that can be inhibited by rG-CSF.[19] Among low-risk MDS specimens studied, this effect was most pronounced in erythroid progenitors from RARS patients.

Recombinant erythropoietin

In patients with MDS, EPO levels may be suboptimally elevated for the degree of anemia. The rationale of rEPO treatment is to provide supraphysiological doses of the cytokine in order to raise serum EPO levels and to enhance the proliferation and differentiation of marrow erythroid progenitors. The clinical aim is to improve hemoglobin levels and anemia-associated fatigue, and to reduce the risks associated with RBC transfusions, such as infection, red cell alloimmunization, and secondary hemochromatosis.

A significant amount of variability in the frequency and dosing of sc rEPO exists among published studies. Although various criteria have been used to define response to rEPO therapy, and the proportion of low- and high-risk FAB subtypes differs in each study, the cumulative response rate of numerous published trials (≥ 20 patients enrolled) is approximately 20% (Table 8.1).[20–28]

To date, the only double-blind, placebo-controlled, randomized study of sc rEPO in MDS has been performed by the Italian Cooperative Study Group.[26] Patients with $< 10\%$ marrow blasts received either placebo or sc rEPO 150 U/kg per day for 8 weeks. A statistically significant hemoglobin response was observed in the rEPO arm, but benefit was limited to the refractory anemia (RA) subtype, and patients with either no prior transfusion requirements or basal EPO levels < 200 U/l. Other non-randomized studies have cited serum EPO levels < 100 U/l, female gender, or normal karyotype as predictors of response to EPO.[22,24] A recent study found that baseline serum EPO levels also predicted survival.[28] Patients with EPO levels > 50 U/l experienced a median survival of 17 months compared to 65 months in patients with EPO levels < 50 U/l.

Using RBC transfusion-independence as the minimal criterion for response, one meta-analysis of 115 patients from 10 trials[29] and a second meta-analysis of 205 patients from 17 published reports[30] reported response rates of 24% and 16%, respectively. In the latter study, patients with RARS

Table 8.1 Clinical trials of recombinant erythropoietin (rEPO) ± recombinant granulocyte colony-stimulating factor (rG-CSF) in myelodysplastic syndrome[a]

Year	Authors	EPO and G-CSF doses	no. of Patients	%	Reference
rEPO alone					
1992	Adamson *et al.*	450–900 U/kg per week	20	50%	[20]
1993	Aloe Spiriti *et al.*	800 U/kg per week	23	30%	[21]
1993	Stenke *et al.*	150 U/kg 3 × per week	27	26%	[22]
1994	Stone *et al.*	300–1200 U/kg per week	20	35%	[23]
1995	Rose *et al.*	450–900 U/kg per week	100	28%	[24]
1997	Stasi *et al.*	450–900 U/kg per week	41	32%	[25]
1998	Italian Cooperative Study Group	1050 U/kg per week	38	37%	[26]
2002	Terpos *et al.*	150 U/kg 3 × per week	281	45%	[27]
2002	Wallvik *et al.*	150–200 U/kg 3 × per week	66	33%	[28]
Meta-analyses					
1994	Rodriguez *et al.*[c]	Various doses and schedules	110	24%	[29]
1995	Hellström-Lindberg[d]	Various doses and schedules	205	16%	[30]
rEPO + rG-CSF					
1993	Negrin *et al.*	G-CSF 1 μg/kg per day; EPO 150–300 U/kg per day	24	42%	[38]
1993	Hellström-Lindberg *et al.*	G-CSF 0.3–3.0 μg/kg per day; EPO 60–120 U/kg per day	21	38%	[39]
1996	Negrin *et al.*	G-CSF 1 μg/kg per day; EPO 150–300 U/kg per day	44	48%	[40]
1997	Hellström-Lindberg *et al.*	G-CSF 0.3–3.0 μg/kg per day; EPO 60–300 U/kg per day	98	36%	[41]
1998	Hellstrom-Lindberg *et al.*	G-CSF 30–150 μg/day; EPO 5000–10 000 U/day	47	38%	[42]
2000	Mantovani *et al.*	G-CSF 1.5 μg/kg per day; EPO 200–400 U/kg 3 × per week	25, 28[g]	61%, 80%[g]	[45]
2003	Hellström-Lindberg *et al.*	G-CSF 75–300 μg/day; EPO 10 000 U 5 × per week	53	42%	[43]
2003	Jadersten *et al.*[e]	Median doses: G-CSF 225 μg/week EPO 30 000 U per week	128	39%	[47]
2004	Casadevall *et al.*[f]	G-CSF 105 μg 3 × per week; EPO 20 000 U 3 × per week	24	42%	[46]

[a] Clinical trials enrolling 20 or more patients are shown.

[b] Response criteria differ between studies.

[c] Meta-analysis of 10 studies.

[d] Meta-analysis of 17 studies.

[e] 129 patients enrolled in three Nordic MDS studies between 1990 and 1999.

[f] Randomized trial of rEPO + rG-CSF versus supportive care

[g] 25 patients evaluated in 12-week follow-up with 61% response rate; 28 evaluated in 36-week follow-up with 80% response rate.

showed a significantly lower response rate (8%) than all other patients (21%). Other factors predictive of response were the absence of transfusion need (44% versus 10%) and serum EPO concentration $\leq$ 200 U/l. Patients without an RBC transfusion requirement and MDS patients other than RARS showed a response rate > 50% irrespective of their serum EPO level. There was no dose–response relationship, and no correlation between maximal dose and time to response. The optimal rEPO dose was generally in the range of 450–1000 U/kg per week. The limited clinical efficacy of rEPO in these trials likely partly reflects the suboptimal numbers or responsiveness of myelodysplastic BFU-E to rEPO.[9,10]

Durability of the EPO response has been studied in two trials. In a small study of 18 primarily low-risk MDS patients treated with sc rEPO 10 000 U thrice weekly, 3 patients were still responding at 30, 41, and 56 months.[31] Two of these patients were maintained on a lower rEPO dose, and one was still responding 48 months after rEPO had been stopped. In 7 patients, anemia recurred with tapering of the initial rEPO dose, and a second course of rEPO resulted in responses in 5 of 6 retreated patients. The remaining 8 patients died during or soon after the initial treatment period, 3 from transformation to AML. At the time of follow-up, 5 patients maintained hemoglobin responses with a median duration of 36+ months.

A larger phase II study of 281 patients evaluated whether response rates to rEPO increased with prolonged administration.[27] Using a dose of 150 U/kg sc thrice weekly, the overall erythroid response rate was 18% at 3 months, and increased to 45% at 6 months. The median duration of response was 17 months. Significant predictors of response included EPO level < 150 U/l, good cytogenetic risk group by International Prognostic Scoring System (IPSS) criteria, and RA compared to RARS and RAEB French–American–British (FAB) subtypes.

Two studies with small numbers of MDS patients have evaluated the efficacy of once-weekly dosing of rEPO. Musto *et al.* treated 13 low- to intermediate-risk anemic MDS patients with rEPO 40 000 U sc weekly for at least 8 weeks.[32] Five patients (38%) exhibited major erythroid responses which were ongoing for 3–11+ months at the time of publication, without the need for dose modification. One of these patients had previously received rEPO 10 000 U sc thrice weekly for at least 2 months without a significant improvement in the hemoglobin.

In a study by Garypidou and colleagues,[33] 4 of 10 (40%) MDS patients (3 RA, 1 RAEB) achieved a major erythroid response to rEPO 40 000 U sc weekly after 2–3 months of therapy. After a median follow-up time of 21.5 months (range 9–44 months), all 4 patients had maintained their responses. One additional patient from the Musto *et al.* study and 2 patients from the latter trial manifested major erythroid responses at 3 months of therapy, indicating that prolonged administration of weekly rEPO may improve response rates. Although once-weekly rEPO injections would likely have a beneficial impact on patient compliance and quality of life, randomized comparisons with more conventional dosing regimens (e.g., thrice-weekly or daily dosing) in a larger cohort of patients are needed to compare the response rates and durability.

Recombinant granulocyte colony-stimulating factor

In a pilot 6–8-week dose-escalation phase I/II trial of sc rG-CSF at doses of 0.1–3.0 μg/kg per day,[34] 16 of 18 patients demonstrated a rise in the absolute neutrophil count from five- to 40-fold. Cessation of treatment resulted in return of counts to baseline values over a 2–4-week period. Bone marrow myeloid maturation improved in 16 of 18 patients. Significant responses in other lineage responses were not observed. Eleven patients from this initial cohort were subsequently enrolled in a long-term maintenance trial of rG-CSF.[35] Ten patients responded with persistent improvements in neutrophil counts for up to 16 months. In a retrospective analysis, there was a significant reduction in bacterial infection risk during periods with an ANC > 1500/mm^3 with rG-CSF therapy compared to periods with an ANC < 1500/mm^3. Enhancement of in vitro neutrophil function (phagocytosis and chemotaxis) persisted during the maintenance phase. Of 10 anemic patients, 2 non-RBC transfusion-requiring patients had a > 20% impovement in the hemoglobin, and another 2 patients had decreases in their RBC transfusion requirements. Cytogenetic abnormalities, when present, persisted after rG-CSF treatment, indicating differentiation of the abnormal clone. Three patients progressed to AML after 3–16 months of treatment. Chronic rG-CSF administration was well tolerated without clinically significant toxicities.

A phase III multi-institutional randomized trial of 102 patients with high-risk MDS was performed to determine the impact of rG-CSF on the natural history of the disease.[36] Fifty patients with RAEB or RAEB-T were treated with sc rG-CSF 1–5 µg/kg daily, and 52 patients received only supportive care. rG-CSF was well tolerated with a low incidence of minor side-effects. The rate and time to progression to AML were similar in RAEB and RAEB-T patients in both arms of the study. The survival of RAEB-T patients was also comparable in both arms; however, the median survival of RAEB patients was significantly shorter in patients receiving rG-CSF (10.4 versus 21.4 months), due to a higher rate of disease-related non-leukemic deaths, primarily from bleeding. A retrospective analysis found that RAEB patients receiving rG-CSF had a median survival comparable to previously reported RAEB survival data in the literature; in contrast, RAEB patients in the supportive-care group had prolonged survival. An increased proportion of RAEB patients receiving rG-CSF (29% versus 14%) were in the high-prognostic-risk category, using a scoring system that stratified MDS patients according to the percentage of bone marrow blasts, platelets, and age. Decreased survival was only observed in this subgroup of poor-risk RAEB patients receiving rG-CSF. The survival differences in RAEB patients may therefore be attributed to either the increased number of high-risk patients in the rG-CSF arm, or the unusually long survival of high-risk patients receiving just supportive measures. rG-CSF was not shown to alter the rate of infections in these patients.

rEPO + rG-CSF

Synergy between rEPO and rG-CSF has been demonstrated in vitro for the production of both normal and MDS marrow BFU-E numbers.[37] rG-CSF enhances the development of early precursors into EPO-responsive hematopoietic progenitors.[37] Two phase II studies confirmed improved in vivo erythroid responses to combined rEPO + rG-CSF treatment compared to either agent alone.[38,39] These trials initially used rG-CSF at doses of 1 µg/kg (0.3–3 µg/kg) sc daily to normalize or double the neutrophil count. rEPO 100 U/kg per day sc was then administered and the dose was escalated to 150–300 U/kg per day every 4 weeks, or maintained at 120 U/kg per day in the other study, while continuing rG-CSF. Ten (42%) of 24 patients in one study[38] and 8 (38%) of 21 patients in the second study[39] had substantial erythroid responses, characterized by increased hemoglobin values and decreased transfusion requirements. Nearly all patients had improvements

Table 8.2 Model for predicting erythroid responses to granulocyte colony-stimulating factor and erythropoietin (EPO) in myelodysplastic syndrome patients

	Scores[a]					
Variable	−3	−2	−1	0	+1	+2
Serum EPO (U/l)	> 500				100–500	< 100
Transfusions (U/month)	≥ 2			< 2		

		Response group	
Predictive score	Type	% Responders (patients)	
> +1	High	74 (22/29)	
±	Intermediate	23 (7/31)	
< −1	Low	7 (3/34)	

[a] Multivariate logistic regression analysis; weighted logistic coefficients.
From Hellström-Lindberg et al.[41] with permission from Blackwell.

in neutrophil counts. Factors predicting response included lower endogenous serum EPO levels (< 200–500 U/l), less advanced pancytopenia, and less pretreatment RBC transfusion needs. Responses were seen in all FAB subtypes; the best rate (60%) was observed in RARS patients who respond poorly to rEPO alone. A subsequent study of maintenance rG-CSF treatment showed that approximately one-half of the patients lost their response upon rG-CSF withdrawal and regained it when rG-CSF was resumed.[40]

In a multi-institutional Scandinavian–American trial of 98 MDS patients treated with rEPO + rG-CSF, a similar erythroid response rate of 36% was observed.[41] Multivariate analysis showed that baseline serum EPO levels and initial transfusion needs predicted responses to combination therapy. Using pretreatment serum EPO levels as a ternary variable (< 100, 100–500, or > 500 U/l) and RBC transfusion requirement as a binary variable (< 2 or ≥ 2 units per month), a scoring system was devised as a means of predicting erythroid response (Table 8.2). Patients were divided into three groups: one group with a high probability of erythroid responses (74%), one intermediate group (23%), and one group with poor responses to treatment (7%). A subsequent randomized phase II study corroborated the results of the Scandinavian–American trial, and established a durable median response time of 24 months.[42] Response rates were identical in two treatment groups primed with either rG-CSF (4 weeks) or rEPO (8 weeks), indicating that initial treatment with rG-CSF was not necessary.

The Scandinavian MDS Group has recently provided further data validating the Scandinavian–American model defining subgroups of patient with good, intermediate, and poor erythroid responses to the combination of rEPO + rG-CSF. This study also indicated improved quality of life for responding patients.[43] The Scandinavian–American score was useful in predicting erythroid responses in a Spanish multicenter study of 32 MDS patients with RA or RARS and serum EPO levels at study entry of ≤ 250 U/l.[44] A 50% erythroid response rate was observed among the subset of 14 patients treated with rG-CSF 1 μg/kg in addition to rEPO 300 U/kg thrice weekly. In a phase II study from Germany, Mantovani and colleagues assessed a prolonged schedule of combined rEPO + rG-CSF treatment.[45] After 12 weeks of treatment, the erythroid response rate was 61%, and increased to 80% after 36 weeks. After 1 and 2 years of ongoing combined cytokine treatment, 50% of the initial responders showed continuing responses.

Casadevall and colleagues recently published the first randomized trial comparing treatment with rEPO (20 000 units thrice weekly) + rG-CSF (150 μg thrice weekly) versus supportive care.[46] Using stringent response criteria, 10/24 (42%) in the rEPO + rG-CSF group exhibited erythroid responses after 3 months compared to no hemoglobin responses in the supportive-care arm. The response rates were 50%, 46%, and 20% in RA, RARS, and RAEB patients, respectively. Of the 10 responders, 8 continued on to a 40-week maintenance phase of rEPO alone. Anemia recurred in 6 of these patients, and re-addition of G-CSF in 4 patients corrected the anemia in all cases. These response rates corroborate the findings of earlier nonrandomized studies of rEPO + rG-CSF in MDS patients. However, rEPO + rG-CSF treatment was threefold more expensive than supportive care, primarily related to the cost of these medications.

Long-term rEPO + rG-CSF treatment: the Nordic MDS experience

Long-term follow-up data from 129 MDS patients treated with rEPO + rG-CSF enrolled in three Nordic MDS Group studies between 1990 and 1999 were recently presented.[47] Outcomes (e.g., survival, evolution to AML) were compared to untreated patients from the International MDS Risk Analysis Workshop (IMRAW) database[48] for MDS. Among their treated patients, 129 individuals were stratified by the FAB classification (30 RA, 41 RARS, 58 RAEB) and 118 patients by IPSS[48] subgroupings (30 low, 57 intermediate 1, 22 intermediate 2, and 5 high). Patients were followed for a median of 30 months (range 2–142 months). An overall erythroid response rate of 39% was observed with rEPO + rG-CSF therapy (RA 39%, RARS 50%, RAEB 31%). The median duration of response was 23 months (range 3–116 months), with 20% of erythroid responses lasting > 4 years. Erythroid responses were significantly more durable in RA/RARS versus RAEB patients (median 28 versus 12 months). The lowest effective median maintenance dose of rEPO was 30 000 U/week (range 5000–50 000 U/week), and the median dose for rG-CSF was 225 μg/week (range 0–900 μg/wk). When comparing a cohort of these patients who had a short time from diagnosis to treatment (< 3 months) with patients in the IPSS database, there was no statistical difference in the odds ratio for risk of death. Also, there was no difference in the time it took for 25% of the patients to evolve to AML. These results indicated that rEPO + rG-CSF elicited durable erythroid responses, predominantly in low-risk MDS patients, and had no adverse impact on the long-term outcomes of survival and transformation to leukemia.

Recombinant granulocyte-macrophage colony-stimulating factor

Despite the use of different schedules and routes of administration, numerous phase I/II studies have shown that rGM-CSF produces dose-dependent increases in neutrophil counts in the majority of MDS patients.[49–62] A European Organization for Research and Treatment of Cancer (EORTC) randomized multicenter study evaluated the effects of up to 2 months rGM-CSF treatment in MDS patients with fewer than 10% bone marrow blasts.[60] Approximately two-thirds of patients responded at dose levels of 108 or 216 μg sc daily. The small number of patients and limited duration of treatment precluded determination of the effects of rGM-CSF therapy on disease progression and infection frequency. Another multicenter study randomized MDS patients to rGM-CSF 3 μg/kg sc daily for 3 months versus observation.[61] After 3 months of therapy, patients could cross over from the observation to rGM-CSF arm if infections were documented. A marked increase in neutrophils and fewer infections were observed in the rGM-CSF group. rGM-CSF was not associated with an increased rate of conversion to leukemia. Survival benefit could not be assessed because of the study's cross-over design.

These multicenter trials of rGM-CSF have generally shown no clinically significant erythroid responses, and many thrombocytopenic patients developed lower platelet counts during treatment, necessitating more platelet transfusions.[60,61] In addition, a significant proportion of patients discontinued treatment with rGM-CSF because of side-effects, including pulmonary infiltrates, flu-like syndromes, hyperleukocytosis, and bone pain.[60–62]

rEPO + rGM-CSF

Similar to trials of rEPO + rG-CSF, investigators have assessed the clinical efficacy of combined rEPO + rGM-CSF treatment in MDS patients. In small phase II trials of concurrent or sequential rEPO + rGM-CSF treatment, increases in hemoglobin levels or decreased transfusion requirements occurred in 23–46% of patients.[63–66] A 12-week randomized, placebo-controlled trial of rGM-CSF (0.3–5.0 μg/kg per day) and rEPO therapy (150 U/kg thrice weekly) stratified 66 MDS patients to endogenous EPO levels of < 500 or > 500 U/l.[67] Combined rGM-CSF and EPO therapy significantly improved neutrophil counts, but platelet counts were unaffected. A trend toward reduced RBC transfusion requirements was observed in patients with EPO levels lower than 500 U/l, but only 9% of patients in the combined cytokine group achieved a hemoglobin response ≥ 2 g/dl. In a study of 19 low-risk MDS patients, sequential rGM-CSF (3 μg/kg) and rEPO (60–120 U/kg) were administered weekly for 3 months.[68] Ten of 19 (53%) responded, with 7 patients achieving a good response, and 3 patients a partial response. All responding RARS patients continued to demonstrate erythroid responses during 3–24 months of follow-up, whereas 1 RA and 2 RAEB patients did not have continuing responses at 2–12 months. Although these studies of rGM-CSF and rEPO treatment demonstrate some clinically important erythroid responses, the combination of rG-CSF and rEPO is at least as effective and is generally better tolerated because of the greater toxicity associated with rGM-CSF.

rEPO plus other agents

In recent phase II trials, amifostine added to sc rEPO $\pm$ rGSF has generally not resulted in clinically significant erythroid reponses or improvements in other blood lineages.[69–72] Sustained but limited multilineage responses (11%) were noted with *all*-trans retinoic acid plus rEPO in low- and intermediate-risk MDS patients.[73] Further study is warranted to evaluate this combination.

Recombinant interleukins (rILs)

rIL-3

Three phase I/II studies have evaluated the efficacy of short-term rIL-3 treatment in MDS patients.[74–76] These preliminary studies indicated that rIL-3 could increase neutrophil counts, but not as prominently as rGM-CSF or rG-CSF. Although rIL-3 transiently improved thrombocytopenia in some patients, erythropoiesis was rarely stimulated. A longer-term study of 3-month rIL-3 therapy elicited improvements in 2 of 5 patients with initial platelet counts lower than 50 000/mm³, without other lineage responses.[77] The issue as to whether hematopoietic growth factor support with a combination of rIL-3 and rEPO could augment erythroid responses was evaluated in 22 MDS patients.[78] The combination produced increased reticulocyte counts in 5 patients, but only 2 patients experienced a decreased need for RBC transfusions. The erythroid response was comparable to studies of rEPO alone, but rIL-3-related side-effects prompted dose reduction in the majority of patients.

rIL-6

The in vitro stimulatory effect of rIL-6 on thrombopoiesis prompted its evaluation in a phase I study of 22 low-risk MDS patients with thrombocytopenia.[79] Eight (36%) patients experienced a transient rise in platelet counts, but only 3 were classified as major responders. rIL-6 increased the frequency of higher-ploidy megakaryocytes without increasing the number of megakaryocyte progenitors, consistent with its known maturation-inducing effect. Non-dose-dependent anemia developed in most patients, and no neutrophil responses were documented. Constitutional symptoms and anemia were experienced by most patients, precluding all but 3 patients from receiving maintenance therapy. The marginal activity and significant therapy-related toxicity of rIL-6 make it of limited value as a thrombopoietic agent in MDS.

rIL-11

Because of rIL-11-associated toxicity (e.g., peripheral and pulmonary edema) at doses of 50 μg/kg per day, Kurzrock and coworkers studied lower-dose rIL-11 at 10 μg/kg per day in patients with bone marrow failure.[80] Six (38%) of 16 patients showed clinically significant platelet responses to rIL-11. The median increase in peak platelet counts was 95 000/mm^3 above baseline (range increase of 55 000–130 000/mm^3 above baseline). Responses were seen in 5 of 11 MDS patients and in 1 patient with aplastic anemia. Responses lasted for 3–8.5+ months. Side-effects of rIL-11 were mild in severity and included peripheral edema, conjunctival injection, and myalgias. Further investigation of rIL-11 is warranted to determine whether the cytokine can elicit clinically relevant improvements in the platelet count in MDS patients with severe thrombocytopenia or thrombocytopenia-related bleeding.

Thrombopoietin

Biologic studies

In 1994 the ligand of the *c-mpl* receptor was cloned and found to be thrombopoietin (TPO, *c-mpl* ligand).[81–85] TPO acts as a lineage-specific HGF by promoting the proliferation and differentiation of megakaryocytes into platelets.[86] TPO has also been found to have effects on hematopoietic stem cells, promoting their survival and stimulating their growth in combination with other cytokines such as IL-3 or stem cell factor.[87,88] Preclinical studies in animals and several phase I/II studies in humans have shown that TPO can reduce the severity and duration of thrombocytopenia after chemotherapy-induced myelosuppression.[89–94] There has been great interest in using recombinant TPO (rTPO) to improve the thrombocytopenia and multilineage responses in MDS patients.

Plasma TPO levels are inversely correlated with platelet count and bone marrow megakaryocyte mass.[95] Plasma TPO levels have generally been found to be higher in MDS patients than in normal individuals.[96] RA patients had higher plasma TPO levels than RAEB/RAEB-T patients, irrespective of similar platelet counts in these groups. The plasma TPO level was upregulated and inversely correlated with the platelet count in RA patients, but not in RAEB/RAEB-T or CMML patients.[97,98] These findings suggest that the physiological pathways for TPO production and metabolism are intact in low-risk MDS patients, but may be deranged in the advanced stages of MDS where the leukemic clone has progressed. One study found the number of TPO receptors (*c-mpl*) was decreased in MDS marrow cells compared to normals, and was similar across all MDS FAB subtypes.[98] Reduced numbers of TPO receptors, in addition to thrombocytopenia, may contribute to the increased plasma TPO levels found in MDS patients.

In vitro studies have assessed the effects of rTPO on the proliferation and differentiation of MDS and AML bone marrow progenitor cells. In short-term liquid cultures and progenitor assays, recombinant megakaryocyte growth and development factor (rMGDF) (a modified TPO) stimulated DNA synthesis and potentiated leukemic cluster growth of marrow mononuclear cells in approximately 25% of MDS cases.[99] rMGDF-induced blast cell proliferation correlated with elevated expression of *c-mpl*. rMGDF stimulated CFU-Mk growth in 45% of these cases. In another study, rTPO increased blast number from cultured marrow cells from high-risk MDS patients, but not lower-risk individuals (RA/RARS).[100] High lactate dehydrogenase value was associated with TPO-induced blast proliferation in high-risk patients. In a study of 7-day suspension cultures, rMGDF increased CFU-Mk growth in 1 of 10 AML and 6 of 16 MDS marrows, and CD61+ (a marker of megakaryocytes) cell numbers were increased in 9 of 13 AML and 12 of 15 MDS samples.[101] In this series, rMGDF did not increase CFU-GM colony or cluster growth. Stimulation of in vitro megakaryopoiesis by rMGDF in MDS samples could be augmented by rIL-3 and stem cell factor.[102] When fetal calf serum and rEPO were added to MDS marrow samples, TPO induced MDS CFU-GM and BFU-E cell proliferation in a dose-dependent manner by up to 100%.[103] These in vitro effects were comparable to previous results obtained with rG-CSF, rGM-CSF, and rIL-3. rTPO also augmented the stimulatory effects of these cytokines on MDS marrow cells. These in vitro studies indicate that TPO can induce differentiation of MDS megakaryocyte precursors. However, the potential for fostering leukemic cell growth also exists, a concern that needs to be carefully scrutinized in future clinical trials of rTPO in MDS.

Clinical trials

A phase I/II, open-label cohort sequential dose escalation study evaluated the effects of a 14-day course of intravenous pegylated rMGDF in MDS and aplastic anemia patients with average baseline platelet counts < 30 000/mm^3 without transfusion.[104] Preliminary data indicated that the drug was well tolerated, but only modest increases in platelet counts were observed in the dose range of 1.25–5.0 μg/kg per day.

Recently, a provocative report described long-term use of intravenous pegylated rMGDF in a female patient with RBC transfusion-dependence and severe thrombocytopenia (platelet count < 10 000/mm^3).[105] She had the RARS subtype of MDS (65% ringed sideroblasts) and a karyotype consisting of 46,XX, add(11)(p11). A limited 14-day course of 10 μg/kg per day resulted in a transient improvement in the platelet count to 64 000/mm^3 on day 21, which returned to baseline levels by day 35. However, reinitiation of pegylated rMGDF on a continuous basis resulted in RBC transfusion-independence by day 105. A repeat bone marrow examination revealed less dysplasia, a decrease in ringed sideroblasts to 18%, and a marked reduction in the abnormal karyotype. The cytogenetic response and bicytopenic improvement to rMGDF in this case of MDS bears out in vitro observations of TPO's capacity to support the self-renewal and expansion of normal human hemopoietic stem cells.

Further studies assessing rTPO or rMGDF are still required to establish whether these thrombopoietic substances can elicit clinically meaningful increases of the platelet count in MDS patients with severe thrombocytopenia or thrombocytopenia-related bleeding, whether multilineages are feasible, and the proportion of patients who develop neutralizing antibodies to rTPO.

Iron overload in MDS

Although high doses of rEPO alone or in conjunction with rG-CSF or rGM-CSF or various experimental therapies may alleviate the need for RBC transfusions, a large proportion of patients with MDS who do not respond to these treatments subsequently develop iron overload and are at risk for organ damage from tissue siderosis.

β-Thalassemia major provides a model to understand the pathophysiology and negative effects of chronic transfusional iron overload on cardiac, hepatic, and endocrine function.[106] When plasma iron exceeds transferrin's

Table 8.3 Comparison of red blood cell transfusion-dependent states

Marrow abnormalities	Thalassemia major	Myelodysplastic syndromes
Ineffective erythropoiesis	++++	++++ → ++
Intramedullary hemolysis	++++	++++ → ++
Apoptosis	++++	++++ → ++
Mitochondrial dysfunction	+++	+++
Genetic lesions	Globin	Multiple
Cellular target	Erythroid progeny	Hemopoietic stem cell, progeny
Leukemic potential	–	+ → ++++
Oxidative damage	NTBI	NTBI, TNF-α, Ox-pyrimidine NT
Stromal anomalies: (↑ inhibitory, ↓ stimulatory cytokines)	–	+++

NTBI, non-transferrin-bound iron; TNF-α, tumor necrosis factor-α; Ox-pyrimidine NT, oxidized pyrimidine nucleotides.
From Greenberg, P. L., Iron Overload in Hematologic Disorders Symposium, American Society of Hematology 2003.

binding capacity, the increased non-transferrin-bound iron (NTBI) combines with oxygen to form hydroxyl radicals.[107] These toxic elemental byproducts can cause lipid peroxidation and damage to cell membranes, protein, and DNA.[108]

MDS and β-thalassemia major are two RBC transfusion states that exhibit a number of similarities which relate in part to the presence of high levels of oxidant-damaging substances such as NTBI (Table 8.3). These common features include ineffective erythropoiesis with intramedullary hemolysis, and enhanced apoptosis of marrow progeny with dysfunctional mitochondria.[106,108] However, the oxidant-damaging effects have differing genotoxic effects on MDS patients' marrow cells because of the different nature of their stem cells (multipotent, clonal, often with multiple cytogenetic abnormalities and stromal derangements; Fig. 8.1).[108] These stromal abnormalities include increased elaboration of inhibitory cytokines, including tumor necrosis factor-α and interferon-γ, decreased stimulatory cytokines such as EPO and G-CSF, and increased angiogenesis.[109]

Desferroxiamine, also known as Desferal, is currently the only drug approved by the US Food and Drug Administration for the treatment of RBC transfusion-related iron overload. It is the standard of therapy against which

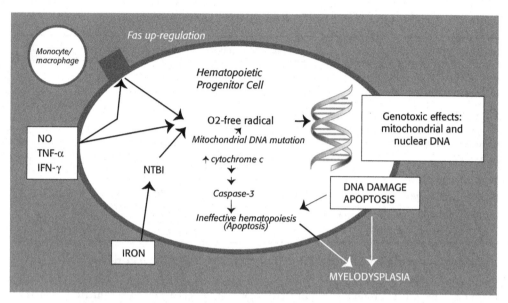

Fig. 8.1   Oxidative stress mechanisms in myelodysplastic syndromes (MDS). NO, nitric oxide; TNF-α, tumor necrosis factor-α; IFN-γ, interferon-γ; NTBI, non-transferrin-bound iron. Reprinted from Farquhar & Bowen,[108] courtesy of *International Journal of Hematology*.

other iron chelators are compared. Studies in β-thalassemia have established the ability of desferroxiamine to reduce morbidity and mortality related to iron overload, particularly as it relates to cardiac disease.[110–112]

Reversal of some of the consequences of iron overload in MDS by iron chelation therapy has been addressed by few studies. A study by Jensen and colleagues carefully evaluated a cohort of MDS patients who had undergone effective desferroxiamine chelation for up to 60 months.[113] Iron body stores were reduced as measured by serial serum ferritin levels and magnetic resonance imaging of liver iron content. With prolonged treatment, iron chelation also resulted in the improvement of cytopenias. For example, improvement in transfusion-dependence by $\geq 50\%$ was seen in 7 of 11 (64%) patients, and 5 patients (46%) became RBC transfusion-independent. Platelet counts increased in 7 of 11 (64%) patients and the neutrophil counts improved in 7 of 9 (78%) evaluable patients. This study suggests that iron overload and its oxidative damaging effects through NTBI may contribute to ineffective hematopoiesis in MDS, and some of these adverse consequences may be reversed by prolonged iron chelation.

In a study of 27 patients with iron overload, including 10 patients with MDS, desferroxiamine given by a 12-h continuous subcutaneous infusion was compared to twice-daily bolus sc injection.[114] The two methods of administration yielded similar rates of urinary iron excretion after 48 h. The longer-term efficacy of bolus desferroxiamine was evaluated in a 20-month extension study. Ferritin concentrations fell below 1000 μg/l and 500 μg/l in 73% and 42% of patients, respectively, and normalized in 26% of individuals. Optimal results were achieved in patients no longer receiving RBC transfusions at the time that chelation therapy was begun. In a more recent 4-year update of 15 regularly transfused patients, 7 had died from disease progression; 3 of the remaining 8 patients experienced painful, postinjection swelling lasting 12–24 h, prompting change of therapy to standard sc desferroxiamine infusion.[115] The 5 remaining patients, along with an additional 7 cases (8 of these 12 patients had MDS) were followed for a mean of 47 months. In this cohort, there was a decrease in the mean ferritin value from 1670 to 914 μg/l. These initial encouraging results merit larger trials evaluating the efficacy of long-term sc continuous versus bolus desferroxiamine injection. Such studies should help clarify the tolerability of large-volume bolus injections.

Due to the logistic difficulties of chronic sc desferroxiamine infusions in the predominantly elderly population, such therapy is often begun late in the course of iron overload and with limited enthusiasm by both clinicians and patients. Its cumbersome mode of administration often engenders poor patient compliance, which has been shown to contribute to decreased long-term efficacy and survival in patients with β-thalassemia.[111,112]

With an aim to overcoming the logistical drawbacks of desferroxiamine therapy, several oral iron chelators have entered clinical testing in humans. The oral iron chelator deferiprone (L1, Ferriprox) is approved in Europe, India, and other countries for second-line use in desferroxiamine-intolerant patients with β-thalassemia. It is cleared renally, with a standard dose being 75 mg/kg per day divided three times daily.[116] Some of the more common side-effects associated with therapy include nausea/vomiting, abdominal pain, arthralgias, and, more rarely, neutropenia or idiosyncratic agranulocytosis.[116,117] Although an initial study suggested a link between deferiprone and an increased incidence of hepatic fibrosis, this finding has not been validated in additional studies.[118–123]

Deferiprone can reduce the liver iron concentration in patients with β-thalassemia, but some studies suggest that it may not be as effective as desferroxiamine.[116–119,124,125] In a Dutch multicenter trial, deferiprone was studied in patients with predominantly hematologic malignancies characterized by transfusion-dependence, including 18 cases of MDS.[126] The median duration of treatment was 16 months. Using a definition of negative iron excretion and/or at least a 20% decrease in serum ferritin, a 61% response rate was observed, with a median decrease in ferritin of 25%. The most serious side-effect was agranulocytosis in 1 patient, observed after several months of treatment. Studies of deferiprone in MDS are clearly warranted, as this oral agent may prove to be a convenient and effective alternative for these patients. Studies in β-thalassemia intermedia/hemoglobin E patients have also shown the efficacy of deferiprone in decreasing liver iron content and serum ferritin levels.[127] A portion of these patients also had improved hemoglobin levels.

ICL670 is an orally active tridentate iron chelator which has high affinity and specificity for iron.[128] The efficacy and safety of ICL670 were demonstrated in animal models and then in phase I clinical trials. Iron chelated by ICL670 is processed through the hepatic/biliary route and is mainly excreted in the feces, with < 10% excreted in the urine.[129] ICL670 was well tolerated at doses up to 40 mg/kg, with diarrhea, nausea, abdominal pain, and rash being the most common toxicities.[129] The frequency of adverse events was proportional to the dose.

ICL670 was evaluated in a phase II, open-label, randomized trial of 71 β-thalassemia patients with transfusional iron overload.[130] Patients were distributed among two ICL670 dose levels, 10 or 20 mg/kg per day, and desferroxiamine 40 mg/kg per day was given as a sc infusion 5 days weekly. The trial duration was 12 months, after which all patients randomized to desferroxiamine were offered therapy with ICL670 as part of an extension study. At 6 months of follow-up, ICL670 at a dose of 20 mg/kg per day was comparable with 40 mg/kg per day desferroxiamine at reducing the liver iron concentration (measured by SQUID, superconducting quantum interference device). In a more recent 18-month analysis,[131] success in reducing the liver iron concentration (based on pre-specified trial criteria and initial hepatic iron burden), was observed in 33% (5 of 15) of patients in the 10 mg/kg per day ICL670 cohort, compared to 60% (9 of 15) of patients in the ICL670 20 mg/kg arm, and 75% (12 of 16) patients in the desferroxiamine group.

From a safety perspective, ICL670 was well tolerated, with a low frequency of skin rash, and low-grade, dose-related gastrointestinal events. No clinically relevant ophthalmologic, auditory, cardiac, or renal toxicities were noted. Occasional elevations of urinary β_2-microglobulin and mild proteinuria were seen, but the clinical relevance of this is still under investigation. Follow-up multicenter, phase II single-arm trials of ICL670 in β-thalassemia patients who are intolerant of desferroxiamine and patients with MDS and other transfusion-dependent chronic anemias have been initiated.

Summary and future directions

Recombinant HGFs, in particular rEPO $\pm$ rG-CSF, have now been evaluated in MDS patients for over a decade, with both short- and long-term studies providing a detailed picture of their efficacy, safety, and impact on survival and AML evolution. HGFs need evaluation as to whether combination with novel biologically specific therapies for MDS (see Chapter 7) may enhance response rates (e.g., with thalidomide, CC-5013 (lenalidomide, Revlimid), 5-azacytidine/decitabine, farnesyltransferase inhibitors, arsenic trioxide, and histone deacetylase inhibitors).

Newer longer-acting recombinant cytokines such as darbepoetin alfa (and pegfilgrastim) have been approved for cancer patients with anemia due to chronic disease or multicycle chemotherapy. These cytokines are now entering phase I/II trial testing in MDS. The recent establishment of consensus response criteria by the International Working Group should permit better interpretation of the results of trials of these cytokines and other agents in MDS.[132] Quality of life (see Chapter 10) and pharmacoeconomic comparisons between transfusions and both the old and new HGF formulations will assist physician and patient decision-making regarding these treatment options, and will shape the health care debate regarding resource allocation for these diseases.[133]

MDS is a prime example of a disease of transfusional iron overload critically in need of both an effective and practically feasible iron chelator. Similar to trials of deferiprone and ICL670 in β-thalassemia, studies evaluating these oral iron chelators in MDS are now incorporating non-invasive investigational techniques such as magnetic resonance imaging and SQUID as alternative methods of measuring liver iron content. It will be of interest to evaluate other surrogate markers of body iron, including hepcidin, a newly discovered protein found to play a role in iron homeostasis.[134] Since cardiac disease is a primary contributor to iron-related morbidity and mortality, it will also be important to assess the ability of these oral iron chelators to remove cardiac iron.

REFERENCES

1. Greenberg, P. L. (1996). Biologic and clinical implications of marrow culture studies in the myelodysplastic syndromes. *Semin. Hematol.*, **33**, 163–75.
2. Greenberg, P. L. and Mara, B. (1979). The preleukemic syndrome: correlation of in vitro parameters of granulopoiesis with clinical features. *Am. J. Med.*, **66**, 951–8.
3. Chui, D. H. and Clarke, B. J. (1982). Abnormal erythroid progenitor cells in human preleukemia. *Blood*, **60**, 362–7.
4. Juvonen, E., Partanen, S., Knuutila, S., and Ruute, T. (1986). Megakaryocyte colony formation by bone marrow progenitors in myelodysplastic syndromes. *Br. J. Haematol.*, **63**, 331–4.
5. Nagler, A., Ginzton, N., Negrin, R. S. *et al.* (1990). In vitro differentiative and proliferative effects of human recombinant colony-stimulating factors on marrow hemopoiesis in myelodysplastic syndromes. *Leukemia*, **4**, 193–202.
6. Schipperus, M. R., Sonneveld, P., Lindemans, J. *et al.* (1990). The combined effects of IL-3, GM-CSF, and G-CSF on the in vitro growth of myelodysplastic myeloid progenitor cells. *Leuk. Res.*, **14**, 1019–25.
7. Greenberg, P. L., Mackichan, M. L., and Negrin, R. (1990). Production of granulocyte colony-stimulating factor by normal and myelodysplastic syndrome peripheral blood cells. *Blood*, **76** (suppl. 1), 146a (abstract).
8. Nagler, A., Binet, C., Mackichan, M. L. *et al.* (1990). Impact of marrow cytogenetics and morphology on in vitro hemopoiesis in the myelodysplastic syndromes: comparison between recombinant human granulocyte colony-stimulating factor and granulocyte-monocyte colony-stimulating factor. *Blood*, **76**, 1299–307.
9. Merchav, S., Nielsen, O. J., Rosenbaum, H. *et al.* (1990). In vitro studies of erythropoietin-dependent regulation of erythropoiesis in myelodysplastic syndromes. *Leukemia*, **4**, 771–4.
10. Greenberg, P. L., Negrin, R. S., and Ginzton, N. (1991). G-CSF synergizes with erythropoietin for enhancing erythroid colony-formation in myelodysplastic syndromes. *Blood*, **78** (suppl. 1), 38a (abstract).
11. Sawada, K., Sato, N., Tarumi, T. *et al.* (1993). Proliferation and differentiation of myelodysplastic CD34+ cells in serum-free medium: response to individual colony-stimulating factors. *Br. J. Haematol.*, **83**, 349–58.

12. Budel, L. M., Dong, F., Lowenberg, B., and Touw, I. P. (1995). Hematopoietic growth factor receptors: structure variations and alternatives of receptor complex formation in normal hematopoiesis and in hematopoietic disorders. *Leukemia*, **9**, 553–61.

13. Hoefsloot, L. H., van Amelsvoort, M. P., Broeders, L. C. *et al.* (1997). Erythropoietin-induced activation of STAT5 is impaired in the myelodysplastic syndrome. *Blood*, **89**, 1690–700.

14. NCCN Myelodysplastic Syndromes Panel (2003). Myelodysplastic syndromes – clinical practice guidelines in oncology. *J.N.C.C.N.*, **1**, 456–71.

15. Fontenay-Roupie, M., Bouscary, D., Guesnu, M. *et al.* (1999). Ineffective erythropoiesis in myelodysplastic syndromes: correlation with Fas expression but not with lack of erythropoietin receptor signal transduction. *Br. J. Haematol.*, **106**, 464–73.

16. Claessens, Y. E., Bouscary, D., Dupont, J. M. *et al.* (2002). In vitro proliferation and differentiation of erythroid progenitors from patients with myelodysplastic syndromes: evidence for *Fas*-dependent apoptosis. *Blood*, **99**, 1594–601.

17. Rigolin, G. M., Della Porta, M., Bigoni, R. *et al.* (2002). rHuEPO administration in patients with low-risk myelodysplastic syndromes: evaluation of erythroid precursors' response by fluorescence in situ hybridization on May-Grunwald-Giemsa-stained bone marrow samples. *Br. J. Haematol.*, **119**, 652–9.

18. Schmidt-Mende, J., Tehranchi, R., Forsblom, A. M. *et al.* (2001). Granulocyte colony-stimulating factor inhibits *Fas*-triggered apoptosis in bone marrow cells isolated from patients with refractory anemia with ringed sideroblasts. *Leukemia*, **15**, 742–51.

19. Tehranchi, R., Fadeel, B., Forsblom, A. M. *et al.* (2003). Granulocyte colony-stimulating factor inhibits spontaneous cytochrome c release and mitochondria-dependent apoptosis of myelodysplastic syndrome hematopoietic progenitors. *Blood*, **101**, 1080–6.

20. Adamson, J. W., Schuster, M., Allen, S., and Haley, N. R. (1992). Effectiveness of recombinant human erythropoietin therapy in myelodysplastic syndromes. *Acta Haematol.*, **87** (suppl. 1), 20–4.

21. Aloe Spiriti, M. A., Petti, M. C., Latagliata, R. *et al.* (1993). Is recombinant human erythropoietin treatment in myelodysplastic syndromes worthwhile? *Leuk. Lymphoma*, **9**, 79–83.

22. Stenke, L., Wallvik, J., Celsing, F., and Hast, R. (1993). Prediction of response to treatment with human recombinant erythropoietin in myelodysplastic syndromes. *Leukemia*, **7**, 1324–7.

23. Stone, R. M., Bernstein, S. H., Demetri, G. *et al.* (1994). Treatment with recombinant human erythropoietin in patients with myelodysplastic syndromes. *Leuk. Res.*, **18**, 769–76.

24. Rose, E. H., Abels, R. I., Nelson, R. A., McCullough, O. M., and Lessin, L. (1995). The use of r-HuEPO in the treatment of anaemia related to myelodysplasia (MDS). *Br. J. Haematol.*, **89**, 831–7.

25. Stasi, R., Brunetti, M., Bussa, S. *et al.* (1997). Response to recombinant human erythropoietin in patients with myelodysplastic syndromes. *Clin. Cancer Res.*, **3**, 733–9.

26. Italian Cooperative Study Group for rHuEpo in Myelodysplastic Syndromes (1998). A randomized double-blind placebo-controlled study with subcutaneous recombinant human erythropoietin in patients with low-risk myelodysplastic syndromes. *Br. J. Haematol.*, **103**, 1070–4.

27. Terpos, E., Mougiou, A., Kouraklis, A. *et al.* (2002). Prolonged administration of erythropoietin increases erythroid response rate in myelodysplastic syndromes: a phase II trial in 281 patients. *Br. J. Haematol.*, **118**, 174–80.

28. Wallvik, J., Stenke, L., Bernell, P. *et al.* (2002). Serum erythropoietin (EPO) levels correlate with survival and independently predict response to EPO treatment in patients with myelodysplastic syndromes. *Eur. J. Haematol.*, **68**, 180–5.

29. Rodriguez, J. N., Dieguez, J. C., Muniz, R. *et al.* (1994). [Human recombinant erythropoietin in the treatment of myelodysplastic syndromes anemia. Meta-analytic study.] *Sangre (Barc.)*, **39**, 435–9 (in Spanish).

30. Hellström-Lindberg, E. (1995). Efficacy of erythropoietin in the myelodysplastic syndromes: a meta-analysis of 205 patients from 17 studies. *Br. J. Haematol.*, **89**, 67–71.

31. Hast, R., Wallvik, J., Folin Abernell, P., and Stenke, L. (2001). Long-term follow-up of 18 patients with myelodyplastic syndromes responding to recombinant erythropoietin treatment. *Leuk. Res.*, **25**, 13–18.

32. Musto, P., Falcone, A., Sanpaolo, G. *et al.* (2003). Efficacy of a single, weekly dose of recombinant erythropoietin in myelodysplastic syndromes. *Br. J. Haematol.*, **122**, 267–71.

33. Garypidou, V., Verrou, E., Vakalopoulou, S. *et al.* (2003). Efficacy of a single, weekly dose of recombinant erythropoietin in myelodysplastic syndromes. *Br. J. Haematol.*, **123**, 958.

34. Negrin, R. S., Haeuber, D. H., Nagler, A. *et al.* (1989). Treatment of myelodysplastic syndromes with recombinant human granulocyte colony-stimulating factor. *Ann. Intern. Med.*, **110**, 976–84.

35. Negrin, R. S., Haeuber, D. H., Nagler, A. *et al.* (1990). Maintenance treatment of patients with myelodysplastic syndromes using recombinant human granulocyte colony-stimulating factor. *Blood*, **76**, 36–43.

36. Greenberg, P., Taylor, K., Larson, R. *et al.* (1993). Phase III randomized multicenter trial of recombinant human G-CSF in MDS. *Blood*, **82** (suppl. 1), 196a (abstract).

37. Greenberg, P. L., Negrin, R. S., and Ginzton, N. (1992). In vitro–in vivo correlations of erythroid responses to G-CSF plus erythropoietin in myelodysplastic syndromes. *Exp. Hematol.*, **20**, 733 (abstract).

38. Negrin, R. S., Stein, R., Doherty, K. *et al.* (1993). Treatment of the anemias of MDS using recombinant human granulocyte colony-stimulating factor in combination with erythropoietin. *Blood*, **82**, 737–43.

39. Hellström-Lindberg, E., Birgegard, G., Carlsson, M. *et al.* (1993). A combination of granulocyte colony-stimulating factor and erythropoietin may synergistically improve the anaemia in patients with myelodysplastic syndromes. *Leuk. Lymphoma*, **11**, 221–8.

40. Negrin, R. S., Stein, R., Doherty, K. *et al.* (1996). Maintenance treatment of the anemia of myelodysplastic syndromes with recombinant human granulocyte colony-stimulating factor and erythropoietin: evidence for in vivo synergy. *Blood*, **87**, 4076–81.

41. Hellström-Lindberg, E., Negrin, R., Stein, R. *et al.* (1997). Erythroid response to treatment with G-CSF plus erythropoietin for the anaemia of patients with myelodysplastic syndromes: proposal for a predictive model. *Br. J. Haematol.*, **99**, 344–51.

42. Hellström-Lindberg, E., Ahlgren, T., Beguin, Y. *et al.* (1998). Treatment of anemia in myelodysplastic syndromes with granulocyte colony-stimulating factor plus erythropoietin; results from a randomized phase II study and long-term follow-up of 71 patients. *Blood*, **92**, 68–75.

43. Hellström-Lindberg, E., Gulbrandsen, N., Lindberg, G. *et al.* (2003). A validated decision model for treating the anaemia of myelodysplastic syndromes with erythropoietin + granulocyte colony-stimulating factor: significant effects on quality of life. *Br. J. Haematol.*, **120**, 1037–46.

44. Remacha, A. F., Arrizabalaga, B., Villegas, A. *et al.* (1999). Erythropoietin plus granulocyte colony-stimulating factor in the treatment of myelodysplastic syndromes. Identification of a subgroup of responders. *Haematologica*, **84**, 1058–64.

45. Mantovani, L., Lentini, G., Hentschel, B. *et al.* (2000). Treatment of anaemia in myelodysplastic syndromes with prolonged administration of recombinant human granulocyte colony-stimulating factor and erythropoietin. *Br. J. Haematol.*, **109**, 367–75.

46. Casadevall, N., Durieux, P., Dubois, S. *et al.* (2004). Health, economic, and quality-of-life effects of erythropoietin and granulocyte colony-stimulating factor for the treatment of myelodysplastic syndromes: a randomized, controlled trial. *Blood*, **104**, 321–7.

47. Jadersten, M., Montgomery, S. M., Astermark, J. *et al.* (2003). Treatment of anemia in myelodysplastic syndromes with granulocyte colony-stimulating factor and erythropoietin: response and impact on survival in a long-term follow-up of 129 patients. *Blood*, **102** (suppl. 1), 184a–5a (abstract).

48. Greenberg, P., Cox, C., Le Beau, M. M. *et al.* (1997). International scoring system (IPSS) for evaluating prognosis in myelodysplastic syndrome. *Blood*, **89**, 2079–88.

49. Vadhan-Raj, S., Keating, M., LeMaistre, A. *et al.* (1987). Effects of recombinant human granulocyte-macrophage colony-stimulating factor in patients with myelodysplastic syndromes. *N. Engl. J. Med.*, **317**, 1545–52.

50. Antin, J. H., Weinberg, D. S., and Rosenthal, D. S. (1990). Variable effect of recombinant human granulocyte-macrophage colony-stimulating factor on bone marrow fibrosis in patients with myelodysplasia. *Exp. Hematol.*, **18**, 266–70.

51. Ganser, A., Volkers, B., Greher, J. *et al.* (1989). Recombinant human-granulocyte-macrophage colony-stimulating factor in patients with myelodysplastic syndromes – a phase I/II trial. *Blood*, **73**, 31–7.

52. Hermann, F., Lindemann, A., Klein, H. *et al.* (1989). Effect of recombinant human granulocyte-macrophage colony-stimulating factor in patients with myelodysplastic syndrome with excess blasts. *Leukemia*, **3**, 335–8.

53. Hoelzer, D., Ganser, A., Greher, J., Volkers, B., and Walther, F. (1988). Phase I/II study with GM-CSF in patients with myelodysplastic syndromes. *Behring Inst. Mitt.*, **83**, 134–8.

54. Thompson, J. A., Douglas, J. L., Kidd, P. *et al.* (1989). Subcutaneous granulocyte macrophage colony-stimulating factor in patients with myelodysplastic syndrome: toxicity, pharmacokinetics, and hematological effects. *J. Clin. Oncol.*, **7**, 629–37.

55. Estey, E. H., Kurzrock, R., Talpaz, M. *et al.* (1991). Effects of low doses of recombinant human granulocyte-macrophage colony-stimulating factor (GM-CSF) in patients with myelodysplastic syndromes. *Br. J. Haematol.*, **77**, 291–5.

56. Rosenfeld, C. S., Sulecki, M., Evans, C., and Shadduck, R. K. (1991). Comparison of intravenous versus subcutaneous recombinant human granulocyte-macrophage colony-stimulating factor in patients with primary myelodysplasia. *Exp. Hematol.*, **19**, 273–7.

57. Gradishar, W. J., Le Beau, M. M., O'Laughlin, R., Vardiman, J. W., and Larson, R. A. (1992). Clinical and cytogenetic responses to granulocyte-macrophage colony-stimulating factor in therapy-related myelodysplasia. *Blood*, **80**, 2463–70.

58. Takahashi, M., Yoshida, Y., Kaku, K. *et al.* (1993). Phase II study of recombinant granulocyte-macrophage colony-stimulating factor in myelodysplastic syndrome and aplastic anemia. *Acta Haematol.*, **89**, 189–94.

59. Rose, C., Wattel, E., Bastion, Y. *et al.* (1994). Treatment with very low-dose GM-CSF in myelodysplastic syndromes with neutropenia. A report on 28 cases. *Leukemia*, **8**, 1458–62.

60. Willemze, R., Van Der Lely, N., Zwierzina, H. *et al.* (1992). A randomized phase-I/II multicenter study of recombinant human granulocyte-macrophage colony-stimulating factor (GM-CSF) therapy for patients with myelodysplastic syndromes and a relatively low risk of acute leukemia. *Ann. Hematol.*, **64**, 173–80.

61. Schuster, M. W., Thompson, J. A., Larson, R. *et al.* (1995). Randomized phase II study of recombinant granulocyte macrophage-colony stimulating factor (rGM-CSF) in patients with neutropenia secondary to myelodysplastic syndrome (MDS). *Blood*, **86** (suppl. 1), 338a (abstract).

62. Yoshida, Y., Nakahata, T., Shibata, A. *et al.* (1995). Effects of long-term treatment with recombinant human granulocyte-macrophage colony-stimulating factor in patients with myelodysplastic syndrome. *Leuk. Lymphoma*, **18**, 457–63.

63. Runde, V., Aul, C., Ebert, A., Grabenhorst, U., and Schneider, W. (1995). Sequential administration of recombinant human granulocyte-macrophage colony-stimulating factor and human erythropoietin for treatment of myelodysplastic syndromes. *Eur. J. Haematol.*, **54**, 39–45.

64. Hansen, P. B., Johnsen, H. E., Hippe, E., Hellstrom-Lindberg, E., and Ralfkiaer, E. (1993). Recombinant human granulocyte-macrophage colony-stimulting factor plus recombinant human erythropoietin may improve anemia in selected patients with myelodysplastic syndromes. *Am. J. Hematol.*, **44**, 229–36.

65. Bernell, P., Stenke, L., Wallvik, J., Hippe, E., and Hast, R. (1996). A sequential erythropoietin and GM-CSF schedule offers clinical benefits in the treatment of anemia in myelodysplastic syndromes. *Leuk. Res.*, **20**, 693–9.

66. Stasi, R., Pagano, A., Terzoli, E., and Amadori, S. (1999). Recombinant human granulocyte-macrophage colony-stimulating factor plus erythropoietin for the treatment of cytopenias in patients with myelodysplastic syndromes. *Br. J. Haematol.*, **105**, 141–8.

67. Thompson, J., Gilliland, G., Prchal, J. *et al.* (1995). The use of GM-CSF+ r-HuEPO for the treatment of cytopenias associated with myelodysplastic syndromes. *Blood*, **86** (suppl. 1), 337a (abstract).

68. Economopoulos, T., Mellou, S., Papageorgiou, E. *et al.* (1999). Treatment of anemia in low risk myelodysplastic syndromes with granulocyte-macrophage colony-stimulating factor plus recombinant human erythropoietin. *Leukemia*, **13**, 1009–12.

69. Tefferi, A., Elliott, M. A., Steensma, D. P. *et al.* (2001). Amifostine alone and in combination with erythropoietin for the treatment of favorable myelodysplastic syndrome. *Leuk. Res.*, **25**, 183–5.

70. Neumeister, P., Jaeger, G., Eibl, M. *et al.* (2001). Amifostine in combination with erythropoietin and G-CSF promotes multilineage hematopoiesis in patients with myelodysplastic syndrome. *Leuk. Lymphoma*, **40**, 345–9.

71. Tsiara, S. N., Kapsali, H. D., Panteli, K., Christou, L., and Bourantas, K. L. (2001). Preliminary results of amifostine administration in combination with recombinant human erythropoietin in patients with myelodysplastic syndromes. *J. Exp. Clin. Cancer Res.*, **20**, 35–8.

72. Grossi, A., Musto, P., Santini, V. *et al.* (2002). Combined therapy with amifostine plus erythropoietin for the treatment of myelodysplastic syndromes. *Haematologica*, **87**, 322–3.

73. Stasi, R., Brunetti, M., Terzoli, E., and Amadori, S. (2002). Sustained response to recombinant human erythropoietin and intermittent *all*-trans retinoic acid in patients with myelodysplastic syndromes. *Blood*, **99**, 1578–84.

74. Ganser, A., Seipelt, G., Lindemann, A. *et al.* (1990). Effects of recombinant human interleukin-3 in patients with myelodysplastic syndromes. *Blood*, **76**, 455–62.

75. Kurzrock, R., Talpaz, M., Estrov, Z., Rosenblum, M. G., and Gutterman, J. U. (1991). Phase I study of recombinant human interleukin-3 in patients with bone marrow failure. *J. Clin. Oncol.*, **9**, 1241–50.

76. Nimer, S. D., Paquette, R. L., Ireland, P. *et al.* (1994). A phase I/II study of interleukin-3 in patients with aplastic anemia and myelodysplasia. *Exp. Hematol.*, **22**, 875–80.

77. Ganser, A., Ottmann, O. G., Seipelt, G. *et al.* (1993). Effect of long-term treatment with recombinant human interleukin-3 in patients with myelodysplastic syndromes. *Leukemia*, **7**, 696–701.

78. Miller, A. M., Noyes, W. E., Taetle, R., and List, A. F. (1999). Limited erythropoietic response to combined treatment with recombinant human interleukin 3 and erythropoietin in myelodysplastic syndrome. *Leuk. Res.*, **23**, 77–83.

79. Gordon, M. S., Nemunaitis, J., Hoffman, R. *et al.* (1995). A phase I trial of recombinant human interleukin-6 in patients with myelodysplastic syndromes and thrombocytopenia. *Blood*, **85**, 3066–76.

80. Kurzrock, R., Cortes, J., Thomas, D. A. *et al.* (2001). Pilot study of low-dose interleukin-II in patients with bone marrow failure. *J. Clin. Oncol.*, **19**, 4165–72.

81. Lok, S., Kaushansky, K., Holly, R. D. *et al.* (1994). Cloning and expression of murine thrombopoietin cDNA and stimulation of platelet production in vivo. *Nature*, **369**, 565–8.

82. De Sauvage, F. J., Hass, P. E., Spencer, S. D. *et al.* (1994). Stimulation of megakaryocytopoiesis and thrombopoiesis by the *c-mpl* ligand. *Nature*, **369**, 533–8.

83. Kaushansky, K., Lok, S., Holly, R. D. *et al.* (1994). Promotion of megakaryocyte progenitor expansion and differentiation by the *c-mpl* ligand thrombopoietin. *Nature*, **369**, 568–71.

84. Wendling, F., Maraskovsky, E., Debili, N. *et al.* (1994). cMpl ligand is a humoral regulator of megakaryocytopoieisis. *Nature*, **369**, 571–4.

85. Bartley, T. D., Bogenberger, J., Hunt, P. *et al.* (1994). Identification and cloning of a megakaryocyte and development factor that is a ligand for the cytokine receptor *mpl*. *Cell*, **77**, 1117–24.

86. Debili, N., Wendling, F., Katz, A. *et al.* (1995). The Mpl-ligand or thrombopoietin of megakaryocyte growth and differentiative factor has both direct proliferative and differentiative activities on human megakaryocyte progenitors. *Blood*, **86**, 2516–25.

87. Sitnicka, E., Lin, N., Priestley, G. V. *et al.* (1996). The effect of thrombopoietin on the proliferation and differentiation of murine hematopoietic stem cells. *Blood*, **87**, 4998–5005.

88. Katayama, N., Itoh, R., Kato, T. *et al.* (1997). Role for *C-MPL* and its ligand thrombopoietin in early hematopoiesis. *Leuk. Lymphoma*, **28**, 51–6.

89. Molineaux, G., Hartley, C., McElroy, P., McCrea, C., and McNiece, I. K. (1996). Megakaryocyte growth and development factor accelerates platelet recovery in peripheral blood progenitor cell transplant recipients. *Blood*, **88**, 366–76.

90. Farese, A. M., Hunt, P., Grab, L. B., and MacVittie, T. J. (1996). Combined administration of recombinant human megakaryocyte growth and development factor and granulocyte colony-stimulating factor enhances multilineage hematopoietic reconstitution in non-human primates after radiation-induced marrow aplasia. *J. Clin. Invest.*, **97**, 2145–51.

91. Basser, R. L., Rasko, J. E., Clarke, K. *et al.* (1996). Thrombopoietic effects of pegylated recombinant human megakaryocyte growth and development factor (PEG-rHuMGDF) in patients with advanced cancer. *Lancet*, **348**, 1279–81.

92. Vadhan-Raj, S., Murray, L. J., Bueso-Ramos, C. *et al.* (1997). Stimulation of megakaryocyte and platelet production by a single dose of recombinant human thrombopoietin in patients with cancer. *Ann. Intern. Med.*, **126**, 673–81.

93. Basser, R. L., Rasko, J. E., Clarke, K. *et al.* (1997). Randomized, blinded, placebo-controlled phase I trial of pegylated recombinant human megakaryocyte growth and development factor with filgrastim after dose-intensive chemotherapy in patients with advanced cancer. *Blood*, **89**, 3118–28.

94. Fanucchi, M., Glaspy, J., Crawford, J. *et al.* (1997). Effects of polyethylene glycol-conjugated recombinant human megakaryocyte growth and development factor on platelet counts after chemotherapy for lung cancer. *N. Engl. J. Med.*, **336**, 404–9.

95. Emmons, R. V., Reid, D. M., Cohen, R. L. *et al.* (1996). Human thrombopoietin levels are high when thrombocytopenia is due to megakaryocyte deficiency and low when due to increased platelet destruction. *Blood*, **87**, 4068–71.

96. Wang, W., Matsuo, T., Yoshida, S. *et al.* (2000). Colony-forming unit-megakaryocyte (CFR-meg) numbers and serum thrombopoietin concentrations in thrombocytopenic disorders: an inverse correlation in myelodysplastic syndromes. *Leukemia*, **14**, 1751–6.

97. Zwierzina, H., Rollinger-Holzinger, I., Nuessler, V., Herold, M., and Meng, Y. G. (1998). Endogenous serum thrombopoietin concentrations in patients with myelodysplastic syndromes. *Leukemia*, **12**, 59–64.

98. Tamura, H., Ogata, K., Luo, S. *et al.* (1998). Plasma thrombopoietin (TPO levels) and expression of TPO receptor on platelets in patients with myelodysplastic syndromes. *Br. J. Haematol.*, **103**, 778–84.

99. Fontenay-Roupie, M., Dupont, J. M., Picard, F. *et al.* (1998). Analysis of megakary-ocyte growth and development factor (thrombopoietin) effects on blast cell and megakaryocyte growth in myelodysplasia. *Leuk. Res.*, **22**, 527–35.

100. Luo, S. S., Ogata, K., Yokose, N., Kato, T., and Dan, K. (2000). Effect of throm-bopoietin on proliferation of blasts from patients with myelodysplastic syndromes. *Stem Cells*, **18**, 112–19.

101. Adams, J. A., Liu Yin, J. A., Brereton, M. L. *et al.* (1997). The in vitro effect of pegy-lated recombinant human megakaryocyte growth and development factor (PEG rHuMGDF) on megakarypoiesis in normal subjects and patients with myelodys-plasia and acute myeloid leukemia. *Br. J. Haematol.*, **99**, 139–46.

102. Liu Yin, J. A., Adams, J. A., Brereton, M. L. *et al.* (2000). Megakaryopoiesis in vitro in myelodysplastic syndromes and acute myeloid leukemia: effect of pegylated recom-binant human megakaryocyte growth and development factor in combination with other growth factors. *Br. J. Haematol.*, **108**, 743–6.

103. Ferrajoli, A., Talpaz, M., Kurzrock, R. *et al.* (1998). Thrombopoietin stimulates myelodysplastic syndrome granulocyte-macrophage and erythroid progenitor pro-liferation. *Leuk. Lymphoma*, **30**, 279–92.

104. Komatsu, N., Okamoto, T., Yoshida, T. *et al.* (2000). Pegylated recombinant human megakaryocyte growth and development factor (PEG-rHuMGDF) increased platelet counts (PLT) in patients (pts) with aplastic anemia (AA) and myelodys-plastic syndrome (MDS). *Blood*, **96**, 296a (abstract).

105. Kizaki, M., Yoshitaka, M., and Ikeda, Y. (2003). Long-term administration of pegy-lated recombinant human megakaryocyte growth and development factor dra-matically improved cytopenias in a patient with myelodysplastic syndrome. *Br. J. Haematol.*, **122**, 764–7.

106. Olivieri, N. F. (1999). The beta-thalassemias. *N. Engl. J. Med.*, **341**, 99–109.

107. Hershko, C., Graham, G., Bates, G. W., and Rachmilewitz, E. A. (1978). Non-specific serum iron in thalassemia: an abnormal serum iron fraction of potential toxicity. *Br. J. Haematol.*, **40**, 255–63.

108. Farquhar, M. J. and Bowen, D. T. (2003). Oxidative stress and the myelodysplastic syndromes. *Int. J. Hematol.*, **77**, 342–50.

109. Gotlib, J. and Greenberg, P. L. (2002). Myelodysplastic syndromes. In *Leukemia*, 7th Edn, ed. E. Henderson, T. Lister, M. F. Greaves. New York: Churchill Livingstone, pp. 545–82.

110. Olivieri, N. F., Nathan, D. G., MacMillan, J. H. *et al.* (1994). Survival in medi-cally treated patients with homozygous beta-thalassemia. *N. Engl. J. Med.*, **331**, 574–8.

111. Brittenham, G. M., Griffith, P. M., Nienhuis, A. W. *et al.* (1994). Efficacy of defer-oxamine in preventing complications of iron overload in patients with thalassemia major. *N. Engl. J. Med.*, **331**, 567–73.

112. Olivieri, N. F. and Brittenham, G. M. (1997). Iron-chelating therapy and the treatment of thalassemia. *Blood*, **89**, 739–61.

113. Jensen, P. D., Heickendorff, L., Bendix-Hansen, K. *et al.* (1996). The effect of iron chelation on haemopoiesis in MDS patients with transfusional iron overload. *Br. J. Haematol.*, **94**, 288–99.

114. Franchini, M., Gandini, G., de Gironcoli, M. *et al.* (2000). Safety and efficacy of subcutaneous bolus injection of deferoxamine in adult patients with iron overload. *Blood*, **95**, 2776–9.

115. Franchini, M., Gandini, G., Veneri, D., and Aprili, G. (2004). Safety and efficacy of subcutaneous bolus injection of deferoxamine in adult patients with iron overload: an update. *Blood*, **103**, 747–8.

116. Hoffbrand, A. V., Cohen, A., and Hershko, C. (2003). Role of deferiprone in chelation therapy for transfusional iron overload. *Blood*, **102**, 17–24.

117. Cohen, A. R., Galanello, R., Piga, A., De Sanctis, V., and Tricta, F. (2003). Safety and effectiveness of long-term therapy with the oral iron chelator deferiprone. *Blood*, **102**, 1583–7.

118. Olivieri, N. F., Brittenham, G. M., McLaren, C. E. *et al.* (1998). Long-term safety and effectiveness of iron-chelation therapy with deferiprone for thalassemia major. *N. Engl. J. Med.*, **339**, 417–23.

119. Hoffbrand, A. V., Al-Refaie, F., Davis, B. *et al.* (1998). Long-term trial of deferiprone in 51-transfusion-dependent iron overloaded patients. *Blood*, **91**, 295–300.

120. Stella, M., Pinzello, G., and Maggio, A. (1998). Iron chelation with oral deferiprone in patients with thalassemia. *N. Engl. J. Med.*, **339**, 1710–11.

121. Tondury, P., Zimmermann, A., Nielsen, P., and Hirt, A. (1998). Liver iron and fibrosis during long-term treatment with deferiprone in Swiss thalassaemic patients. *Br. J. Haematol.*, **101**, 413–15.

122. Berdoukas, V., Bohane, T., Eagle, C. *et al.* (2000). The Sidney Children's Hospital experience with the oral iron chelator deferiprone (L1). *Transfus. Sci.*, **23**, 239–40.

123. Wanless, I. R., Sweeney, G., Dhillon, A. P. *et al.* (2002). Lack of progressive hepatic fibrosis during long-term therapy with deferiprone in subjects with transfusion-dependent beta-thalassemia. *Blood*, **100**, 1566–9.

124. Addis, A., Loebstein, R., Koren, G., and Einarson, T. R. (1999). Meta-analytic review of the clinical effectiveness of oral deferiprone (L1). *Eur. J. Clin. Pharmacol.*, **55**, 1–6.

125. Barman Balfour, J. A. and Foster, R. H. (1999). Deferiprone: a review of its clinical potential in iron overload in beta-thalassaemia major and other transfusion-dependent diseases. *Drugs*, **58**, 553–78.

126. Kersten, M. J., Lange, R., Smeets, M. E. *et al.* (1996). Long-term treatment of transfusional iron overload with the oral iron chelator deferiprone (L1): a Dutch multicenter trial. *Ann. Hematol.*, **73**, 247–52.

127. Pootrakul, P., Sirankapracha, P., Sankote, J. *et al.* (2003). Clinical trial of deferiprone iron chelation therapy in beta-thalassaemia/haemoglobin E patients in Thailand. *Br. J. Haematol.*, **122**, 305–10.

128. Nick, H., Acklin, P., Lattmann, R. *et al.* (2003). Development of tridentate iron chelators: from desferrithiocin to ICL670. *Curr. Med. Chem.*, **10**, 1065–76.

129. Nisbet-Brown, E., Olivieri, N. F., Giardina, P. J. *et al.* (2003). Effectiveness and safety of ICL670 in iron-loaded patients with thalassaemia: a randomised, double-blind, placebo-controlled, dose-escalation trial. *Lancet*, **361**, 1597–602.

130. Piga, A., Galanello, R., Cappellini, M. D. *et al.* (2002). Phase II study of oral chelator ICL670 in thalassaemia patients with transfusional iron overload: efficacy, safety, pharmacokinetics (PK) and pharmacodynamics (PD) after 6 months of therapy. *Blood*, **100** (suppl. 1), 5a (abstract).

131. Piga, A., Galanello, R., Cappellini, M. D. *et al.* (2003). Phase II study of ICL670, an oral chelator, in adult thalassaemia patients with transfusional iron overload: efficacy, safety, pharmacokinetics (PK) and pharmacodynamics (PD) after 18 months of therapy. *Blood*, **102** (suppl. 1), 121a (abstract).

132. Cheson, B. D., Bennett, J. M., Kantarjian, H. *et al.* (2000). Report of an international working group to standardize response criteria for myelodysplastic syndromes. *Blood*, **96**, 3671–4.

133. Bowen, D. T. and Hellstrom-Lindberg, E. (2001). Best supportive care for the anaemia of myelodysplasia: inclusion of recombinant erythropoietin therapy? *Leuk. Res.*, **25**, 19–21.

134. Nicolas, G., Bennoun, M., Devaux, I. *et al.* (2001). Lack of hepcidin gene expression and severe tissue iron overload in upstream stimulatory factor 2 (USF2) knockout mice. *Proc. Natl Acad. Sci. U.S.A.*, **98**, 8780–5.

9

Hematopoietic cell transplantation for myelodysplastic syndromes

H. Joachim Deeg and Bart Scott

Fred Hutchinson Cancer Research Center, and the University of Washington, Seattle, WA, USA

Introduction

Hematopoietic cell transplantation (HCT) provides effective therapy for various malignant and non-malignant disorders. The indications are relatively clear for some diseases, but are less well defined for others such as the myelodysplastic syndromes (MDS).

MDS are clonal stem cell disorders that are characterized by ineffective hematopoiesis and a propensity to transform into acute myeloid leukemia (tAML).[1,2] The median age at diagnosis of MDS is about 70–72 years; approximately half of the patients with de novo MDS have clonal cytogenetic abnormalities detectable by conventional cytogenetics.[1] Details of disease classification are discussed elsewhere in this volume. According to the French–American–British (FAB) classification, MDS includes refractory anemia (RA; <5% marrow blasts), RA with ringed sideroblasts (RARS; > 15% marrow ringed sideroblasts), RA with excess blasts (RAEB; 5–20% marrow blasts), RAEB in transformation (RAEBT; 21–30% marrow blasts) and chronic myelomonocytic leukemia (CMML).[3] The World Health Organization (WHO) defined MDS subgroups more narrowly in a revised classification including RA, RARS, refractory cytopenia with multilineage dysplasia (RCMD), del 5q syndrome, RAEB 1 (5–10% marrow blasts) and 2 (11–20% marrow blasts), and unclassifiable MDS. Furthermore, the threshold for the diagnosis of AML was reduced to >20% myeloblasts, effectively eliminating RAEB-T as a diagnostic category.[4] In addition, CMML was reclassified as a myeloproliferative disorder.

Myelodysplastic Syndromes: Clinical and Biological Advances, ed. Peter L. Greenberg. Published by Cambridge University Press. © Cambridge University Press 2006.

Table 9.1 International Prognostic Scoring System (IPSS) for myelodysplastic syndrome: survival and acute myeloid leukemia evolution[5]

Prognostic variable	Score value				
	0	0.5	1.0	1.5	2.0
Bone marrow blasts (%)	< 5	5–10	–	11–20	21–30
Karyotype[a]	Good	Intermediate	Poor		
Cytopenias	0/1	2/3			

Cumulative scores for risk groups are as follows: low, 0; intermediate-1, 0.5–1.0; intermediate-2, 1.5–2.0; high, ≥ 2.5.

[a] Good: normal, $-Y$, del(5q), del(20q); poor: complex ($\geq$ three abnormalities) or chromosome 7 anomalies; intermediate: other abnormalities.

The incorporation of cytogenetic findings and the number of cytopenias, in addition to the blast count, into a new risk scoring system termed the International Prognostic Scoring System (IPSS) provides improved prognostic precision,[5] not only for the natural history of the disease, but also for results with HCT. See Chapters 1 and 2 for expanded discussion of MDS classification.

General considerations for HCT

As the clinical course of MDS is highly variable, an accurate prognostic assessment at the time of diagnosis is essential before deciding upon therapy (Tables 9.1 and 9.2). Patients in IPSS risk groups low or intermediate-1 may have life expectancies in the range of 5–10 years with supportive care only or low-intensity therapy. These considerations are particularly important if the clinical course is stable or performance status or age (>65 years) precludes these patients from undergoing HCT. However, reassessment in regard to transplantation is indicated in any patient with disease progression, and it is important to emphasize that HCT may be available to patients up to 65 (or even 70) years of age. For patients with intermediate-2 or high-risk MDS by IPSS, HCT is likely to be the treatment of choice if they are less than 65 years old and have good performance status. In patients more than 65 years of age with adequate performance

Table 9.2 Factors to be considered for hematopoietic cell transplant in myelodysplastic syndrome patients

Disease stage
   Bone marrow blast count
   Cytogenetic abnormalities   } Reflected by IPSS score
   Peripheral blood cytopenia(s)
Patient age
   Children
   Older patients
Donor availability
Clinical evidence of disease progression
Comorbid conditions
Availability of alternative treatment options

IPSS, International Prognostic Scoring System.

status, low-intensity (non-transplant) therapy may be preferable unless they qualify for a non-myeloablative (NMA)/reduced-intensity conditioning (RIC) transplant.

While originally based on survival in non-transplanted patients, recent reports show that IPSS scores also impact on survival after HCT. Among 251 patients transplanted at the Fred Hutchinson Cancer Research Center (FHCRC), the 5-year relapse-free survival (RFS) was 60% with low and intermediate 1 risk, 36% for intermediate 2 risk, and 28% for patients with high-risk disease.[6] Similar results have been reported by Nevill *et al.*, who showed 7-year RFS for patients in the good, intermediate, and poor-risk cytogenetic subgroups (as determined by IPSS) to be 51%, 40%, and 6%, respectively.[7] The corresponding figures for actuarial relapse were 19%, 12%, and 82%, respectively. There was no difference for non-relapse mortality (NRM) between the three groups. In addition to single or multiorgan failure, the major causes of NRM after allogeneic HCT are graft-versus-host disease (GvHD) and associated complications, in particular, infections. Figure 9.1 illustrates the impact of acute GvHD on RFS among 277 patients with MDS transplanted from unrelated donors.[8]

Taking into consideration the IPSS information and transplant results, Cutler *et al.*, in an analysis involving patient data from multiple institutions,

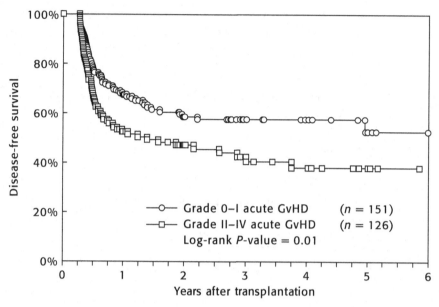

Fig. 9.1   Impact of acute graft-versus-host disease (GvHD) on disease-free survival (DFS). This research was originally published in *Blood*. Castro-Malaspina, H., Harris, R. E., Gajewski, J., *et al.* Unrelated donor marrow transplantation for myelodysplastic syndromes: outcome analysis in 510 transplants facilitated by the National Marrow Donor Program. *Blood*, 2002; **99**, 1943–51. © the American Society of Hematology.

suggested that patients in risk groups intermediate 2 and high, who are transplant candidates, will have the best overall life expectancy if they proceed to transplantation without delay. Conversely, patients with low to intermediate 1 risk disease may have the longest life expectancy if HCT is delayed.[9]

The role of intensive remission induction and consolidation chemotherapy before HCT in patients with MDS has remained controversial. De Witte *et al.* reported on 184 patients who received one or two remission induction courses followed by consolidation (in patients in complete remission). Patients who did not achieve a complete remission with induction were advised to undergo HCT as salvage therapy or receive high-dose cytosine avabinoside. Following consolidation, patients then proceeded to either allogeneic or autologous HCT depending on donor availability. Four-year overall survival in the entire cohort was 26%, and RFS was

29%.[10] Yakoub-Agha *et al.* have shown that patients who achieve remissions with pretransplant chemotherapy have a substantially better outcome after transplantation than patients who do not.[11] Our own data suggest that patients whose MDS has advanced to AML may derive an advantage from pretransplant induction chemotherapy, but no benefit was observed among patients with RAEB or RAEB-T.[12] Controlled studies comparing HCT with and without prior chemotherapy are necessary to address these questions.

Transplant strategies

Myeloablative ("conventional") HCT

"Less advanced" MDS

The best results with allogeneic HCT are achieved in patients with low myeloblast counts, i.e., RA/RARS (or RCMD; refractory cytopenia with ring sideroblasts (RCRS)), at transplantation, and patients without high-risk cytogenetic abnormalities (less advanced MDS) (Table 9.1).

The European Group for Blood and Marrow Transplantation (EBMT) reported on 131 patients, most conditioned with total body irradiation (TBI)-based regimens (70%) and given HCT from human leukocyte antigen (HLA)-identical siblings. Five-year RFS was 52%, and relapse incidence was 13% for patients with RA/RARS.[13] In a cohort of 510 patients with MDS transplanted from unrelated donors under the auspices of the National Marrow Donor Program (NMDP), patients conditioned with busulfan (BU)/cyclophosphamide (CY) fared better than patients prepared with other regimens.[8] RFS and relapse rate in patients with RA were 40% and 5%, respectively.[8] BU/CY regimens have been used by several transplant teams,[7,14] some adding cytosine arabinoside to BU/CY (BAC).[15] Despite encouraging results, NRM due to infections, GvHD, and single- and multi organ toxicity was in the range of 30–54%.[7,8,13] The team at the FHCRC reported results achieved with a BU/CY regimen in which the BU dose was adjusted to maintain steady-state plasma levels of 800–900 ng/ml (targeted BU)[16] (Table 9.3). Among 69 patients with RA/RARS the 3-year probability of RFS was 68% with HLA-identical sibling donors, and 70% with unrelated donors. The incidence of NRM among all patients was 12% at 100 days, and 31% at 3 years; relapse occurred in 5% of patients. Outcomes

Table 9.3 Transplant outcome in patients with myelodysplastic syndromes (MDS) conditioned with a regimen of "targeted" busulfan and cyclophosphamide[16]

MDS risk group	Transplant outcome (proportion)[a]		
	RFS	Relapse	NRM
All patients (n = 109)	0.57	0.13	0.31
IPSS			
Low	0.80	0.00	0.20
Intermediate-1	0.64	0.06	0.30
Intermediate-2	0.40	0.29	0.31
High	0.29	0.42	0.29

[a] At 3 years after transplantation

RFS, relapse-free survival; NRM, non-relapse mortality; IPSS, International Prognostic Scoring System.

tended to be superior in patients transplanted with granulocyte colony-stimulating factor (G-CSF)-mobilized peripheral blood progenitor cells (PBPC) rather than marrow.

A retrospective survey of the EBMT compared results with marrow and G-CSF-mobilized PBPC for allogeneic HCT from HLA-identical siblings (with either TBI- or chemotherapy-based conditioning regimens) and confirmed that the incidence of treatment failure in all MDS subgroups was lower with PBPC as a source of stem cells.[17] The only subgroup for which NRM was not reduced with PBPC were patients with RA and high-risk cytogenetics. The incidences of acute GvHD were comparable; however, chronic GvHD occurred more frequently with PBPC. Nevertheless, these studies show excellent overall results with allogeneic HCT in less advanced MDS with up to 70% RFS, and suggest that the lack of a suitably matched related donor should not be cause to abandon plans for transplantation.

"Advanced" MDS

The risk of posttransplant relapse increases with the proportion of marrow blasts present at the time of transplantation (advanced MDS (RAEB/RAEB-T)).[8,16,18] Relapse rates in the range of 15–50% have been reported.[8,13,16,19] Studies in the 1980s using CY and TBI-containing regimens reported RFS in the range of 30–40%.[19] To determine if more intensive conditioning would improve results, 31 patients with RAEB, RAEB-T, or CMML were prepared with a BU/CY/TBI regimen before HLA-identical or non-identical related or unrelated donor marrow transplants.[20] Compared to historical controls conditioned with CY/TBI, relapse rates were lower (28% versus 54%), but NRM was markedly increased (68% versus 36%), and RFS at 3 years was not improved (23% versus 30%).

The EBMT study cited above also included 63 patients with RAEB/RAEB-T, and 18 patients with tAML and showed 5-year RFS of 34%, 19%, and 26% for patients with RAEB, RAEB-T, and tAML, respectively.[13] The majority of patients (70%) received TBI as part of the conditioning regimen. The relapse rate was 44% for RAEB, 52% for RAEB-T, and 50% for tAML. NRM was highest in patients with RAEB-T (60%), followed by tAML (48%), and RAEB (38%). Younger age, absence of excess blasts, and a shorter interval from diagnosis to HCT were associated with better outcome. Another EBMT trial including 105 patients (69 conditioned with TBI) who received HLA-matched unrelated donor transplants showed RFS of 27%, 8%, and 27% for RAEB, RAEB-T and tAML patients, respectively.[21] A recent report from the International Bone Marrow Transplant Registry (IBMTR) on 452 patients transplanted from HLA-identical siblings (44% conditioned with TBI regimens) between 1989 and 1997 showed a RFS of 40% at 3 years.[18] Corresponding figures for relapse incidence and NRM were 23% and 37%, respectively. The proportion of marrow blasts at transplantation was the strongest predictor for relapse and RFS, and younger age correlated with higher probability of survival.

CY is not stem cell-toxic but contributes to non-hematopoietic toxicity. Thus, in another study, 60 patients with RAEB, RAEB-T, CMML, or tAML (20 patients with related and 40 with unrelated donors) were conditioned with BU/TBI without the use of CY.[22] The Kaplan–Meier estimate of survival at 3 years was 26% with a cumulative incidence of relapse of 25%. The incidence of NRM at 100 days was 38%. The relapse rate was comparable to that observed previously with a regimen combining BU/TBI with CY. Despite the omission of CY, NRM was considerable, particularly with transplants from unrelated donors. While these data showed that CY was not required for successful transplantation in either related or unrelated recipients, they also suggested that TBI may not be the best modality to prepare patients with MDS for transplantation. In conceptual agreement with this notion, the NMDP analysis cited above showed that patients in all FAB categories prepared with non-TBI regimens had a higher probability of overall survival and RFS than patients conditioned with TBI.[8]

As with less advanced MDS, the use of PBPC was associated with a lower treatment failure incidence than the use of marrow in all patients with advanced MDS.[17] In a recent FHCRC trial using a regimen of targeted BU/CY, RFS at 3 years among patients with RAEB was 45% with transplants from HLA-identical siblings, and 40% with transplants from unrelated donors.[16] The corresponding figures for RAEB-T/tAML were 33%/17%. This trial also confirmed that the IPSS score correlated with posttransplant relapse and transplant outcome after a non-TBI-containing regimen (Fig. 9.2).

Another pilot study evaluated toxicity and efficacy of a conditioning regimen in which targeted BU was combined with fludarabine (rather than CY).[23] That trial included 38 patients with advanced MDS (or RA with high-risk cytogenetics) who were transplanted with PBPC from HLA-matched siblings or unrelated donors. The day-100 NRM was 7%, the incidence of acute GvHD of grades II–IV was 54%, and the 1-year RFS was 45%. These preliminary data suggest excellent tolerability of this regimen, although longer follow-up is needed to assess relative risk.

Non-myeloablative (reduced-intensity) conditioning (NMA/RIC) regimens

The recent development of NMA or RIC or transplant regimens ("mini-transplants") has met with considerable interest.[24] The rationale of this approach is that reduced-intensity conditioning will also reduce NRM. Post-transplant administration of immunosuppressive drugs (e.g., cyclosporin plus mycophenolate mofetil) will facilitate donor cell engraftment and enhance the effect of donor lymphocytes against the patients' clonal cells (graft-versus-MDS effect).[25] In view of the generally high incidence of NRM in older patients, such an approach is attractive for the treatment of patients with MDS. RIC regimens might also be of interest in patients with comorbid conditions or with relapse after a conventional transplant, particularly if debulking with chemotherapy before such a transplant is successful. The field is developing rapidly.[18,26–31] Kroger et al. used a regimen of fludarabine combined with BU and showed an RFS of 38% at 3 years among 37 patients

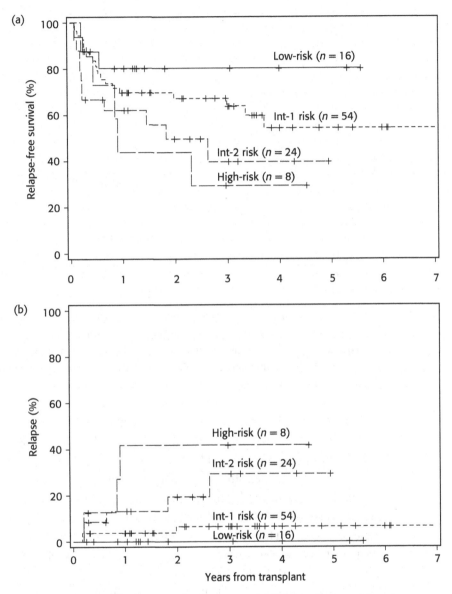

Fig. 9.2   Impact of pretransplant International Prognostic Scoring System risk category on (a) relapse-free survival and (b) relapse after allogeneic hematopoietic cell transplant for IPSS. Int-1, intermediate-1; int-2, intermediate-2 patients.

This research was originally published in *Blood*. Deeg, H. J., Storer, B. *et al*. Conditioning with targeted busulfan and cyclophosphamide for hemopoietic stem cell transplantation from related and unrelated donors in patients with myelodysplastic syndrome. *Blood*, 2002;**100**, 1201–7. © the American Society of Hematology.

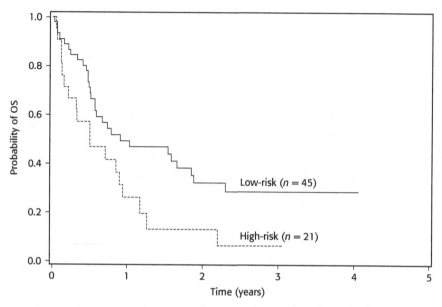

Fig. 9.3   Overall survival (OS) of patients conditioned with a reduced-intensity regimen (fludarabine plus 200 cGy of total body irradiation (TBI)) and transplanted from related or unrelated donors. Shown separately are outcomes for high-risk International Prognostic Scoring System (IPSS) (intermediate 2 and high) and low-risk (IPSS low and intermediate 1)
disease. (Courtesy of M. J. Stuart, Stanford University Medical Center.)

with MDS or tAML (transplanted from related ($n = 19$) or unrelated HLA-
matched ($n = 18$) donors).[31] The cumulative incidence of relapse was 32%.

A recent update on RIC/NMA transplants includes 78 patients with MDS
(45 related, 33 unrelated; 46 were IPSS low/intermediate 1, and 32 intermediate 2/high or unknown).[28] These patients were conditioned with fludarabine
plus 200 cGy of TBI. Graft failure occurred in 6% of patients, and 42% of
patients relapsed. The NRM was 14% at day-100, and 25% at 1 year. Approximately 20% of patients were surviving at 3 years (25% with low-risk, and
less than 10% with high-risk disease) (Fig. 9.3).[28] Parker *et al.* reported on
23 patients conditioned with RIC regimens (fludarabine/BU/campath).[29]
They observed that about 65% sustained engraftment, and 9% had
procedure-related mortality. The 2-year RFS was 39%. An increased relapse
rate in patients with MDS prepared with RIC was also reported by Martino
et al.[32] It is important to note, of course, that patients prepared with RIC
regimens tended to be older and often had significant comorbid conditions.

Thus, RIC regimens are one approach to the reduction of regimen-related mortality. However, additional work is needed to secure sustained engraftment and a potent anti-MDS effect.

Autologous HCT

Autologous HCT is associated with lower treatment-related mortality than allogeneic transplants and may hold promise in patients in whom a "pure" population of normal hemopoietic stem cells is obtainable. The EBMT reported results in 79 patients with MDS and showed a 2-year RFS of 28% after autologous HCT.[33] NRM was 39% in patients >40 years of age. These results were restricted to patients who achieved complete remissions after induction chemotherapy. Wattel *et al.* prospectively assessed feasibility of autologous HCT (either with bone marrow or PBPC) after conditioning with BU/CY in 24 of 39 patients who achieved complete remissions after induction chemotherapy. Among these, 50% were alive 8–55 months after HCT.[34]

De Witte and colleagues presented data on 184 patients with MDS/tAML who received induction chemotherapy.[10] Among these, 56 had HLA-identical related donors available, and 128 did not. One hundred patients achieved remission, and 39 were transplanted with allogeneic, and 61 with autologous stem cells. The rate of continuous complete remission was 33% for allogeneic and 31% for autologous HCT. The 4-year survival in remission (expressed as a proportion of the total cohort) was 25% for allogeneic, and 15% for autologous transplants.[10]

The same authors recently reported outcomes in patients with and without an HLA-identical sibling donor on an intention-to-treat basis.[35] There were 159 patients included in the analysis, all of whom received remission induction and consolidation chemotherapy. Sixty-five patients did not have a donor available; of these, 33 ultimately received an autologous transplant. RFS was 23.1% for patients with a donor and 21.5% for patients without a donor. Alternative donor transplants did not significantly alter the survival of the group without a donor. This intention-to-treat analysis failed to show a survival advantage for patients with donors compared to those without an available donor. The data suggest, however, that outcome with autologous HCT in these patient populations is superior to that without intervention.

Special considerations

The "older" patient

Is HCT an option for "older" patients with MDS? Fifty patients with MDS, 55–66 years of age, were transplanted at the FHCRC after conditioning with either BU/CY plus fractionated TBI or BU/CY alone.[36] Donors were HLA-identical siblings in 34, HLA-non-identical family members in 4, identical twins in 4, and unrelated volunteers in 6 patients. The Kaplan–Meier estimates of RFS at 3 years were 53% for RA, 46% for RAEB, and 33% for RAEB-T/tAML or CMML.[36] When only transplants from HLA-identical siblings were considered, RFS for patients with RA was 67%. Survival in all FAB categories was highest among patients conditioned with targeted BU/CY. A recent analysis in a larger cohort of patients confirmed those results and showed no significant impact of age (up to 66 years) on HCT outcome.[16]

Childhood MDS

MDS accounts for less than 10% of all childhood leukemias.[37,38] Childhood MDS may be associated with constitutional abnormalities, such as Down or Pearson syndrome, and 60% of children have cytogenetic abnormalities, most commonly monosomy 7.[39] Children with RA/RARS are generally younger than those with advanced MDS stages.[39] The FAB criteria, primarily established to classify adult MDS, are of limited value for children, since some subtypes of MDS (e.g., RARS) are extremely rare in childhood, and other hematologic syndromes, such as juvenile chronic myelomonocytic leukemia (JMML) or the infantile monosomy-7 syndrome, are not considered in the FAB classification.

A retrospective analysis by the European Working Group on MDS in Childhood (EWOG-MDS), involving 29 patients, showed RFS, NRM, and relapse incidence of 58%, 21%, and 26%, respectively, after HCT from HLA-identical siblings.[40] A survey of results in 100 children with MDS and partial or complete monosomy 7 suggests that HCT without prior chemotherapy is the treatment of choice for children with MDS and JMML.[41] Children with RA, RAEB, or JMML treated with HCT alone achieved a 3-year survival of 73%. The Children's Cancer Group trial 2891 included 90 children with various forms of MDS, JMML, and AML. Patients were treated with a five-drug induction regimen and, if they achieved remission, allocated to one of three postremission therapies (allogeneic or autologous HCT or intensive chemotherapy).[42] There was a trend towards improved survival with allogeneic HCT over the two other strategies.[42] In other trials, using different preparative protocols and matched or mismatched related or unrelated donors, RFS ranged from 38% to 69%.[43–46] As for adult patients, the IPSS score was a powerful predictor of posttransplant outcome.[37] Without transplantation, outcome is extremely poor in children with JMML, with a probability of extended survival of 6%. A recent European study suggests that with HCT the 5-year RFS may be 55%.[47] Therefore, HCT should be offered to all children with JMML who have a suitable donor.[48]

Secondary MDS

Treatment-related (secondary) MDS occurs after therapy for various disorders. Incidence figures of 1.1–19.8% have been reported at 10 years after autologous HCT for Hodgkin's disease (HD) and non-Hodgkin's lymphoma (NHL).[49–51] The median time from primary disease to secondary MDS ranges from 4 to 9 years.[1,50] Abnormal, usually high-risk karyotypes (monosomy 7; complex abnormalities) are present in 80–90% of patients.[49–51] Exposure to irradiation and chemotherapy, as given for the patient's original disease, is thought to be causative. As prior therapy is expected to result in tissue damage, the sequelae are likely to predispose the patient to substantial morbidity and mortality with a transplant for secondary MDS.

Among 552 patients who had received autologous HCT for NHL, Friedberg *et al.* observed 41 who developed MDS at a median of 47 months, for an actuarial incidence of 19.8% at 10 years.[50] Thirteen patients underwent allogeneic HCT, and all died with a median survival of 1.8 months. These results are in agreement with an earlier report by the EBMT group which showed a 5-year survival of 0% in patients with secondary MDS.[52] A French group reported on 70 patients receiving allogeneic HCT (various conditioning regimens) for therapy-related MDS and AML.[11] Overall, 54 patients died, 19 of relapse, 34 of NRM, and 1 of relapse of the primary disease. Age greater than 37 years, absence of complete remission at HCT, and intensive schedules for conditioning were associated with poor outcome. RFS, relapse incidence, and NRM rates at 2 years were 28%, 42%, and 49%, respectively.[11] It is of note, however, that all these patients had been given pretransplant induction chemotherapy, and patients who achieved remissions had a substantially higher chance of RFS than patients who were not in remission.

We evaluated the outcome of 111 consecutive patients with secondary MDS transplanted at the FHCRC between 1971 and 1998 from either related or unrelated donors using the same conditioning regimens as employed for patients with de novo MDS.[53] The primary diagnoses included HD, NHL, breast carcinoma, aplastic anemia, multiple myeloma, polycythemia vera, and other malignancies or immunologic disorders. The 5-year RFS was 8% for patients prepared with TBI, 19% for those given BU/CY, and 30% for those prepared with targeted BU/CY. The 5-year relapse rate was 40% for tAML, 40% for RAEB-T, 26% for RAEB, and 0% for RA and RARS.[53] Thus, as with de novo MDS, disease stage was the most important risk factor for outcome, and the conditioning regimen had a major impact. Ballen *et al.* reported an RFS of 14% and NRM of 50% at 3 years for 18 patients with secondary MDS treated with HCT from HLA-matched related or unrelated donors after preparation with various conditioning regimens.[54] Leahey *et al.* have presented similar results for pediatric patients.[55]

Thus, results obtained with allogeneic HCT for treatment-related MDS are currently not satisfactory, although HCT may be the only viable option for many of these patients. Efforts must be directed firstly at the prevention of secondary MDS, and secondly at improved tolerability of HCT conditioning. Some preliminary studies with induction chemotherapy followed by RIC regimens have yielded encouraging results.

Posttransplant relapse

Posttransplant relapse remains a problem in patients with advanced MDS or "high-risk" cytogenetics or both. Reports on the efficacy of donor lymphocyte infusions (DLI) in patients with MDS are limited.[5–58] A Japanese series noted complete remissions in 5 of 11 MDS patients.[58] We have given DLI to 7 patients with MDS (5 with RAEB and 2 with RA), and 3 (all with RAEB) achieved complete remissions. Two patients are alive, disease-free, at more than 2 years (M. Flowers *et al.*, unpublished observations). These observations are of interest, but firm conclusions cannot be drawn at this point. Some patients with relapse have undergone successful second HCT.[28] Conceivably,

RIC regimens are effective in these patients, particularly if carried out before disease evolution.

Summary and future directions

Patients with intermediate-2 or high-risk MDS who have suitably HLA-matched related or unrelated donors should be transplanted early in their disease course. About 35–45% and 25–30%, respectively, are surviving in remission after transplantation from related and unrelated donors. The incidence of posttransplant relapse is 10–35%. Patients with less advanced MDS by FAB criteria (<5% marrow blasts) but with high-risk IPSS cytogenetic findings or severe multilineage cytopenias according to IPSS, and transfusion dependence or severe neutropenia, should also be considered for early HCT. Three-year survivals of 65–75% are achievable with HLA-identical related and HLA-matched unrelated donors. The probability of relapse is <5%. Patients with MDS with low-risk IPSS cytogenetic features and without severe cytopenias may do well for extended periods of time with more conservative management. HCT can be carried out successfully, even in the seventh decade of life. It appears that, overall, non-TBI regimens are better tolerated than TBI-containing regimens. Results with a regimen using a combination of BU (targeted to predetermined plasma levels) and CY are particularly encouraging. The use of PBPC may offer an advantage over marrow cells. The place of RIC/NMA transplants, other than for patients of advanced age (older than 65 years), remains to be determined. Improved survival with HCT from unrelated volunteer donors in part reflects selection of donors on the basis of high-resolution (allele-level) HLA typing. Autologous HCTs are an option for patients without a suitable donor if a remission can be induced pretransplant. Investigations in the future will focus on the identification of additional prognostic parameters allowing one to predict prognosis as well as on determination of the optimal timing of HCT.[9,59]

ACKNOWLEDGMENT

This work was supported by National Institutes of Health grants CA87948, CA18029, and HL36444, Bethesda, MD. Bart Scott was also supported by National Institutes of Health training grant T32-CA09515.

REFERENCES

1. Greenberg, P. L. (2000). Myelodysplastic syndrome. In *Hematology: Basic Principles and Practice*, 3rd edn, ed. R. Hoffman, E. J. Benz, S. J. Shattil, B. Furie *et al.* New York: Churchill Livingstone, pp. 1106–29.

2. Sanz, G. F., Sanz, M. A., Vallespì, T. *et al.* (1989). Two regression models and a scoring system for predicting survival and planning treatment in myelodysplastic syndromes: a multivariate analysis of prognostic factors in 370 patients. *Blood*, **74**, 395–408.

3. Bennett, J. M., Catovsky, D., Daniel, M. T. *et al.* (1982). Proposals for the classification of the myelodysplastic syndromes. *Br. J. Haematol.*, **51**, 189–99.

4. Vardiman, J. W., Harris, N. L., and Brunning, R. D. (2002). The World Health Organization (WHO) classification of the myeloid neoplasms (review). *Blood*, **100**, 2292–302.

5. Greenberg, P., Cox, C., Le Beau, M. M. *et al.* (1997). International scoring system for evaluating prognosis in myelodysplastic syndromes. *Blood*, **89**, 2079–88. (published erratum appears in *Blood*, 1998; **91**, 1100).

6. Appelbaum, F. R. and Anderson, J. (1998). Allogeneic bone marrow transplantation for myelodysplastic syndrome: outcomes analysis according to IPSS score. *Leukemia*, **12** (Suppl. 1), S25–9.

7. Nevill, T. J., Fung, H. C., Shepherd, J. D. *et al.* (1998). Cytogenetic abnormalities in primary myelodysplastic syndrome are highly predictive of outcome after allogeneic bone marrow transplantation. *Blood*, **92**, 1910–17.

8. Castro-Malaspina, H., Harris, R. E., Gajewski, J. *et al.* (2002). Unrelated donor marrow transplantation for myelodysplastic syndromes: outcome analysis in 510 transplants facilitated by the National Marrow Donor Program. *Blood*, **99**, 1943–51.

9. Cutler, C., Lee, S., Greenberg, P. *et al.* (2002). A decision analysis of allogeneic stem cell transplantation for MDS: delayed transplantation for low risk MDS is associated with improved outcome. *Blood*, **100** (Part 1), 74a (abstract 270).

10. de Witte, T., Suciu, S., Verhoef, G. *et al.* (2001). Intensive chemotherapy followed by allogeneic or autologous stem cell transplantation for patients with myelodysplastic syndromes (MDSs) and acute myeloid leukemia following MDS. *Blood*, **98**, 2326–31.

11. Yakoub-Agha, I., de La Salmonière, P., Ribaud, P. *et al.* (2000). Allogeneic bone marrow transplantation for therapy-related myelodsyplastic syndrome and acute myeloid leukemia: a long-term study of 70 patients-report of the French Society of bone marrow transplantation. *J. Clin. Oncol.*, **18**, 963–71.

12. Scott, B. L., Deeg, H. J., and Appelbaum, F. R. (2003). Pre-transplant induction chemotherapy and post-transplant relapse in patients with advanced MDS. *Blood*, **102** (Part 1), 152a. (abstract 523).

13. Runde, V., de Witte, T., Arnold, R. *et al.* (1998). Bone marrow transplantation from HLA-identical siblings as first-line treatment in patients with myelodysplastic syndromes: early transplantation is associated with improved outcome. Chronic Leukemia Working Party of the European Group for Blood and Marrow Transplantation. *Bone Marrow Transplant.*, **21**, 255–61.

14. O'Donnell, M. R., Long, G. D., Parker, P. M. *et al.* (1995). Busulfan/cyclophosphamide as conditioning regimen for allogeneic bone marrow transplantation for myelodysplasia. *J. Clin. Oncol.*, **13**, 2973–9.

15. Ratanatharathorn, V., Karanes, C., Uberti, J. *et al.* (1993). Busulfan-based regimens and allogeneic bone marrow transplantation in patients with myelodysplastic syndromes. *Blood*, **81**, 2194–9.

16. Deeg, H. J., Storer, B., Slattery, J. T. *et al.* (2002). Conditioning with targeted busulfan and cyclophosphamide for hemopoietic stem cell transplantation from related and unrelated donors in patients with myelodysplastic syndrome. *Blood*, **100**, 1201–7.

17. Guardiola, P., Runde, V., Bacigalupo, A. *et al.* (2002). Retrospective comparison of bone marrow and granulocyte colony-stimulating factor-mobilized peripheral blood progenitor cells for allogeneic stem cell transplantation using HLA identical sibling donors in myelodysplastic syndromes. *Blood*, **99**, 4370–8.

18. Sierra, J., Pérez, W. S., Rozman, C. *et al.* (2002). Bone marrow transplantation from HLA-identical siblings as treatment for myelodysplasia. *Blood*, **100**, 1997–2004.

19. Appelbaum, F. R., Barrall, J., Storb, R. *et al.* (1990). Bone marrow transplantation for patients with myelodysplasia. Pretreatment variables and outcome. *Ann. Intern. Med.*, **112**, 590–7.

20. Anderson, J. E., Appelbaum, F. R., Schoch, G. *et al.* (1996). Allogeneic marrow transplantation for myelodysplastic syndrome with advanced disease morphology: a phase II study of busulfan, cyclophosphamide, and total-body irradiation and analysis of prognostic factors. *J. Clin. Oncol.*, **14**, 220–6.

21. Arnold, R., de Witte, T., van Biezen, A. *et al.* (1998). Unrelated bone marrow transplantation in patients with myelodysplastic syndromes and secondary acute myeloid leukemia: an EBMT survey. European Blood and Marrow Transplantation Group. *Bone Marrow Transplant.*, **21**, 1213–16.

22. Jurado, M., Deeg, H. J., Storer, B. *et al.* (2002). Hematopoietic stem cell transplantation for advanced myelodysplastic syndrome after conditioning with busulfan and fractionated total body irradiation is associated with low relapse rate but considerable nonrelapse mortality. *Biol. Blood Marrow Transplant.*, **8**, 161–9.

23. Bornhäuser, M., Storer, B., Slattery, J. T. *et al.* (2003). Conditioning with fludarabine and targeted busulfan for transplantation of allogeneic hematopoietic stem cells. *Blood*, **102**, 820–6.

24. Carella, A. M., Champlin, R., Slavin, S., McSweeney, P. and Storb, R. (2000). Mini-allografts: ongoing trials in humans (editorial). *Bone Marrow Transplant.*, **25**, 345–50.

25. McSweeney, P. A. and Storb, R. (1999). Mixed chimerism: preclinical studies and clinical applications (review). *Biol. Blood Marrow Transplant.*, **5**, 192–203.

26. Storb, R., McSweeney, P. A., Sandmaier, B. M. *et al.* (2000). Allogeneic hematopoietic stem cell transplantation: from the nuclear age into the 21st century. *Transplant Proc.*, **32**, 2548–9.

27. Kroger, N., Schetelig, J., Zabelina, T. *et al.* (2001). A fludarabine-based dose-reduced conditioning regimen followed by allogeneic stem cell transplantation from related or unrelated donors in patients with myelodysplastic syndrome. *Bone Marrow Transplant.*, **28**, 643–7.

28. Stuart, M. J., Cao, T. M., Sandmaier, B. M. *et al.* (2003). Efficacy of non-myeloablative allogeneic transplant for patients with myelodysplastic syndrome (MDS) and myeloproliferative disorders (MPD) (except chronic myelogenous leukemia). *Blood*, **102** (Part 1), 185a (abstract 644).

29. Parker, J. E., Shafi, T., Pagliuca, A. *et al.* (2002). Allogeneic stem cell transplantation in the myelodysplastic syndromes: interim results of outcome following reduced-intensity conditioning compared with standard preparative regimens. *Br. J. Haematol.*, **119**, 144–54.

30. Taussig, D. C., Davies, A. J., Cavenagh, J. D. *et al.* (2003). Durable remissions of myelodysplastic syndrome and acute myeloid leukemia after reduced-intensity allografting. *J. Clin. Oncol.*, **21**, 3060–5.

31. Kroger, N., Bornhauser, M., Ehninger, G. *et al.* (2003). Allogeneic stem cell transplantation after a fludarabine/busulfan-based reduced-intensity conditioning in patients with myelodysplastic syndrome or secondary acute myeloid leukemia. *Ann. Hematol.*, **82**, 336–42.

32. Martino, R., van Biezen, A., Iacobelli, S. *et al.* (2003). Reduced-intensity conditioning (RIC) for allogeneic hematopoietic stem cell transplantation (HSCT) from HLA-identical siblings in adults with myelodysplastic syndromes (MDS): a comparison with standard myeloablative conditioning: a study of the EBMT-Chronic Leukemia Working Party (EBMT-CLWP). *Blood*, **102** (Part 1), 184a (abstract 642).

33. de Witte, T., van Biezen, A., Hermans, J. *et al.* (1997). Autologous bone marrow transplantation for patients with myelodysplastic syndrome (MDS) or acute myeloid leukemia following MDS. *Blood*, **90**, 3853–7.

34. Wattel, E., Solary, E., Leleu, X. *et al.* (1999). A prospective study of autologous bone marrow or peripheral blood stem cell transplantation after intensive chemotherapy in myelodysplastic syndromes. *Leukemia*, **13**, 524–9.

35. Oosterveld, M., Suciu, S., Verhoef, G. *et al.* (2003). The presence of an HLA-identical sibling donor has no impact on outcome of patients with high-risk MDS or secondary AML (sAML) treated with intensive chemotherapy followed by transplantation:

results of a prospective study of the EORTC, EBMT, SAKK and GIMEMA Leukemia Groups (EORTC study 06921). *Leukemia*, **17**, 859–68.

36. Deeg, H. J., Shulman, H. M., Anderson, J. E. *et al.* (2000). Allogeneic and syngeneic marrow transplantation for myelodysplastic syndrome in patients 55 to 66 years of age. *Blood*, **95**, 1188–94.

37. Sasaki, H., Manabe, A., Kojima, S. *et al.* (2001). Myelodysplastic syndrome in childhood: a retrospective study of 189 patients in Japan. *Leukemia*, **15**, 1713–20.

38. Hasle, H., Wadsworth, L. D., Massing, B. G., McBride, M., and Schultz, K. R. (1999). A population-based study of childhood myelodysplastic syndrome in British Columbia, Canada. *Br. J. Haematol.*, **106**, 1027–32.

39. Novitzky, N. (2000). Myelodysplastic syndromes in children. A critical review of the clinical manifestations and management. *Am. J. Hematol.*, **63**, 212–22.

40. Locatelli, F., Zecca, M., Niemeyer, C. *et al.* (1996). Role of allogeneic bone marrow transplantation for the treatment of myelodysplastic syndromes in childhood. The European Working Group on Childhood Myelodysplastic Syndrome (EWOG-MDS) and the Austria–Germany–Italy (AGI) Bone Marrow Transplantation Registry (review). *Bone Marrow Transplant.*, **18** (suppl. 2), 63–8.

41. Hasle, H., Arico, M., Basso, G. *et al.* (1999). Myelodysplastic syndrome, juvenile myelomonocytic leukemia, and acute myeloid leukemia associated with complete or partial monosomy 7. *Leukemia*, **13**, 376–85.

42. Woods, W. G., Barnard, D. R., Alonzo, T. A. *et al.* (2002). Prospective study of 90 children requiring treatment for juvenile myelomonocytic leukemia or myelodysplastic syndrome: a report from the Children's Cancer Group. *J. Clin. Oncol.*, **20**, 434–40.

43. Nagatoshi, Y., Okamura, J., Ikuno, Y., Akamatsu, M., and Tasaka, H. (1997). Therapeutic trial of intensified conditioning regimen with high-dose cytosine arabinoside, cyclophosphamide and either total body irradiation or busulfan followed by allogeneic bone marrow transplantation for myelodysplastic syndrome in children. *Int. J. Hematol.*, **65**, 269–75.

44. Davies, S. M., Wagner, J. E., DeFor, T. *et al.* (1997). Unrelated donor bone marrow transplantation for children and adolescents with aplastic anaemia or myelodysplasia. *Br. J. Haematol.*, **96**, 749–56.

45. Casper, J., Camitta, B., Truitt, R. *et al.* (1995). Unrelated bone marrow donor transplants for children with leukemia or myelodysplasia. *Blood*, **85**, 2354–63.

46. Woolfrey, A. E., Gooley, T. A., Sievers, E. L. *et al.* (1998). Bone marrow transplantation for children less than 2 years of age with acute myelogenous leukemia or myelodysplastic syndrome. *Blood*, **92**, 3546–56.

47. Locatelli, F., Noellke, P., Zecca, M. *et al.* (2003). Hematopoietic stem cell transplantation (HSCT) in children with juvenile myelomonocytic leukemia (JMML): results of the EWOG-MDS trial. *Blood*, **102** (Part 1), 186a (abstract 647).

48. Niemeyer, C. M., Arico, M., Basso, G. *et al.* (1997). Chronic myelomonocytic leukemia in childhood: a retrospective analysis of 110 cases. *Blood*, **89**, 3534–43.

49. Sobecks, R. M., Le Beau, M. M., Anastasi, J., and Williams, S. F. (1999). Myelodysplasia and acute leukemia following high-dose chemotherapy and autologous bone marrow or peripheral blood stem cell transplantation. *Bone Marrow Transplant.*, **23**, 1161–5.

50. Friedberg, J. W., Neuberg, D., Stone, R. M. *et al.* (1999). Outcome in patients with myelodysplastic syndrome after autologous bone marrow transplantation for non-Hodgkin's lymphoma. *J. Clin. Oncol.*, **17**, 3128–35.

51. Micallef, I. N. M., Lillington, D. M., Apostolidis, J. *et al.* (2000). Therapy-related myelodsyplasia and secondary acute myelogenous leukemia after high-dose therapy with autologous hematopoietic progenitor-cell support for lymphoid malignancies. *J. Clin. Oncol.*, **18**, 947–55.

52. de Witte, T. (1999). Stem cell transplantation in myelodysplastic syndromes (review). *Forum*, **9**, 75–81.

53. Witherspoon, R. P., Deeg, H. J., Storer, B. *et al.* (2001). Hematopoietic stem-cell transplantation for treatment-related leukemia or myelodysplasia. *J. Clin. Oncol.*, **19**, 2134–41.

54. Ballen, K. K., Gilliland, D. G., Guinan, E. C. *et al.* (1997). Bone marrow transplantation for therapy-related myelodysplasia: comparison with primary myelodysplasia. *Bone Marrow Transplant.*, **20**, 737–43.

55. Leahey, A. M., Friedman, D. L., and Bunin, N. J. (1999). Bone marrow transplantation in pediatric patients with therapy-related myelodysplasia and leukemia. *Bone Marrow Transplant.*, **23**, 21–5.

56. Castagna, L., El Weshi, A., Bourhis, J. H. *et al.* (1998). Successful donor lymphocyte infusion (DLI) in a patient with myelodysplastic syndrome (MDS) after failure of T-cell-depleted bone marrow transplantation (TD-BMT) (letter). *Br. J. Haematol.*, **103**, 284–5.

57. Bader, P., Klingebiel, T., Schaudt, A. *et al.* (1999). Prevention of relapse in pediatric patients with acute leukemias and MDS after allogeneic SCT by early immunotherapy initiated on the basis of increasing mixed chimerism: a single center experience of 12 children. *Leukemia*, **13**, 2079–86.

58. Shiobara, S., Nakao, S., Ueda, M. *et al.* (2000). Donor leukocyte infusion for Japanese patients with relapsed leukemia after allogeneic bone marrow transplantation: lower incidence of acute graft-versus-host disease and improved outcome. *Bone Marrow Transplant.*, **26**, 769–74.

59. Benesch, M., Wells, D. A., Leisenring, W. *et al.* (2002). Prognostic significance of pretransplant multidimensional flow cytometric parameters for posttransplant survival and relapse in 111 patients with myelodysplastic syndrome (MDS). *Blood*, **100** (Part 1), 97a (abstract 358).

10

Health-related quality of life and myelodysplastic syndrome: conceptualization, measurement, and implications for research and practice

Mary Laudon Thomas

Veterans Affairs Palo Alto Health Care System, Palo Alto, CA, USA

As a concept, quality of life (QOL) is difficult to define. As noted by Kurland, "I don't know how to define it, but I know it when I see it."[1] This statement is certainly not quite as poignant as Aristotle's definition: "a virtuous activity of the soul." But it does illustrate the individual nature of QOL, and its subjectivity. QOL is an extremely subjective, dynamic phenomenon. It is highly personal and can incorporate broad concepts, such as one's economic status and position within society. This chapter will describe QOL from both a conceptual and clinical perspective. Issues related to measuring this complex concept will be presented, including examples of commonly used questionnaires and instruments. This background provides a framework for delineating salient issues that can affect a person's QOL when diagnosed with myelodysplastic syndromes (MDS) and reviewing relevant QOL studies in this patient population. The chapter concludes with suggestions for future direction, including the incorporation of patient-reported outcomes in future studies.

QOL: conceptual frameworks

For a long time, QOL was relatively ignored as an important issue in the health care setting. Frequently, clinicians utilized the Biomedical Model as the focus of health care delivery. In this model, the focus is on etiologic agents, pathological processes, and clinical outcomes.[2] (Fig. 10.1). Using

Myelodysplastic Syndromes: Clinical and Biological Advances, ed. Peter L. Greenberg. Published by Cambridge University Press. © Cambridge University Press 2006.

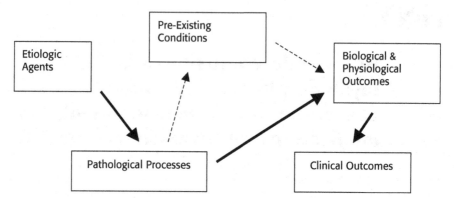

Fig. 10.1 Traditional biomedical model as a focus of health care. This model is based on understanding the causation of illness at a fundamental scientific level. Such understanding is important for the diagnosis and treatment of disease; clinical outcomes are typically disease-related. Pre-existing conditions can also impact the pathologic processes and biological/physiological outcomes (dashed lines). Absent from this model is the human experience of living with the disease. (See text.)

MDS as an example, etiologic agents might be prior chemotherapy or benzene exposure. Pathological processes include increased apoptosis within the marrow, and clinical outcomes include extent of cytopenias, infectious complications, and evolution to acute myeloid leukemia. Obviously a specific disease process, such as MDS, does not necessarily exist in a vacuum. Thus pre-existing conditions impact not only the pathologic processes, but also the biological outcomes of another illness. Given that MDS most frequently occurs in the elderly, concomitant illnesses tend to be commonplace and can have a significant impact on the person's ability to tolerate the outcomes of those illnesses. For example, patients with pre-existing cardiac and pulmonary disease may be more intolerant of anemia associated with MDS.

The Biomedical Model is useful for explaining causation; this in turn is obviously useful to clinicians in guiding diagnosis and treatment.[2] However, a significant limitation of this model, particularly in the context of serious or chronic illness, is that it ignores the human experience of living with the illness – a significant factor in one's QOL. Thus other frameworks are necessary to enhance understanding of this concept.

Health care typically limits its focus to those aspects of QOL that relate to, and are impacted by, an individual's health. Cella & Cherin define this

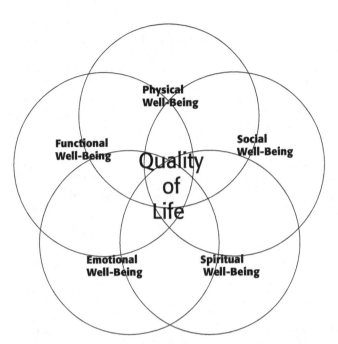

Fig. 10.2   Health-related quality-of-life conceptual framework. The domains of physical, functional, social, emotional, and spiritual well-being are interrelated and have varying degrees of impact on an individual's quality of life.

concept as "patients' appraisal of, and satisfaction with, their current level of functioning compared to what they perceive to be possible or ideal."[3] The Department of Health and Human Services defines health-related quality of life (HRQOL) as "the value assigned to duration of life as modified by impairments, functional states, perceptions, and social opportunities, and as influenced by disease, injury, treatment, or policy."[4] Within the HRQOL concept are several distinct domains. These domains vary among QOL conceptual frameworks, but most commonly include physical, functional, social, emotional, and spiritual well-being.[3,5–9] A simple depiction of the HRQOL conceptual framework is illustrated in Figure 10.2. When reviewing or critiquing HRQOL literature, it is important to remain cognizant that HRQOL remains only a subset (albeit an important one) of QOL.

Wilson & Cleary expanded the HRQOL model to incorporate relationships between characteristics of the individual and the environment as well as biological and physiological variables related to illness, all of which impact

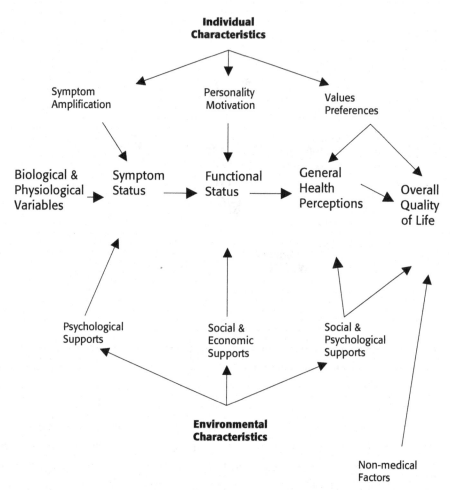

Fig. 10.3   Wilson & Cleary's health-related quality of life (HRQOL) conceptual model: relationships among measures of patient outcomes.[2] This model delineates relationships between individual and environmental characteristics as well as the biological and physiological variables related to illness. All of these components can impact an individual's QOL. (See text.)

QOL[2] (Fig. 10.3). In this model, biological and physiological factors are referred to as those commonly measured in clinical practice and include results of diagnostic tests (e.g., bone marrow analysis, cytogenetics) and disease states (e.g., International Prognostic Scoring System (IPSS) scores, see Chapter 1).[10] Symptoms refer to the *patient's* perception of an abnormal physical, emotional, or cognitive state. In this context, symptoms such as fatigue are often what cause an individual to seek health care. However, the relationships between biological factors and symptoms can be inconsistent. This is often true with hematologic disorders, where a discrepancy between severity of symptoms and severity of illness is common.

Functional status is defined as an assessment of the individual's ability to perform certain defined tasks.[2] At a minimum, there are four domains of function represented here: physical, social, role, and psychological. While symptom status is an important determinant of functioning, it is not the only one. The individual's personality, motivation, and information-processing style can also have a huge impact. For instance, while some individuals with MDS may become obsessed with close monitoring of their blood count results, others may minimize symptoms (such as those related to infection until the infection has progressed to an advanced state). Functional status is also strongly impacted by one's social and economic support systems. Individuals who have extremely limited resources often suffer a greater detriment to their overall level of functioning than those who have more resources available for assistance.

General health perceptions represent an integration of all of the previous health concepts identified in this model. While subjective, it can be the best predictor of the use of health services and even is a strong predictor of mortality.[2] One's own values, as well as social and psychological supports, may have an impact here. If patients do not feel well, they may repeatedly seek intervention, perhaps in the form of expert opinion, or may perhaps be non-compliant with treatment because they do not perceive it as beneficial. In contrast, if patients continue to feel well, they may remain highly functional and their life span may exceed physicians' predictions.

In this model, overall QOL is an assessment of subjective well-being and satisfaction with life. As with general health perceptions, QOL can be impacted by one's social and psychological supports, as well as one's own values. Patient preferences are important factors in influencing individuals' perception of their health and of their QOL. This model is depicted to be linear, with increasing complexity as one moves from the biological variables component to general health perceptions. In actuality, all of its concepts can be impacted by each other, and all have a role in QOL. Guyatt *et al.* argue that each concept within the model can and should be carefully measured.[11]

An important concept related to QOL is that of response shift. Response shift can be defined as: "a change in the meaning of one's self-evaluation of QOL as a result of changes in internal standards, values and the conceptualization of QOL."[12] Response shift can be a significant factor in either a "ceiling effect" (where QOL ratings are higher than anticipated) or a "floor effect" (where QOL ratings are lower than anticipated).

Because QOL is dynamic and subjective, people may change their expectations and hopes as situations change, including those related to health. This, in turn, can impact an individual's rating of QOL. For instance, one's rating of QOL may remain high, despite a rather significant decline in that individual's ability to function. This is particularly true in the setting of a life-threatening illness, or near the end of life, when family and spiritual issues may take precedence over employment and physical functioning.

Clinically, the impact of response shift can be seen within the Wilson & Cleary model depicted in Figure 10.3. Here, dimensions of HRQOL can change in relation to one another. Symptoms, general health perceptions, and overall quality of life are the components most likely to be impacted by response shifts, simply because they are subjective rather than objective, and often broader in scope. In contrast, concepts that are objective, more specific, and discrete are less likely to reflect a response shift.[13] For example, in the MDS patient, objective biological and physiological variables (such as cytogenetic abnormalities and cytopenias) would not likely be impacted by response shift. Yet the resultant fatigue could certainly be so impacted (where patients rate their fatigue higher or lower than would be anticipated based on the extent of anemia). Similarly, over time, patients may become accustomed to the chronic fatigue and modify their lifestyle accordingly. In so doing, the individuals may no longer rate their general health as negatively as prior to making such modifications. Alternatively, individuals may give little importance to the fatigue experienced or may attribute it to normal aging processes. When diagnosed with MDS, the meaning of the fatigue changes, and subsequently, the perception of general health. While the concept of response shift has important clinical implications, it also has important implications for measurement and interpretation of results.

Importance of HRQOL assessment

Why is assessing health-related QOL important? In the setting of chronic illness, such as MDS, curative interventions (with the possible exception of hematopoietic stem cell transplant) are non-existent. Therefore, interventions need to be chosen that either have a positive impact on HRQOL, or provide minimal negative impact. However, for this selection to be successful, patient participation in the decision-making is crucial. Indeed, "increased patient participation in care may well be a critical element of successful chronic illness care."[14] Routine HRQOL assessments can be extremely useful in enhancing communication between patient and physician. Moreover, the information obtained can provide the physician with an increased awareness of patients' perceptions related to their symptoms, functional status, and general health, areas that may not otherwise arise during the brief patient interview. Interventions can then be better targeted at meeting patients' health and functional needs, as opposed to those only related to illness. Thus care truly becomes *patient*-centered, rather than disease-centered.

In the context of clinical trials, HRQOL measurements provide clinicians with very useful data about treatment alternatives beyond the typically reported response rates and grade III–IV toxicity data. These measurements also help patients and clinicians assess the extent to which a treatment designed to control disease is appropriate for that patient given the symptoms or side-effects associated with that therapy. This assessment is also useful when choosing between treatment options. In fact, the American Society of Clinical Oncology purports that, even if an improvement in survival is not possible, a treatment should still be recommended if it improves QOL.[15]

When should HRQOL be measured? Unless a clinician wishes to use the information for targeting interventions as delineated above, HRQOL measurements need not be used in all clinical situations. However, there are certain situations when such measurements are particularly useful and appropriate.[11] For example, a treatment modality can improve how a patient feels when there is no correlating biological measure available. A classic example of this situation is the use of drugs to treat depression where measuring mood is critical for assessing efficacy of therapy. Another illustration is using a biologic surrogate for QOL such as bone-density measurements as a substitute for hip fracture in the setting of bisphosphonate therapy, or granulocyte colony-stimulating factors (G-CSFs) in the setting of neutropenia. A more obvious example of the need to include HRQOL measurement is the situation where a decrease in mortality (or prolongation of survival) comes at the cost of high morbidity. The classic illustration of this situation is the use of high-dose chemotherapy or transplant, such as might be used in patients with high-risk MDS.

Another important situation where HRQOL measurements are important is simply when little is known about the impact of illness on sense of well-being. This situation is true for MDS, a highly complex illness with varied illness trajectory, where HRQOL research has only recently begun. Having actual data will prevent the too-frequent problem of incorrect assumptions about what QOL issues are important to patients and embarking on interventions that are in conflict with patients' real needs and desires.

Methods of HRQOL measurement

A variety of methods are used in measuring HRQOL. Measurements can be a simple, global single assessment such as a Linear Analog Self Assessment where patients rate their QOL on a 100-mm line or using a 0–10 numeric scale, with extreme anchors (e.g., best/worst possible) on either end of the scale. Given that all respondents will use differing factors to rate their own QOL, such measurements are best used for within-patient rather than between-patient measurement.

More global quantitative HRQOL instruments exist, often that measure various functional impairments (such as the 36-Item Short-Form Survey (SF-36)). Other instruments can be specifically designed to capture the more salient domains of HRQOL in a specific disease state, such as cancer or multiple sclerosis. Disease or treatment modality-specific instruments contain items designed to capture areas of specific patient concerns or of specific problems or toxicity. In larger institutions, technology (e.g., touch-screen computers or scanned scoring systems) has afforded clinicians the ability to receive (and hopefully use) data obtained from patients within the clinic setting in real time. A distinct disadvantage to quantitative methods in the research setting is that a large sample is often required, particularly when comparisons are made between groups of patients, or when the effect of a therapeutic modality on QOL is being assessed. Examples of quantitative HRQOL instruments can be found in Table 10.1.

Qualitative methods are another approach to HRQOL measurement. Here, subjects are often asked open-ended questions related to their views about QOL and how their health (or lack thereof) impacts their QOL. Qualitative

Table 10.1 Quantitative health-related quality-of-life (QOL) instruments potentially useful in the myelodysplastic syndrome patient population

Instrument	Format	Domains	Time frame
SF-36[63]	36 items Likert scale[a]	Physical and social functioning; role limitations (physical and emotional); mental health, vitality, pain, general health perceptions	Present, past 4 weeks, previous year
EORTC QLQ C-30[67]	30 items total Likert scale[a] yes/no	Global QOL; five functional domains: physical, social, emotional, role, overall perceived health status Symptoms: pain, nausea, vomiting, dyspnea, fatigue, diarrhea, constipation, sleep disturbance, cognitive disturbance	Past week
FACIT-G (FACT–General)[5]	27 items 5-point Likert scale[a]	Physical, functional, social, emotional well-being; total QOL	Past week
FACIT–Spiritual[62]	12 items 5-point Likert scale[a]	Spiritual well-being	Past week
Thomas Uncertainty Scale[60]	14 items 5-point Likert scale[a]	Impact of uncertainty on QOL	Past 2 weeks
Profile of Mood States (POMS)[74]	65 items; 5-point Likert scale[a]	Mood state: vigor–activity, fatigue–inertia, confusion–bewilderment, tension–anxiety, anger–hostility, depression–dejection; total mood disturbance	Past week
Mental Health Inventory (MHI)[73]	38 items	Five subscales: anxiety, depression, emotional ties, positive affect, loss of behavioral and emotional control Total score (MHI index) Psychological distress subscale Psychological well-being subscale	

[a] Likert scale: a unidimensional scaling method where subjects rate the extent to which they agree or disagree with a particular statement; each degree of agreement is assigned a numerical value.

SF-36, 36-Item Short Form Health Survey; EORTC QLQ C-30, European Organization for Research and Treatment of Cancer Quality of Life Cancer; FACIT-G, Functional Assessment of Chronic Illness Therapy–General; FACT, Functional Assessment of Cancer Therapy.

measurements provide extremely rich data. The disadvantage to their use is the time involved in interviewing subjects, the labor involved in data analysis, and the need to adhere to rigorous analytic methods so as to ensure the results are deemed reliable and valid.

Other methods of measuring HRQOL include utility assessments, which are based on the premise that patients can provide a preference for a state of health even under periods of uncertainty.[16] A detailed description of these methods (e.g., quality-adjusted life-years or QALYs, time trade-off, and standard gamble) is beyond the scope of this paper and the reader is referred elsewhere for descriptions of these methods as well as their usefulness and limitations.[16–21]

Problems with HRQOL data in clinical trials

With many clinical trials, HRQOL measurement is included, but it is not as carefully incorporated into the study design as need be. Consequently, the data obtained may not be as valid, or as clinically useful in answering the questions delineated in the specific aims of the study. For example, the primary study endpoint is typically the impact of a particular therapeutic intervention on response rates, not HRQOL. As such, the study is powered for changes in response rates, not changes in HRQOL, which requires a much smaller sample size. Thus, changes seen in HRQOL may not be statistically significant simply because the sample size is inadequate.

Equally important is the issue of missing data. Sometimes, the cause of missing data is simply the result of a lack of interest on the part of the investigators to ensure the QOL instruments are provided to the subjects in a timely manner. However, a more important issue arises when the subject becomes ill, develops complications from treatment, drops out, or is withdrawn from the study ("treatment failures"). It is in these very situations that it is crucial to capture the QOL data if the impact of therapy on a person's sense of health and well-being is to be truly known; it is in these very situations that QOL data are typically not obtained, or delayed until the subject has recovered. In these situations, the negative impact is not adequately captured vis-à-vis the QOL measurements, thus threatening the validity of the study's findings. Statistical methods now exist to address this important issue partially.[22] (The reader is referred to *Statistics in Medicine*, 1998, **17** (no. 5–7), for detailed information on statistical methods that can be utilized when confronted with missing data in QOL studies.)

Research has documented that symptoms and side-effects are important factors in a patient's HRQOL.[6–7,23–24] Yet typically, there is no specific attention called to side-effect measurement beyond the common toxicity criteria (CTC) or World Health Organization (WHO) toxicity ratings. Measuring pulmonary or cardiac function via cardiac catheterization, echo, or pulmonary function tests does not provide useful information for the patient if dyspnea is also not measured. Similarly, measuring anemia, without concurrently measuring fatigue, is not useful for the patient.

The National Comprehensive Cancer Network MDS Practice Guidelines define supportive care as containing six components: (1) observation (clinical monitoring, psychosocial support, and QOL assessment); (2) transfusions (red cells for "symptomatic" anemia, platelet transfusions for "thrombocytopenic bleeding"); (3) antibiotics for bacterial infection; (4) antifibrinolytic agents for refractory bleeding; (5) iron chelation when transfusions have exceeded 20–30 units of red cells; and (6) cytokine use.[25] Unfortunately, QOL is merely identified as a component of observation without any further delineation.

Within the context of clinical trials, interventions for side-effect management are frequently at "physician discretion." In these situations, particularly when there are multiple investigators involved, much variability exists in interpreting when to intervene, selecting what interventions to use, and in deciding how aggressively such interventions should be implemented. With such variability, the validity of measuring the impact of these interventions on HRQOL becomes suspect. "Physician discretion" is also often used when "supportive care" is a treatment arm, as is often the case in clinical trials for MDS. Here, supportive care is often not strictly defined, but simply the use of transfusions or antimicrobial support as needed. Without specific parameters delineated within the study design (e.g., parameters of when to transfuse and how much to transfuse), the validity of findings within a supportive care arm is threatened.

When including HRQOL in a clinical trial, several issues should be addressed during the development of the study design. Foremost is the careful consideration of the precise question to be addressed as well as the selection of the best method for addressing the question. For example, the investigator

Table 10.2 Reliability of common health measurements

High reliability	Moderate reliability	Low reliability
Survival	Tumor size as measured by imaging studies (CT or MRI)	Spleen size (by physical exam)
Hemoglobin level	FACIT-G scale scores	Tumor measurement over time (inter-observer)
FACIT fatigue scores		Time to progression
Bacterial evidence of septicemia (blood cultures positive for bacteria)		Fungal evidence of septicemia (positive blood cultures)

Modified from Cella et al.[26]
CT, computed tomography; MRI, magnetic resonance imaging; FACIT-G, Functional Assessment of Chronic Illness Therapy–General.

needs to decide if a generic HRQOL questionnaire is adequate to answer the specific question within the study. Often, other components are also needed, such as a comprehensive assessment of fatigue, pain, or psychological distress. Frequently, a quantitative measure of functional status is included and may be a highly relevant study endpoint. However, it is imperative to delineate precisely which areas of functioning are relevant (e.g., cognitive functioning, role function, physical stamina). Furthermore, careful attention should focus on precisely how the symptoms of illness and treatment will be measured.

In clinical trial design, another important factor to consider is the validity and reliability of each measurement used. Typically consideration is given to the psychometric properties of questionnaires – an important consideration. But often, the validity and reliability of other measures commonly used in the clinical trial are not carefully considered. In fact, many commonly used (and important) measurements actually have low reliability.[26] This concept is illustrated in Table 10.2. When analyzing data within patients (e.g., pre- and posttreatment change scores) higher reliability ratings are required than when analyzing data between patients. An alpha coefficient of 0.8 is considered to be a standard level of acceptability for between-group measurements; 0.9 is required for within-group measurements.[26]

Perhaps the most difficult aspect of HRQOL data lies within their interpretation. While the concept of statistically significant differences in HRQOL measurement is easily understood, it can be difficult to interpret that difference as being clinically significant. Clinical significance provides both patient and clinician with a means of evaluating the outcome of therapeutic intervention beyond assuring the difference is not merely caused by chance (i.e., *P*-values) but rather, if the difference has implications for patient care.[27] A variety of methods exist to address this issue and the reader is referred to some excellent reviews on the subject.[28,29] HRQOL data should be portrayed in ways to facilitate interpretation of clinical relevance. Examples of such portrayal include providing percentages of patients who experienced improvements or deterioration in their functioning and the length of time needed to experience what is considered to be a minimally important change in that functioning.

Specific HRQOL issues relevant in the MDS patient population

As a disease state, MDS poses unique problems for those who live with it. Due to the heterogeneity of the disease, the illness trajectory is quite varied and is often confounded by a myriad of other factors, such as comorbid conditions, functional status, and physiological age.[30,31] A brief description of some of the more salient issues will be briefly described.

Fatigue

As is true in the cancer patient population, fatigue is considered to be an important QOL issue in individuals with MDS.[30] There are significant differences in the meaning of fatigue among differing cultures. Glaus[32] notes that, in many countries, laypersons would not understand the term "fatigue" as there is no corresponding word for it in their language. Different cultures have different views as to the cause of fatigue, how it should be managed, and even the willingness of people to report they are experiencing fatigue.

Fatigue is highly complex and multidimensional and therefore, more appropriate to be conceptualized as a syndrome, rather than a symptom.[33] From both a research and clinical perspective, a clear definition of this concept is important. Fatigue is multifactorial and encompasses feelings of lethargy, decreased mental alertness, physical weakness, and diminished concentration.[34] Ream & Richardson[35] define fatigue as subjective and unpleasant, incorporating total body feelings that range from tiredness to exhaustion. However, in the context of malignancy (and other chronic illnesses), fatigue becomes unrelenting and interferes with the individual's ability to function to normal capacity. Glaus[36] defines this type of fatigue as a "multidimensional experience that focuses on biochemical and pathophysiological causes, but also on psychological and behavioral aspects." It is important to note that anemia is absent from any of these definitions of fatigue, yet it is frequently and inappropriately used as a surrogate marker of fatigue.

Clinicians often minimize the severity of fatigue and its impact. An interesting hypothesis for this concerns the role of epinephrine (adrenaline) in the context of a clinic visit. During their interaction with clinicians, patients naturally experience an increased level of excitement with a resultant increased release of epinephrine. As a result, patients may not appear fatigued, nor necessarily voice complaints of fatigue during the clinic visit, but become significantly fatigued afterward. Winningham[37] refers to this as the "white coat syndrome." In other situations, patients try valiantly to describe the impact of the fatigue they are experiencing, but feel their complaints are minimized by their clinicians.[38,39]

Many instruments exist to measure the concept of fatigue, and examples are depicted in Table 10.3. Choice of instrumentation should be based on the specific domains of fatigue of interest (either clinical or research) as well as the instrument's psychometric properties. In the absence of using such instruments, a clinical assessment should be comprehensive, incorporating the many dimensions of fatigue and its complex impact on one's quality of life. Several such clinical assessment guides are available.[28,40,41]

Transfusion support

Transfusion support remains the primary therapeutic intervention used in MDS. Yet the impact of transfusion has not been well studied. In Thomas' qualitative study, patients demonstrated concern about the safety related to transfusions.[24] Others voiced concern about iron overload. But more frequently, patients complained that transfusions interfered with their ability to live their lives. This interference was either due to the complicated logistics involved in simply receiving the transfusion, or to the gradual decline in physical health and functional ability until the hemoglobin dropped to a sufficient level that would warrant transfusion.

Studies rarely use patient symptoms as an outcome variable when studying the impact of transfusions. Gleeson & Spencer[42] studied symptoms in 91 cancer patients who had a chronic transfusion requirement and found

Table 10.3 Examples of quantitative instruments to measure the concept of fatigue

Instrument	Format	Domains	Time frame
FACIT–Fatigue[61]	13 items 5-point Likert scale[a]	Impact of fatigue on QOL	Past week
Schwartz Cancer Fatigue Scale[75]	28 items 7-point Likert scale[a]	Physical, emotional, cognitive, temporal dimensions	Past 2 weeks
Fatigue Symptom Inventory[76]	13 items 11-point Likert scale[a]	Intensity, duration, interference with function	Past week
Multidimensional Fatigue Inventory[65]	20 items	General, physical, and mental fatigue Reduced motivation Reduced activity	Previous days
Multidimensional Fatigue Symptom Inventory SF[77]	30 items 5-point Likert scale[a]	General, physical, emotional, mental, vigor	Past week
Revised Piper Fatigue Scale[78]	22 items 0–10 scale	Behavioral/severity; affective; sensory; cognitive/mood	Present
Brief Fatigue Inventory[79]	9 items 0–10 scale	Intensity; interference with function	Past 24 h

[a] Likert scale: a unidimensional scaling method where subjects rate the extent to which they agree or disagree with a particular statement; each degree of agreement is assigned a numerical value.
FACIT, Functional Assessment of Chronic Illness Therapy; QOL, quality of life; SF, short form.

that weakness, dyspnea, and well-being improved after transfusion; these improvements persisted for only 2 weeks. Jansen and colleagues[43] assert that the decision to transfuse a patient with MDS should include HRQOL data, and not be based solely on hemoglobin levels.

For some patients, the need for transfusion support can be diminished by the administration of growth factors. Many studies have demonstrated that growth factors, particularly erythropoietin (EPO), can have a positive impact on HRQOL.[44–48] Studies using EPO in MDS patient populations will be presented in a subsequent section.

Infection

Surprisingly little is known about the impact of repeated infections on the QOL of those with chronic illness, such as MDS. Even relatively minor infection, such as that seen with influenza, can be associated with prolonged periods of fatigue, including after the infection has clinically resolved.[49] Since many with MDS are elderly, they may have diminished "physiologic reserve," which can result in a more prolonged period of recovery.[50] In the setting of chronic neutropenia, studies have documented an improvement in QOL with the use of G-CSFs,[51,52] but these data have not been replicated in the MDS patient population. Thus the impact of this therapy on HRQOL in the MDS population remains unknown.

Uncertainty

People living with MDS often have difficulty coping with uncertainty. Mishel defines this concept as "the inability of determine the meaning of illness-related events."[53] She posits that uncertainty develops when individuals cannot reach a subjective but meaningful interpretation of illness and its treatment. In the MDS illness trajectory, initial uncertainty can result from the apparent disparity between having a life-threatening illness, yet having only mild, if any, symptoms relating to it. Inadequate understanding of the disease process, being unable to anticipate its likely trajectory and resultant problems, and difficulty deciding what – if any – treatment can, or should be employed, can all result in periods of heightened uncertainty.[31] Moreover, knowing that the disease can evolve into acute myeloid leukemia, which is typically refractory to conventional treatment, can greatly increase one's emotional distress.

Communication and trust in clinicians

Because MDS is such a heterogeneous and complex disease, many clinicians may not have adequate expertise in the management of the illness. From a patient's perspective, the ambiguity of the illness can be highly distressing.

The need for information can be profound, and relates not only to the disease process and treatment options, but most importantly, to how the illness and treatment will impact patients' ability to live their lives in the way they are accustomed.[31] The type and amount of information desired may vary throughout the illness trajectory, based in part on what the patient can emotionally process. Unfortunately, the information provided by clinicians is often not the information desired by the patient. For example, patients with complex symptoms such as fatigue may seek validation of their own explanation for their symptoms,[53] but instead receive information about physiologic processes within the marrow as the etiology for their anemia. In contrast, other patients may desire considerably more information about the pathophysiology of MDS and all available treatment options, but have difficulty obtaining such detailed information from their health care providers. Clinicians have their own concept of the type and amount of information that it is appropriate for patients to have and when it should be given[54]; this may conflict with the patient's informational and emotional needs. Moreover, the ease with which professionals present such information can be highly variable. The result of such incongruence is increased anxiety, frustration, and uncertainty for the patient.[31]

Quality of death

For the vast majority, MDS is not a curable illness; people who have it will often die from it or from its resulting complications. Despite its importance, QOL at the end of life as well as during the dying process remains an area needing research and understanding. Adequate understanding is lacking – not only on the part of the patient and family, but too often on the part of the clinicians caring for that patient and family. A review of this issue is beyond the scope of this paper and the reader is referred to some excellent references, including the Institute of Medicine's report on improving care at the end of life.[55–59]

HRQOL in MDS: research to date

In the MDS patient population, QOL research remains in its infancy. Few studies have explored the QOL among those who have MDS. While HRQOL has been an outcome variable in a few studies, the validity and clinical relevance of the findings may be limited. Nonetheless, the data obtained from these studies provide some important insight into QOL in the MDS patient population and salient studies will be briefly reviewed.

Descriptive studies

Thomas *et al.*[60] have conducted some preliminary descriptive studies of QOL in patients with MDS. The first study explored HRQOL in a sample of 97 Americans beginning a clinical trial using the drug amifostine.[60] In this descriptive study, the Functional Assessment of Cancer Therapy – General (FACT-G, now known as the Functional Assessment of Chronic Illness Therapy – General (FACIT-G)) was used.[5] The FACT-G is designed to measure four distinct QOL domains: physical, functional, social, and emotional well-being. Two additional subscales were added that measure fatigue and spiritual well-being; they use the same format as the FACT.[61,62] For each subscale, higher scores reflect higher levels of well-being. An Uncertainty Scale was developed by Thomas to measure this concept and uses the same format as the FACT, although higher scores reflect greater uncertainty, whereas higher FACT scores reflect higher levels of well-being.[60]

Subjects were predominantly male (two-thirds), elderly (mean age 69 ± 12 years) and had a variety of MDS subtypes (49% refractory anemia with excess blasts (RAEB)). Despite high Karnofsky Performance Status (KPS) ratings (mean = 87, SD 9) patients indicated major elements of fatigue. Fatigue scores correlated strongly with physical and functional domain scores ($r = 0.77$ and 0.70, $P < 0.001$), but only marginally with KPS ($r = 0.31$, $P < 0.001$) and not at all with hemoglobin levels ($r = 0.02$, NS). The specific data obtained from items within the fatigue domain provided a more detailed description of how fatigue impacted the QOL in these patients than that obtained from the other subscales or with the KPS. The Uncertainty Scale scores showed modest correlations with all other domains (except social well-being) and with fatigue ($r = 0.5–0.63$, $P < 0.001$). Patients indicated they were uncertain about the future and worried their illness would worsen. Of a possible score of 28, patients had fairly high physical and social well-being scores (mean $21.3 ± 5.7$; $22.9 ± 4.9$) but not functional well-being scores ($17.1 ± 6.2$; Fig. 10.4).

There were no significant differences in QOL or subscale scores when data were sorted by MDS subtype, length of time since diagnosis, enrollment hemoglobin, neutrophil, or platelet levels. QOL was significantly correlated with fatigue ($r = 0.59$), uncertainty ($r = -0.53$), and spiritual well-being ($r = 0.42$) but much less so with KPS ($r = 0.26$), suggesting that the KPS is an inadequate surrogate marker for QOL.

Thomas further explored HRQOL in the MDS patient population using both quantitative and qualitative approaches.[24] In this pilot study, 13 patients with MDS who were not enrolled in a clinical trial participated. The same quantitative instruments were used as in the previous study; however, a qualitative instrument was also used to validate the findings from the quantitative

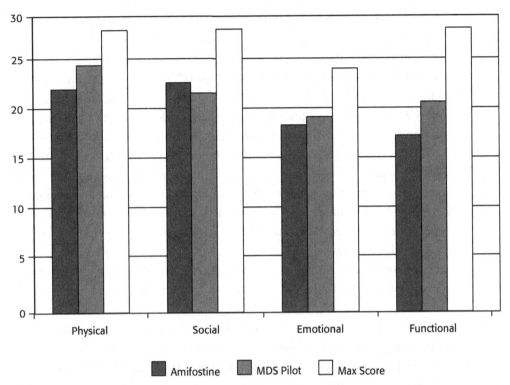

Fig. 10.4   Comparison of Functional Assessment of Cancer Therapy (FACT) subscale scores in two samples of patients with myelodysplastic syndrome (MDS). Max score, maximum possible score for specific subscale. Higher score indicates higher well-being. Difference in physical well-being was significant between the two samples ($P = 0.025$); all other differences were non-significant.[24,60]

measurements.[23] Age was similar to the other sample (mean age 70 years) but more subjects (83%) were male. The average length of time since diagnosis was 18.3 ± 23.5 months. Results from the quantitative instruments were similar here when compared with that from the previous sample; only the physical well-being subscale was significantly different, with lower physical well-being scores obtained from the amifostine study sample (Fig. 10.4).

Fatigue was a significant problem for these people with MDS. Data from the qualitative interviews were rich in providing more detail as to how fatigue impacted these individual's lives. One subject poignantly reported: "I can feel mentally energetic. But the moment I push ahead of doing activity, which is even moderately strenuous, I'm surprised of the adverse reaction which my body feels – for no reason. It would be something like a laborer who had been carrying a very heavy weight. But in my case, I don't need the weight, I just need to get up and start moving and I feel spent."

Another area of concern for those with MDS was uncertainty. Sixty-nine percent of the sample stated they were "quite" or "very much" unsure what the future holds for them. Data from the interviews substantiated several of the individual items from the uncertainty scale. It became apparent that a significant amount of uncertainty centered on an uncertain future – and that may certainly reflect the variable prognosis (ranging from 2 months to several years). Patients' uncertain illness trajectory certainly interfered with their ability to plan – from something as minor as being strong enough to attend a sporting event, to being strong enough to continue working full-time. The need for future treatment was also of concern. One subject reported, "You have only a 30% chance of disease-free survival and that's pretty bad odds." Another said: "It's just the future . . . the unknown – is kind of scary. That's the difficult part; the scary part is not knowing where this will go from here."

Obviously, the sample from this pilot study was very small, limiting the ability to generalize these findings. Nonetheless, the data obtained from the qualitative component of the study provided important insights as to how MDS impacted the lives of these individuals and can serve as a basis for additional research.

Clinical Trials

Jansen and colleagues[43] validated the findings in the initial study by Thomas and colleagues.[60] Here, HRQOL was measured in 50 patients with MDS and its relationship with hemoglobin levels assessed using different instruments. The SF-36[63] is a self-administered generic measurement of various types of functioning and is frequently considered to be a measurement of QOL rather than of health or functional status. Eight scales are measured: (1) mental health; (2) bodily pain; (3) general health perceptions; (4) vitality; and (5) physical, (6) role, (7) emotional, and (8) social functioning. A physical sum score is derived from the physical and role functioning, bodily pain, and general health perceptions scales; a mental sum score is derived from the mental health, vitality, emotional, and social functioning scales. Higher scores indicate a more favorable health state.

The EuroQOL Visual Analog Scale (VAS) depicts a global evaluation on one's "own health today", using a 0–100 visual analog rating scale, where

0 corresponds to worst health and 100 to best health. This single item is taken from the more comprehensive EuroQOL instrument.[64] The Multidimensional Fatigue Inventory (MFI) was designed to measure cancer-related fatigue as well as non-cancer-related fatigue.[65] This questionnaire is designed to measure five dimensions related to fatigue: (1) general, (2) physical, and (3) mental fatigue; (4) reduced motivation; and (5) reduced activity. Higher scores reflect greater fatigue.

Patients completed the three instruments within one day of a clinic visit, at which time the patients' hemoglobin level was measured. Transfusions were not performed within this one-day time period. The findings from this study demonstrated a lower median score of the VAS and SF-36 in the MDS patient population than that of the Dutch population matched for age and gender. This was particularly evident in the following subscales: physical functioning, role functioning, physical sum score, VAS score, and a worse physical fatigue score. There were no significant differences in scores based on MDS type.

Unfortunately, correlations between HRQOL subscale and fatigue scale scores were not provided, but the subscale scores were correlated with hemoglobin levels, often at a statistically significant level ($P < 0.05$). However, these correlations were quite small, thereby reducing the clinical relevance of the association (Table 10.4). The authors conclude that hemoglobin levels can only partially explain HRQOL. While the practice of transfusion is typically based on hemoglobin levels, the authors suggest that findings related to HRQOL should also be included in the decision-making process.

QOL was measured in 36 Scandinavians with MDS[66] using the European Organization for Research and Treatment of Cancer Quality of Life Cancer (EORTC QLQ-C30) instrument.[67] This HRQOL study was conducted within the context of a clinical trial evaluating the efficacy of EPO and G-CSF in 53 patients; HRQOL was measured prior to beginning therapy with EPO and G-CSF and again 12 weeks later. The EORTC QLQ C-30 is designed to measure the following QOL domains: physical, social, role, emotional, and cognitive functioning; it also measures global health and QOL, financial impact, and eight symptoms: (1) nausea/vomiting; (2) pain; (3) fatigue; (4) sleep disturbance; (5) diminished appetite; (6) diarrhea; (7) constipation; and (8) dyspnea. Findings confirm comparable scores when compared to that from the FACT-G (data conversions are required.) Higher scores reflect higher levels of functioning; higher symptom scores reflect higher levels of symptoms.

Table 10.4 Correlations of select health-related quality-of-life variables with hemoglobin (Hb) levels

Instrument	Subscale	Correlation with Hb level	Significance (P)
SF-36	General health	0.15	0.29
	Physical functioning	0.50	0.00
	Role physical	0.35	0.02
	Vitality	0.33	0.02
	Physical sum score	0.35	0.01
VAS		0.29	0.05
MFI	General fatigue	−0.11	0.46
	Physical fatigue	−0.31	0.03
	Mental fatigue	−0.26	0.07
	Reduced activity	−0.34	0.02
	Reduced motivation	−0.27	0.06

Note that, despite high statistical significance, the actual correlations are quite small.
Data from Jansen et al.[43]
SF-36, 36-Item Short-Form Health Survey; VAS, Visual Analog Scale; MFI, Multidimensional Fatigue Inventory.

With the exception of cognitive function, the patients in this sample had significantly lower subscale scores than those seen in gender- and age-matched controls; they also indicated having more fatigue and dyspnea. Virtually all of the subjects who did not respond to therapy did complete the QOL measurements (20 of the 21 non-responders); thus the data reflect the QOL of those individuals who did not benefit from treatment, an important consideration. Patients who responded to therapy indicated higher global QOL ($P < 0.01$) and lower fatigue scores ($P < 0.05$). Given the small number of patients who responded to treatment and provided QOL data ($n = 12$), confirmatory study is warranted.

The effects of EPO and G-CSF in MDS on HRQOL were further studied in a randomized controlled clinical trial.[68] Sixty patients were randomly assigned to receive either EPO and G-CSF or supportive care. Patients assigned to the EPO arm received it and G-CSF for 12 weeks; those who achieved a response (defined as a hemoglobin level of 11.5 g/dl or higher) were then maintained on EPO alone for an additional 40 weeks. Patients randomized to the supportive-care arm received transfusion support aimed at maintaining a hemoglobin level above 8 g/dl. HRQOL was measured with the FACT–Anemia question-naire; it consists of the FACT-G plus 20 additional questions related to fatigue (the fatigue subscale) and seven additional items not related to fatigue.[61,69] Minimal clinically important differences in QOL were used for the QOL anal-ysis; these differences can be considered the "threshold" a patient or clinician would use to determine when to seek or initiate intervention. Direct costs for treatment in both arms were calculated. (Minimally clinically impor-tant differences are a highly complex topic and beyond the scope of this chapter. One definition for this concept is the minimal difference in a specific domain of interest that a patient would perceive as beneficial and that would prompt a change in patient management (barring excessive side-effects and cost).[70] An excellent review of this topic is found in a paper by Sprangers and colleagues.[22])

The data suggest a minimal clinical improvement in FACT–Anemia scores in the treatment arm by week 28 but a return to baseline levels by week 52. Scores from those assigned to the supportive-care arm remained stable through week 28, and then decreased by week 52. There was no increase in transfusion-dependence in those randomized to the supportive-care arm throughout the 52-week study period. Unfortunately, there was a high attri-tion rate in this study, and the amount of missing QOL data was excessive (50–66%); thus it is difficult to interpret these results. Costs were found to be considerably higher in the treatment arm.

The effect of EPO on QOL and brain function was studied in 11 patients with low-risk MDS.[71] QOL was measured by the FACT–Anemia questionnaire. A neurophysiological evaluation (duplex scanning of neck vessels, quantitative electroencephalography, and comprehensive neuropsy-chological evaluation) was performed at baseline and on 8 subjects 24 weeks later. Patients who achieved a response to EPO treatment demonstrated a clinically significant improvement in FACT–Anemia scores. Three of these patients also demonstrated neurophysiological changes; 2 were noted to have abnormalities of brain function in their baseline examination. This study is important in examining neurophysiological function in MDS patients and should be replicated with a larger sample.

The impact of azacitidine or supportive care on the HRQOL of 191 patients with MDS was studied in a Cancer and Leukemia Group B phase III randomized clinical trial.[72] Supportive care was very loosely defined in this study and included transfusions, use of antibiotics, and hospitalizations; moreover, these same interventions were permitted for those randomized to the azacitidine arm. The study design permitted those in the supportive arm to cross over to the azacitidine arm if the MDS progressed. The study hypotheses were that a response to azacitidine would result in improved QOL and less fatigue, which would result in improved social and physical functioning as well as in less psychological distress. Rationale for selecting these specific relationships for evaluation was not provided.

HRQOL was measured by the EORTC QLQ C-30 (previously described above), the Mental Health Inventory (MHI), and a visual analog scale rating disease improvement. The MHI is designed to measure psychological state and contains five subscales: (1) anxiety; (2) depression; (3) emotional ties; (4) positive affect; and (5) loss of emotional and behavioral control.[73] A total score (MHI Index) and two global subscale scores (psychological well-being and psychological distress) are derived from the five subscales. Patients assigned to the azacitidine arm were also asked at each data collection point to rate their assessment as to the extent their condition was improving on a 0–10 visual analog scale (0=not at all, 10=complete improvement); this scale was not used by those still in the supportive-care arm.

QOL assessments were scheduled at four time points during the study; the timing of the assessments was correlated with cycles of azacitidine treatment (prior to randomization, after two cycles of treatment, after completing four cycles of treatment, and 6 months after study initiation). However, in reality, the timing of each assessment varied widely (40–100 days). For those patients assigned to the supportive care arm and then crossed over into the azacitidine arm, QOL assessments began anew from that time point.

In terms of demographic characteristics, the sample was quite evenly distributed between the two groups. However, for unclear reasons, the rate of transformation to AML was considerably higher in the supportive-care arm, raising concern about a possible difference in disease states between groups. Eighty percent of the patients randomized to supportive care were still receiving that care at the time of the second assessment, but only 13% ($n = 12$)

at the time of the fourth assessment. In contrast, 56% of those assigned to azacitidine still received the drug at the time of the fourth assessment, but by this time 22% had dropped from the study, and 16% had died. To control for the high attrition rate, the investigators utilized a pattern mixture model of analysis, which addresses the variation in number of QOL assessments over time.

When compared to those remaining in the supportive-care arm, the patients randomized to receive azacitidine demonstrated a statistically significant improvement in fatigue and in physical function. Further analyses demonstrated an improvement in dyspnea, psychological distress, and positive affect. However, there were no significant relationships identified between response to azacitidine treatment and any of the QOL variables used in this study. As would be anticipated, those subjects who dropped from the study had lower HRQOL scores and higher symptom and distress ratings in the measurement obtained prior to dropping. Furthermore, no QOL assessments were obtained at the time of disease progression, when complications (e.g., hospitalization) occurred. Thus the data obtained may reflect a "ceiling effect" and the potential negative impact of HRQOL in those assigned to the azacitidine arm is unknown.

For those patients who completed all four assessments in the supportive-care arm, all QOL scores remained relatively stable over time, with the exception of a slight decline in physical functioning. These findings may reflect that those patients whose disease remained relatively stable remained in the supportive-care arm; those whose disease progressed may have dropped from the study or were crossed over to the treatment arm. In contrast, those patients assigned to the azacitidine arm demonstrated an improvement in most parameters, but the improvement was typically restricted to those who remained on the study beyond the third assessment.

This is an important study, as it is the first large clinical trial in MDS with an adequate sample size to address relevant HRQOL questions. Yet the methodological and design issues previously identified, as well as the high attrition rate, force the reader to interpret the results with caution. See Chapter 7 for an expanded discussion of other clinical components of this trial.

A summary of the five clinical trials described above, along with relevant study limitations, is presented in Table 10.5.

Table 10.5 Summary of five myelodysplastic syndrome clinical trials using health-related quality of life (HRQOL) as an outcome variable. Brief summations of salient findings are depicted as well as some limitations of each study. See text for details of each study

Study	Sample/design	HRQOL measurements	Findings	Study limitations
Impact of hemoglobin on HRQOL[43]	$n = 50$: descriptive	SF-36 EuroQOL VAS MFI	HRQOL < age- and gender-matched controls. Physical functioning correlated with Hb ($r = 0.50$); other correlations between HRQOL variables and Hb were small, including measures of fatigue	Small sample size. No correlations reported between HRQOL parameters and fatigue scores
Impact of EPO and G-CSF Rx on HRQOL[66]	$n = 36$ (HRQOL) $n = 53$ (EPO) Descriptive, longitudinal Baseline and 12 weeks later	EORTC QLQ C-30	HRQOL < age- and gender-matched controls except cognitive function. ↑ fatigue and dyspnea than controls. Those with CR or PR to EPO had higher HRQOL and lower fatigue ratings	Very small sample, especially those whose disease responded to Rx and who completed HRQOL ($n = 12$)
Effects of EPO + G-CSF versus supportive care on HRQOL[68]	$n = 60$ (30 each arm) Randomized, longitudinal Multiple data points	FACT-An Direct costs	Those in supportive care arm: Stable HRQOL × 28 weeks ($n = 18$); slight ↓ by week 52 ($n = 16$). Those in EPO arm: HRQOL ↑ by week 28 ($n = 15$) but returned to baseline by week 52 ($n = 10$). Costs higher in EPO arm	No reference re: minimal clinically important differences in HRQOL determined. Very high attrition rate over time. No attempt to determine indirect costs

			Response to EPO:	Very small sample
Effect of EPO on HRQOL and brain function[71]	n = 11	FACT-An Neurophysiological evaluation	Response to EPO: ↑ HRQOL scores: Response to EPO: neurophysiological changes (n = 3)	Rationale for specific neurophysiological tests not provided. Clinically significant difference used for analysis but not described, nor referenced
Effect of azacitidine + supportive care versus supportive care alone on HRQOL[72]	n = 191 Azacitidine arm: n = 99 Supportive care arm: n = 92 Randomized, cross-over design Multiple data points (baseline, after 2 cycles of azacitidine (day 50) After 4 cycles azacitidine (day 106) 6 months from entry (day 181)	EORTC QLQ-C30 Mental Health Inventory VAS Self-rating of Improvement (azacitidine arm only)	Those in azacitidine arm indicated: ↓ fatigue ↑ physical function No significant difference in HRQOL in those with response to azacitidine versus those without response ↓ HRQOL, ↑ symptoms, ↑ distress ratings seen in both arms prior to patient dropping out from study	High attrition rate; n = 55 for those in azacitidine day 182 n = 12 for those in supportive care arm day 182 Wide variation in timing of HRQOL assessments No HRQOL measurement during time of disease progression, hospitalization, etc. (Data may demonstrate "ceiling effect")

VAS, Visual Analog Scale; MFI, Multidimensional Fatigue Inventory; Hb, hemoglobin; EPO, erythropoietin; G-CSF, granulocyte-colony-stimulating factor; Rx, prescription; EORTC QLQ C-30, European Organization for Research and Treatment of Cancer Quality of Life Cancer; CR, complete response; PR, partial response; FACT-An, Functional Assessment of Clinical Therapy–Anemia.

Summary and future directions

HRQOL remains a crucial component of quality patient care and deserves to be declared an important outcome variable in clinical trials. Study designs need to incorporate such measurements so that the data obtained are not only valid, but also clinically relevant and easily interpretable.

A useful method for such assurance is the incorporation of relevant patient-reported outcomes as part of the clinical trial. While the number of outcomes need not be excessive, considerable care and attention should be used in their selection and measurement. Patient-reported outcomes should include a careful assessment of symptoms (e.g., fatigue) and functional status, as well as HRQOL. In addition, they should include some measurement of the patient's satisfaction with therapy. These outcomes, in combination with conventional toxicity ratings, response rates, and disease-free or overall survival rates, provide a much more comprehensive view of that survivorship. Moreover, they are useful for both clinician and patient when considering using the study treatment for their own use.

A systematic assessment of HRQOL is equally important in clinical practice. While technological advances have afforded the busy clinician with results of HRQOL assessment in real time, such options may not be realistic or feasible for many. However, on an individual level, technology is completely unnecessary when spending a few moments with patients and asking them to articulate their distress and issues that are of concern. Active listening is an important skill that promotes communication, diminishes acting on false assumptions, and provides the patient with a sense that the care received is based on a concerted effort to meet the needs and desires of the patient as opposed to those of the clinician. In so doing, disease-specific care becomes more patient-centered care, and HRQOL is maintained, even improved.

REFERENCES

1. Kurland, G. (2003). Setting the stage: putting our mission into perspective. In *Quality of Life III: Translating the Science of QOL Assessment into Clinical Practice.* Scottsdale, AZ: Mayo School of Continuing Medical Education.
2. Wilson, I. B. and Cleary, P. D. (1995). Linking clinical variables with health-related quality of life: a conceptual model of patient outcomes. *J.A.M.A.*, **273**, 59–65.

3. Cella, D. and Cherin, E. A. (1988). Quality of life during and after cancer treatment. *Comp. Ther.*, **14**, 69–75.

4. Public Health Service National Institutes of Health (1990). *Quality of Life Assessment in Cancer Clinical Trials.* Bethesda, MD: US Department of Health and Human Services.

5. Cella, D. R., Tulsky, D. S., Gray, G. *et al.* (1993). The Functional Assessment of Cancer Therapy Scale; development and validation of the general measure. *J. Clin. Oncol.*, **11**, 570–9.

6. Jacobsen, P. B. and Weitzner, M. A. (1999). Evaluation of palliative endpoints in oncology clinical trials. *Cancer Control*, **6**, 471–7.

7. Ferrell, B. R. (1996). The quality of lives: 1525 voices of cancer. *Oncol. Nursing Forum*, **23**, 909–16.

8. Ferrell, B. R. (1993). To know suffering. *Oncol. Nursing Forum*, **20**, 1471–7.

9. Dow, K. H., Ferrell, B. R., Haberman, M. R., and Eaton, L. (1999). The meaning of quality of life in cancer survivorship. *Oncol. Nursing Forum*, **26**, 519–28.

10. Greenberg, P. L., Cox, C., Le Beau, M. M. *et al.* (1997). International scoring system for evaluating prognosis in myelodysplastic syndromes. *Blood*, **89**, 2079–88.

11. Guyatt, G., Ferrans, C., Halyard, M. *et al.* (2003). Value of HRQOL to clinicians from clinical research and in clinical practice. In *Quality of Life III: Translating the Science of QOL Assessment into Clinical Practice.* Scottsdale, AZ: Mayo School of Continuing Medical Education.

12. Sprangers, M. and Schwartz, C. (2000). Integrating response shift into health-related quality of life research: a theoretical model. In *Adaptation to Changing Health: Response Shift in Quality-of-Life Research*, ed. C. Schwartz and M. Spangers. Washington, DC: American Psychological Association, pp. 11–23.

13. Wilson, I. B. (2000). Clinical understanding and implications. In *Adaptation to Changing Health: Response Shift in Quality of Life Research*, ed. C. Schwartz and M. Spangers. Washington, DC: American Psychological Association, pp. 73–77.

14. Wagner, E. D., Austin, B. T., and VonKorf, M. (1996). Improving outcomes in chronic illness. *Managed Care Q.*, **4**, 12–25.

15. American Society of Clinical Oncology Committee. (1996). Outcomes of cancer treatment for technology assessment and cancer treatment guidelines. *J. Clin. Oncol.*, **14**, 671–9.

16. Kattan, M. W. (2003). Comparing treatment outcomes using utility assessment for health-related quality of life. *Oncology*, **17**, 1687–93.

17. Cella, D. and Dobrez, D. (2003). The Kattan article reviewed. *Oncology*, **17**, 1697–1701.

18. Weeks, J. C., Cook, E. F., O'Day, S. J. *et al.* (1998). Relationship between cancer patients' prediction of prognosis and their treatment preferences. *J.A.M.A.*, **279**, 1709–14.

19. Bennett, K. J. and Torrance, G. W. (1996). Measuring health state preferences and utilities: rating scale, time trade-off, and standard gamble techniques. In *Quality of Life and Pharmacoeconomics in Clinical Trials*, ed. B. Spilker. Philadelphia: Lippincott-Raven, pp. 253–65.

20. Ross, P. L., Littenberg, B., Fearn, P. *et al.* (2003). Paper standard gamble: a paper-based measure of standard gamble utility for current health. *Int. J. Technol. Assess. Health Care*, **19**, 135–47.

21. Torrance, G. W. (1987). Utility approach to measuring health-related quality of life. *J. Chron. Dis.*, **40**, 593–603.

22. Sprangers, M., Moinpour, C., Moynihan, T. *et al.* (2002). Assessing meaningful change in quality of life over time: a user's guide for clinicians. *Mayo Clin. Proc.*, **77**, 561–71.

23. Ferrell, B. R., Grant, M., Dean, G. E., Funk, B., and Ly, J. (1996). "Bone tired": the experience of fatigue and its impact on quality of life. *Oncol. Nursing Forum*, **23**, 1539–47.

24. Thomas, M. L. (2001). Quality of life in myelodysplastic syndromes: measurement issues in research and clinical practice. *Leuk. Res.*, **25**, S11.

25. NCCN (2004). *NCCN Practice Guidelines in Oncology V. Myelodysplastic Syndromes.* Available online at: www.NCCN.org.

26. Cella, D., Chassany, O., Fairclough, D. *et al.* (2003). A guide for clinicians to compare the precision of health-related quality of life data relative to other measures. In *Quality of Life III: Translating the Science of QOL Assessment into Clinical Practice.* Scottsdale, AZ: Mayo School of Continuing Education.

27. Sloan, J. A., Cella, D., Frost, M. H. *et al.* (2002). Assessing clinical significance in measuring oncology patient quality of life: introduction to the symposium, content overview, and definition of terms. *Mayo Clin. Proc.*, **77**, 367–70.

28. Guyatt, G., Osoba, D., Wu, A. *et al.* (2002). Methods to explain the clinical significance of health status measures. *Mayo Clin. Proc.*, **77**, 371–83.

29. Cella, D., Bullinger, M., Scott, C. *et al.* (2002). Group vs individual approaches to understanding the clinical significance of differences or changes in quality of life. *Mayo Clin. Proc.*, **77**, 384–92.

30. Thomas, M. L. (2002). Quality of life in individuals with MDS: impact of fatigue. In *7th International Symposium on Myelodysplastic Syndromes.* Paris, France.

31. Thomas, M. L. (1998). Quality of life and psychosocial adjustment in patients with myelodysplastic syndromes. *Leuk. Res.*, **22**, S41–7.

32. Glaus, A. (1998). Fatigue in patients with cancer: analysis and assessment. *Rec. Results Cancer Res.*, **145**, 1–168.

33. Winningham, M. L. (2000). The puzzle of fatigue: how do you nail pudding to the wall? In *Fatigue in Cancer: A Multidimensional Approach*, ed. M. L. Winningham and M. Barton-Burke. Sudbury, MA: Jones and Bartlett, pp. 3–29.

34. Sobrero, A., Puglisi, F., Guglielmi, A. *et al.* (2001). Fatigue: a main component of anemia symptomatology. *Semin. Oncol.*, **28** (suppl. 8), 15–18.

35. Ream, E. and Richardson, A. (1997). Fatigue in patients with cancer and chronic obstructive airways disease: a phenomenological inquiry. *Int. J. Nursing Studies*, **34**, 44–53.

36. Glaus, A. (1993). Assessment of fatigue in cancer and non-cancer patients. *Support. Care Cancer*, **1**, 305–15.

37. Winningham, M. L. (2000). The foundations of energetics: fatigue, fuel, and functioning. In *Fatigue in Cancer: A Multidimensional Approach*, ed. M. L. Winningham and M. Barton-Burke. Sudbury, MA: Jones and Bartlett, pp. 31–53.

38. Winningham, M. L. and Barton-Burke, M. (2000). *Fatigue in Cancer: A Multidimensional Approach*. Sudbury, MA: Jones and Bartlett.

39. Gilbert, M. (2003). A survivor's journey: one woman's experience with cancer-related fatigue. *Support. Care Cancer*, **10**, 389–98.

40. Winningham, M. L. and Bookbinder, M. (2000). Assessing manifestations: quality of life from a quality improvement perspective. In *Fatigue in Cancer: A Multidimensional Approach*, ed. M. L. Winningham and M. Barton-Burke M. Sudbury, MA: Jones and Bartlett, pp. 279–93.

41. NCCN (2003). Supportive care practice guidelines: cancer-related fatigue. In *National Comprehensive Cancer Network*. Available online at: www.nccn.org/professionals/physician_glsPDF/fatigue.pdf.

42. Gleeson, C. and Spencer, D. (1995). Blood transfusion and its benefits in palliative care. *Palliative Med.*, **9**, 307–13.

43. Jansen, A. J., Essink-Bot, M. L., Beckers, A. M. *et al.* (2003). Quality of life measurement in patients with transfusion-dependent myelodysplastic syndromes. *Br. J. Hematol.*, **121**, 270–4.

44. Jones, M., Ibels, L., Schenkel, B., and Zagari, M. (2004). Impact of epoetin alfa on clinical end points in patients with chronic renal failure: a meta-analysis. *Kidney Int.*, **65**, 757–67.

45. Shasha, D., George, M. J., and Harrison, L. B. (2003). Once-weekly dosing of epoetin-alpha increases hemoglobin and improves quality of life in anemic cancer patients receiving radiation therapy either concomitantly or sequentially with chemotherapy. *Cancer*, **98**, 1072–9.

46. Littlewood, J. L., Nortier, J., Rapoport, B. *et al.* (2003). Epoetin alfa corrects anemia and improves quality of life in patients with hematologic malignancies receiving non-platinum chemotherapy. *Hematol. Oncol.*, **21**, 169–80.

47. Ross, S. D., Fahrbach, K., Frame, D. *et al.* (2003). The effects of anemia treatment on selected health-related quality-of-life domains: a systematic review. *Clin. Ther.*, **25**, 1786–805.

48. Quirt, I., Roveson, C., Lau, C. *et al.* (2001). Epoetin alfa therapy increases hemoglobin levels and improves quality of life in patients with cancer-related anemia who are not

receiving chemotherapy and patients with anemia who are receiving chemotherapy. *J. Clin. Oncol.*, **19**, 4126–34.

49. Hickie, I., Lloyd, A., Wakefield, D., and Ricci, C. (1996). Is there a postinfection fatigue syndrome? *Aust. Family Phys.*, **25**, 1847–52.

50. Cohen, H. J. (1994). Biology of aging as related to cancer. *Cancer*, **74**, 2092–100.

51. Jones, E. A, Bolyard, A. A., and Dale, D. C. (1993). Quality of life with severe chronic neutropenia receiving long-term treatment with granulocyte colony-stimulating factor. *J.A.M.A.*, **270**, 1132–3.

52. Fazio, M. T. and Glaspy, J. A. (1991). The impact of granulocyte colony stimulating factor on quality of life in patients with severe chronic neutropenia. *Oncol. Nursing Forum*, **18**, 1411–14.

53. Mishel, M. H. (1988). Uncertainty in illness. *Image*, **20**, 225–32.

54. Cohen, S. R., Mount, B. M., Tomas, J., and Mount, L. F. (1996). Existential well-being is an important determinant of quality of life. *Cancer*, **77**, 577–86.

55. Field, M. J. and Cassel, C. K. (eds) (1997). *Approaching Death: Improving Care at the End of Life*. Washington, DC: National Academies Press.

56. Lynn, J. (1997). Measuring quality of care at the end of life: a statement of principles. *J. Am. Geriatr. Soc.*, **45**, 526–7.

57. Singer, P. A., Martin, D. K., and Kelner, M. (1999). Quality end-of-life care: patients' perspectives. *J.A.M.A.*, **281**, 163–8.

58. Steinhauser, K. E., Clipp, E. C., McNeilly, M., McIntyre, L. M., and Tulsky, J. A. (2000). In search of a good death: observations of patients, families, and providers. *Ann. Inter. Med.*, **132**, 825–32.

59. Teno, J. M., Byock, I., and Field, M. J. (1999). Research agenda for developing measures to examine quality of care and quality of life of patients diagnosed with life-limiting illness. *J. Pain Symptom Manage.*, **17**, 75–82.

60. Thomas, M. L., Zhang, J., and Greenberg, P. L. (1999). Quality of life in individuals with myelodysplastic syndromes (MDS): a descriptive study. *Blood*, **94** (suppl. 1), 662a.

61. Yellen, S. B., Cella, D., Webster, K., Blendowski, C., and Kaplan, E. (1997). Measuring fatigue and other anemia-related symptoms with the Functional Assessment of Cancer Therapy (FACT) measurement system. *J. Pain Symptom Manage.*, **13**, 63–74.

62. Brady, M. J., Peterman, A. H., Fitchett, G., Mo, M., and Cella, D. (1999). A case for including spirituality in quality of life measurement in oncology. *Psycho-Oncol.*, **8**, 417–28.

63. Ware, J. E. and Sherbourne, C. D. (1992). The MOS 36 Item Short-Form Health Survey (SF 36). *I*. Conceptual framework and item selection. *Med. Care*, **30**, 473–83.

64. Brooks R. (1996). EuroQoL: the current state of play. *Health Policy*, **37**, 53.

65. Smets, E. M. A., Garssen, B., Bonke, B., and de Haes, J. C. J. M. (1995). Multidimensional Fatigue Inventory (MFI): psychometric qualities of an instrument to assess fatigue. *J. Psychosom. Res.*, **39**, 315–25.

66. Hellstrom-Lindberg, E., Gulbrandsen, N., Lindberg, G. *et al.* (2003). A validated decision model for treating the anaemia of myelodysplastic syndromes with erythropoietin + granulocyte colony-stimulating factor: significant effects of quality of life. *Br. J. Haematol.*, **120**, 1037–346.

67. Aaronson, N. K., Ahmedzai, S., Bergman, B. *et al.* (1993). The European Organization for Research and Treatment of Cancer QLQ C-30: a quality of life instrument for use in international clinical trials in oncology. *J. Natl Cancer Inst.*, **85**, 365–76.

68. Casadevall, N., Durieux, P., Dubois, S. *et al.* (2004). Health, economic, and quality-of-life effects of erythropoietin and granulocyte colony-stimulating factor for the treatment of myelodysplastic syndromes: a randomized, controlled trial. *Blood*, **104**, 321–7.

69. Cella, D. (1997). The Functional Assessment of Cancer Therapy – Anemia (FACT-An) scale: a new tool for the assessment of outcomes in cancer anemia and fatigue. *Semin. Hematol.*, **34** (suppl. 2), 13–19.

70. Jaeschke, R., Singer, J., and Guyatt, G. (1989). Measurement of health status: ascertaining the minimally important difference. *Control Clinical Trials*, **10**, 407–15.

71. Clavio, M., Nobili, F., Balleari, E. *et al.* (2004). Quality of life and brain function following high-dose recombinant human erythropoietin in low-risk myelodysplastic syndromes: a preliminary report. *Eur. J. Haematol.*, **72**, 113–20.

72. Kornblith, A. B., Herndon, J. E., Silverman, L. R. *et al.* (2002). Impact of azacytidine on the quality of life of patients with myelodysplastic syndrome treated in a randomized phase III trial: a Cancer and Leukemia Group B study. *J. Clin. Oncol.*, **20**, 2441–52.

73. Veit, C. T. and Ware, J. E. (1983). The structure of psychological distress and well-being in general populations. *J. Consult. Clin. Psychol.*, **51**, 730–42.

74. McNair, D. M., Lorr, M., and Droppleman, L. F. (1971). *Profile of Moods States*. San Diego, CA: Education and Industrial Testing Service.

75. Schwartz, A. L. (1998). The Schwartz Cancer Fatigue Scale: testing reliability and validity. *Oncol. Nursing Forum*, **25**, 711–17.

76. Hann, D. M., Jacobsen, P. B., Azzarello, L. M. *et al.* (1998). Measurement of fatigue in cancer patients: development and validation of the Fatigue Symptom Inventory. *Qual. Life Res.*, **7**, 301–10.

77. Stein, K. D., Jacobsen, P. B., Blanchard, C. M., and Thors, C. (2004). Further validation of the Multidimensional Fatigue Symptom Inventory-Short Form. *J. Pain Symptom Manage.*, **27**, 14–23.

78. Piper, B. F., Dibble, S. L., Dodd, M. L. *et al.* (1998). The revised Piper Fatigue Scale: psychometric evaluation in women with breast cancer. *Oncol. Nursing Forum*, **25**, 677–84.

79. Mendoza, T. R., Wang, X. S., Cleeland, C. S. *et al.* (1999). The rapid assessment of fatigue severity in cancer patients. *Cancer*, **85**, 1186–96.

Index